Advances in ICD Therapy

Guest Editors

PAUL J. WANG, MD
AMIN AL-AHMAD, MD

CARDIAC ELECTROPHYSIOLOGY CLINICS

www.cardiacEP.theclinics.com

Consulting Editors
RANJAN K. THAKUR, MD, MPH, MBA, FHRS
ANDREA NATALE, MD, FACC, FHRS

September 2011 • Volume 3 • Number 3

SAUNDERS an imprint of ELSEVIER, Inc.

W.B. SAUNDERS COMPANY
A Division of Elsevier Inc.

1600 John F. Kennedy Boulevard • Suite 1800 • Philadelphia, Pennsylvania 19103-2899

http://www.theclinics.com

CARDIAC ELECTROPHYSIOLOGY CLINICS Volume 3, Number 3
September 2011 ISSN 1877-9182, ISBN-13: 978-1-4557-0424-8

Editor: Barbara Cohen-Kligerman
Developmental Editor: Donald Mumford

Cardiac Electrophysiology Clinics (ISSN 1877-9182) is published quarterly by Elsevier Inc., 360 Park Avenue South, New York, NY 10010-1710. Months of issue are March, June, September, and December. Subscription prices are $167.00 per year for US individuals, $250.00 per year for US institutions, $88.00 per year for US students and residents, $187.00 per year for Canadian individuals, $279.00 per year for Canadian institutions, $239.00 per year for international individuals, $299.00 per year for international institutions and $126.00 per year for Canadian and foreign students/residents. To receive student/resident rate, orders must be accompanied by name of affiliated institution, date of term, and the signature of program/residency coordinator on institution letterhead. Orders will be billed at individual rate until proof of status is received. Foreign air speed delivery is included in all Clinics subscription prices. All prices are subject to change without notice. **POSTMASTER:** Send address changes to Cardiac Electrophysiology Clinics, Elsevier Health Sciences Division, Subscription Customer Service, 3251 Riverport Lane, Maryland Heights, MO 63043. **Customer Service: 1-800-654-2452 (US and Canada). From outside of the US and Canada, call 314-477-8871. Fax: 314-447-8029. E-mail: JournalsCustomerService-usa@elsevier.com (for print support); JournalsOnlineSupport-usa@elsevier.com (for online support).**

Reprints. For copies of 100 or more of articles in this publication, please contact the Commercial Reprints Department, Elsevier Inc., 360 Park Avenue South, New York, NY 10010-1710. Tel.: 212-633-3812; Fax: 212-462-1935; E-mail: reprints@elsevier.com.

Printed in the United States of America.

The cover illustration shows capacitor shock waveforms. Classic monophasic and biphasic waveforms are depicted. The tilt of the shock waveform is also illustrated (see Hsia et al "Defibrillation Threshold: Testing, Upper Limit of Vulnerability, and Methods for Reduction" in this issue of *Cardiac Electrophysiology Clinics* for details).

Contributors

CONSULTING EDITORS

RANJAN K. THAKUR, MD, MPH, MBA, FHRS
Professor of Medicine, and Director,
Arrhythmia Service, Thoracic and
Cardiovascular Institute, Sparrow Health
System, Michigan State University, Lansing,
Michigan

ANDREA NATALE, MD, FACC, FHRS
Executive Medical Director of the Texas
Cardiac Arrhythmia Institute at St David's
Medical Center, Austin, Texas; Consulting
Professor, Division of Cardiology, Stanford
University, Palo Alto, California; Clinical
Associate Professor of Medicine, Case
Western Reserve University, Cleveland, Ohio;
Senior Clinical Director, EP Services, California
Pacific Medical Center, San Francisco,
California; Department of Biomedical
Engineering, University of Texas, Austin, Texas

GUEST EDITORS

PAUL J. WANG, MD
Professor, Department of Medicine, Stanford
University School of Medicine, Stanford,
California

AMIN AL-AHMAD, MD
Assistant Professor, Department of Medicine,
Stanford University School of Medicine,
Stanford, California

AUTHORS

KARIN K.M. CHIA, MBBS
Staff Cardiac Electrophysiologist, Department
of Cardiology, Royal Brisbane and Women's
Hospital, Herston, Australia

KATHERINE E. CUTITTA, BA
Department of Psychology, East Carolina
University, Greenville, North Carolina

THOMAS A. DEWLAND, MD
Clinical Fellow, Division of Cardiology,
University of California, San Francisco,
San Francisco, California

ANNE M. DUBIN, MD
Associate Professor, Division of Pediatric
Cardiology, Stanford University, Palo Alto,
California

**KENNETH A. ELLENBOGEN, MD, FACC,
FAHA, FHRS**
Cardiac Electrophysiology, Division of
Cardiology, Medical College of Virginia/
Virginia Commonwealth University,
Richmond, Virginia

LAURENCE M. EPSTEIN, MD
Associate Professor, Cardiovascular Division,
Harvard Medical School Brigham and
Women's Hospital, Boston, Massachusetts

JOHN C. EVANS, MD
Pacific Heart Associates, Portland, Oregon

JESSICA FORD, MA
Department of Psychology, East Carolina
University, Greenville, North Carolina

JAMES V. FREEMAN, MD, MPH, MS
Division of Cardiovascular Medicine, Department of Medicine, Stanford University School of Medicine, Stanford, California

PAUL A. FRIEDMAN, MD
Professor of Medicine, Division of Cardiovascular Diseases, Mayo Clinic, Rochester, Minnesota

JOSEPH J. GARD, MD
Fellow, Division of Cardiovascular Diseases, Mayo Clinic, Rochester, Minnesota

ALLISON C. HILL, MD
Pediatrics Resident, Department of Pediatrics, Stanford University, Palo Alto, California

HENRY H. HSIA, MD, FACC, FHRS
Associate Professor of Medicine, Stanford University, Cardiac Electrophysiology and Arrhythmia Service, Stanford University Medical Center, Stanford, California

JOSE F. HUIZAR, MD
Cardiac Electrophysiology, Division of Cardiology, Medical College of Virginia/Virginia Commonwealth University; Cardiac Electrophysiology, Division of Cardiology, McGuire Veterans Affairs Medical Center, Medical College of Virginia, Richmond, Virginia

KAROLY KASZALA, MD, PhD
Cardiac Electrophysiology, Division of Cardiology, Medical College of Virginia/Virginia Commonwealth University; Cardiac Electrophysiology, Division of Cardiology, McGuire Veterans Affairs Medical Center, Medical College of Virginia, Richmond, Virginia

KARI KIRIAN, MA
Department of Psychology, East Carolina University, Greenville, North Carolina

JAYANTHI N. KONERU, MBBS
Cardiac Electrophysiology, Division of Cardiology, Medical College of Virginia/Virginia Commonwealth University, Richmond, Virginia

BYRON K. LEE, MD, MAS
Assistant Professor of Medicine, Electrophysiology and Arrhythmia Service, Division of Cardiology, University of California, San Francisco, San Francisco, California

MELANIE MAYTIN, MD
Fellow in Clinical Medicine, Cardiovascular Division, Brigham and Women's Hospital, Boston, Massachusetts

JEFFREY E. OLGIN, MD
Professor of Medicine and Chief, Electrophysiology and Arrhythmia Service, Division of Cardiology, University of California, San Francisco, San Francisco, California

JEANNE E. POOLE, MD
Professor of Medicine, Director of Arrhythmia Service, Division of Cardiology, University of Washington, Seattle, Washington

JORDAN M. PRUTKIN, MD, MHS
Assistant Professor of Medicine, Division of Cardiology, University of Washington, Seattle, Washington

ROBERT F. REA, MD
Professor of Medicine, Consultant in Cardiovascular Diseases, Internal Medicine, Mayo Clinic and Foundation, Rochester, Minnesota

MARWAN REFAAT, MD
Cardiovascular Institute, University of Pittsburgh, Pittsburgh, Pennsylvania

SAMIR SABA, MD, FACC, FHRS
Director, Cardiovascular Electrophysiology Section, University of Pittsburgh, Pittsburgh, Pennsylvania

JOHN A. SCHOENHARD, MD, PhD
Clinical Cardiac Electrophysiology Fellow, Division of Cardiovascular Medicine, Stanford University Medical Center, Stanford, California

SAMUEL F. SEARS, PhD
Professor, Departments of Psychology and Cardiovascular Sciences, East Carolina University, East Carolina Heart Institute, Greenville, North Carolina

MINTU P. TURAKHIA, MD, MAS
Division of Cardiovascular Medicine, Department of Medicine, Stanford University School of Medicine, Stanford; Veterans Affairs Palo Alto Health Care System, Stanford University, Palo Alto, California

ADITYA ULLAL, BA
Veterans Affairs Palo Alto Health Care System,
Stanford University, Palo Alto; University of
California at Berkeley, Berkeley, California

NIRAJ VARMA, MA, DM, FRCP
Consultant, Cardiac Pacing and
Electrophysiology, Cleveland Clinic,
Cleveland, Ohio

PAUL J. WANG, MD
Professor, Department of Medicine, Stanford
University School of Medicine, Stanford,
California

BRUCE L. WILKOFF, MD, FHRS
Consultant, Cardiac Pacing and
Electrophysiology, Cleveland Clinic,
Cleveland, Ohio

LAWRENCE K. WOODROW, MA
Department of Psychology, East Carolina
University, Greenville, North Carolina

PAUL C. ZEI, MD, PhD
Clinical Associate Professor, Division of
Cardiovascular Medicine, Stanford University
Medical Center, Stanford, California

Contents

The wearable cardioverter-defibrillator (WCD) is an alternative antiarrhythmic device that provides continuous cardiac monitoring and defibrillation capabilities through a noninvasive electrode-based system. Although the WCD has been shown to be highly effective at restoration of sinus rhythm in patients with a ventricular tachyarrhythmia, randomized trials using the WCD in patient populations at elevated risk for arrhythmic death have not been reported. Clinical indications for WCD use are varied and continue to evolve as further experience with this relatively new technology emerges.

The use of implantable cardioverter–defibrillators in children has increased significantly over the last 10 years. The indications for their use have expanded to include primary prevention for at-risk pediatric patients. Because these devices are made for adults, the design does not account for small body habitus, growth, long life expectancy, strenuous physical activity, or congenital heart disease. Pediatric cardiologists are faced with several challenges in their placement and management. This article reviews the indications, safety, and efficacy of implantable cardioverter–defibrillators in children, followed by special consideration of the variety of placement and lead options.

Implantable cardioverter-defibrillator therapy is a lifesaving technology that has undergone tremendous development. Transvenous implantable cardioverter-defibrillator lead was a major breakthrough, allowing for expanded indications. With expanded cardiovascular implantable electronic device use and indications for device therapy, complications have increased. More frequent device system revisions for complications and system upgrade and/or lead malfunction and longer patient life expectancies have mandated a paradigm shift toward premeditated lead management strategies from implant to removal or replacement. The decision to extract a lead in any patient must involve an individualized process considering all patient variables and the experience and outcomes of the extraction program.

Shocks delivered by implantable cardioverter defibrillators (ICDs) can be lifesaving but are also a source of patient morbidity and mortality. The cascade of events that leads to an ICD shock can be interrupted at many points with comprehensive patient care and thoughtful programming. This article reviews the approach to minimizing shocks, with a special emphasis on the role of supraventricular tachycardia–ventricular tachycardia discriminators.

In large clinical trials, implantable cardioverter-defibrillators have improved mortality in various patient populations. Complications during implantation can occur—related to the implant procedure or to the acuity of the patient's medical illness. In addition, many patients require at least one generator change over their lifetime, increasing the possibility of complications. Lead failure and late presentations of infections add to the possible adverse events. The impact of complications on heath care economics is not fully understood. Nevertheless, efforts directed at minimizing device-related complications are critical. This article summarizes the incidence and variety of complications that have been reported.

Implantable cardioverter-defibrillators (ICDs) constitute an effective therapy for protection against death in survivors of sudden cardiac arrest and in those at risk for sudden cardiac death based on poor left ventricular function. In this article, the authors discuss the totally subcutaneous ICD (SC-ICD) system that was designed to provide an alternative to transvenous electrodes in patients who do not require cardiac pacing. The authors also discuss the promises and shortcomings of this new device technology compared with the conventional transvenous implantable defibrillator system and review the experience up-to-date with the SC-ICD.

Transvenous implantable cardiac defibrillators (ICD) have saved many lives. However, ICD leads are also the "weakest link" in an ICD system and lead fracture is one of the principal reasons for system failure. Inappropriate shocks or asystole in a pacemaker-dependent patient, secondary to oversensing, are severe consequences of lead fracture. In the future, improvements in lead design and development of downloadable algorithms will aid in tackling this very important clinical problem. This article discusses the incidence and causes of lead fracture, diagnostic strategies, and therapeutic options for this important clinical problem.

Trials have shown significant benefit with implantable cardioverter-defibrillators (ICDs) for primary and secondary prevention of sudden cardiac death (SCD). Trials have also shown that cardiac resynchronization therapy with (CRT-D) and without (CRT-P) defibrillator function improves quality of life and survival in patients with symptomatic systolic heart failure and prolonged QRS duration. Studies have shown that ICD and CRT-P therapy are generally cost-effective, but there is uncertainty in the cost-effectiveness of CRT-D, because of the cost associated with these devices. This article provides an overview of cost-effectiveness analysis and reviews the literature on the cost-effectiveness of ICD and CRT devices.

Implantation of cardioverter-defibrillators can be challenging owing to congenital abnormalities of vascular or cardiac anatomy or acquired, often iatrogenic, impediments to passage of leads. This article reviews several approaches to the difficult lead implant. Novel peripheral venous access techniques, novel intrathoracic lead positions, and novel surgical techniques, especially in pediatric and congenital heart disease patients, are described.

Professionals charged with the care of patients with implantable cardioverter-defibrillators (ICDs) are faced with the unique challenge of managing device and cardiac care as well as patients' responses to treatment. Defibrillators reduce mortality by preventing sudden cardiac arrest without decrement to quality of life. However, patients with ICDs have greater risk of psychological morbidity. Identifying risk and resilience factors and addressing critical events in clinical encounters can reduce normative and pathologic distress related to device acceptance, defibrillation, recall, and end of life. Further, treatment from mental health professionals has demonstrated efficacy in treating patients with ICDs.

Cardiac implantable electronic devices are becoming more prevalent. Postimplant follow-up is important for monitoring device function and patient condition. However, practice is inconsistent. For example, ICD follow-up schedules vary widely according to facility and physician preference and availability of resources. Recommended follow-up schedules represent a significant burden, with no surveillance between visits. In contrast, implantable devices with automatic remote monitoring capability allow constant surveillance, with the ability to identify salient patient or system problems rapidly, thus reducing the number of device clinic visits. Recent trial results have significant implications for managing patients receiving all forms of implantable electronic cardiac devices.

Defibrillation efficacy is best measured by the sigmoidal dose-response curve that describes the probability for successful defibrillation versus shock energies. The probability curve provides an estimation of the energy margins between the defibrillator output and the energy required for successful defibrillation. Many methods are available to determine the defibrillation threshold (DFT). The upper limit of vulnerability (ULV) has been closely correlated to the DFT in humans and provides a simple, reliable estimate of the ability to defibrillate with a predictable relationship to the dose-response curve. In patients with increased DFTs, implantable cardioverter-defibrillator system modification, alteration of drug therapy, and correction of patients' underlying substrate are required to achieve an adequate defibrillation margin of safety.

Cardiac Electrophysiology Clinics

READ THE CLINICS ONLINE!

Access your subscription at:
www.theclinics.com

Foreword

Advances in ICD Therapy: "Ripples of the Past"

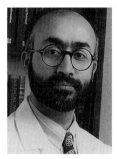

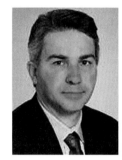

Ranjan K. Thakur, MD, MPH, MBA, FHRS   Andrea Natale, MD, FHRS

Consulting Editors

To appreciate the advances in ICD therapy, it's important to reflect on the past and ask the question, "advances from what?" Today's advances owe their origins to the proverbial pebble dropped in the pond many years ago.

In 1956 Paul Zoll used alternating current defibrillation on post-heart surgery patients and in 1960 Bernard Lown introduced the first DC current defibrillator. While Mirowski and Mower were trying to develop an *implantable* defibrillator in the 1960s, it is the height of irony that it was Bernard Lown, who was the most vocal opponent advancing the charge (pun intended) that "...implanted defibrillator system represents an imperfect solution in search of a plausible and practical application."[1] While this establishment view slowed the development of the ICD, it could not stall it for it was championed by indomitable individuals.

In 1985 the FDA approved the first automatic implanted defibrillator. To qualify for an implant, the patient had to survive *two* episodes of cardiac arrest; contrast that to primary prevention widely practiced today. The initial implanted device envisioned by Mirowski and Mower was a nonthoracotomy device, which delivered the energy via a transducer-tipped catheter, sensing pulsatile pressure, introduced through a peripheral vein into the right ventricle. Technological challenges prevented intracardiac defibrillation in the early years, and the first approved system was implanted by cardiac surgeons, used epicardial patches, and required a thoracotomy for implantation. Transvenous, nonthoracotomy defibrillation became possible a few years later, as shown by Bardy et al, and the implant procedures could be done by electrophysiologists. Innumerable advances, small and large, have occurred since 1985.

Despite these advances, both clinical and technological challenges remain. So, we congratulate Drs Wang and Al-Ahmad for their superb editing of this issue of the *Cardiac Electrophysiology Clinics* focused on "Advances in ICD Therapy." They have selected topics that are relevant to today's technology and clinical practice and they have followed the ripples a little further to glimpse into the future.

Ranjan K. Thakur, MD, MPH, MBA, FHRS
Thoracic and Cardiovascular Institute
405 West Greenlawn, Suite 400
Lansing, MI 48910, USA

Andrea Natale, MD, FHRS
Texas Cardiac Arrhythmia Institute
Center for Atrial Fibrillation at
St David's Medical Center
1015 East 32nd Street, Suite 516
Austin, TX 78705, USA

E-mail addresses:
thakur@msu.edu (R.K. Thakur)
andrea.natale@stdavids.com (A. Natale)

REFERENCE

1. Lown B, Axelrod P. Implanted Standby Defibrillators. Circulation 1972;46:637–9.

doi:10.1016/j.ccep.2011.07.004

Preface
Advances in ICD Therapy

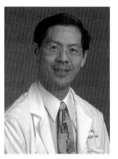 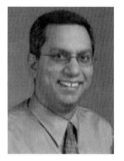

Paul J. Wang, MD   Amin Al-Ahmad, MD
Guest Editors

We are honored and privileged to serve as editors for this volume on advances in ICD therapy. Since the introduction of the first transvenous ICD systems, there have been numerous advances that have made significant improvements in ICD performance and safety. We have invited experts in the field to discuss many of these important developments.

Drs Dewland, Olgin, and Lee lead off the issue with a discussion of the indications for a novel technology, the wearable cardioverter defibrillator. Drs Hill and Dubin then discuss the role of the implantable cardioverter defibrillator in pediatric patients and patients with congenital heart disease. Drs Maytin and Epstein provide a thorough overview of the indications, techniques, and outcomes of ICD lead extraction.

Drs Gard and Friedman review the role of supraventricular tachycardia–ventricular tachycardia discriminators to reduce ICD shocks. Drs Prutkin and Poole discuss the topic of complications of ICD generator change and implantations. Drs Refaat and Saba introduce a new technology, the subcutaneous defibrillator.

Drs Koneru, Kaszala, Huizar, and Ellenbogen focus on the topic of ICD lead fracture and review its incidence, diagnosis, and strategies to prevent inappropriate ICD therapy. Drs Freeman, Ullal, and Turakhia review the analysis of cost effectiveness of implantable cardioverter defibrillators and cardiac resynchronization therapy. Dr Rea provides insights into novel and unusual methods for ICD lead access.

Drs Ford, Cutitta, Woodrow, Kirian, and Sears discuss caring for the heart and mind in ICD patients. Drs Varma and Wilkoff focus on important advances in the remote monitoring of implantable cardiac devices. Drs Hsia, Chia, and Evans discuss the testing of the upper limit of vulnerability and methods of assessing defibrillation threshold. Drs Schoenhard and Zei review methods of reducing ICD shocks for ventricular arrhythmias. Dr Wang discusses new developments in ICD leads and ICD lead configurations.

The articles in this issue are designed to highlight the advances in ICDs and how they may translate into improved outcomes and care of patients with ICDs.

Paul J. Wang, MD
Department of Medicine
Stanford Arrhythmia Service and Cardiac
Electrophysiology
Stanford University School of Medicine
300 Pasteur Drive, Stanford
CA 94305-5233, USA

Amin Al-Ahmad, MD
Department of Medicine
Stanford University School of Medicine
300 Pasteur Dr H2146 MC 5233
Stanford, CA 94305-5233, USA

E-mail addresses:
Paul.J.Wang@stanford.edu (P.J. Wang)
aalahmad@cvmed.stanford.edu (A. Al-Ahmad)

Card Electrophysiol Clin 3 (2011) xv
doi:10.1016/j.ccep.2011.07.005
1877-9182/11/$ – see front matter © 2011 Elsevier Inc. All rights reserved.

Indications for a Wearable Cardioverter-Defibrillator

Thomas A. Dewland, MD[a], Jeffrey E. Olgin, MD[b],
Byron K. Lee, MD, MAS[b],*

KEYWORDS

- Wearable external defibrillator • Sudden cardiac arrest
- Ventricular tachycardia • Fibrillation • Arrhythmia

Since the first description of ventricular fibrillation (VF) termination by means of an externally applied electric shock over half a century ago,[1] substantial progress has been made in the treatment of unstable tachyarrhythmias. The advent of microprocessor technology and improvements in battery storage have enabled the development of compact implantable devices capable of continuous cardiac rhythm monitoring and automated delivery of electrical energy to the myocardium. The modern implantable cardioverter-defibrillator (ICD) has evolved into an efficacious and widely used therapy for the treatment of patients who are at the highest risk for ventricular arrhythmias.

Heightened understanding and awareness of the public health burden imposed by sudden cardiac arrest (SCA) has paralleled advances in device-based antiarrhythmic therapies. Although a staggering 166,000 patients suffer an out-of-hospital SCA in the United States every year, the median survival to hospital discharge after such an event is only 6.4%.[2] Because most of these SCA events are caused by ventricular tachycardia (VT) or VF, improved mechanisms to deliver prompt defibrillation are critical in addressing this low survival rate.

Multiple randomized trials have demonstrated the clinical efficacy of ICDs for the treatment of ventricular arrhythmias and for the primary and secondary prevention of sudden cardiac death.[3–6] Notably, the primary-prevention ICD trials enrolled fairly homogenous patient populations and used low ejection fraction (EF) to identify patients at increased risk for arrhythmic death. It remains unclear how to best treat patients with an elevated risk of SCA who are not among the presently identified groups proved to benefit from an ICD. It is also uncertain how to manage individuals with an accepted indication for device therapy who are unable or unwilling to undergo device implantation.

The use of nonimplantable defibrillation devices, including automated external defibrillators (AEDs), may lead to improvements in witnessed out-of-hospital cardiac arrest outcomes. Uncontrolled studies have demonstrated improved survival after cardiac arrest when AEDs are placed in busy public locations such as casinos and airports.[7–10] AEDs are noninvasive, portable, and relatively inexpensive devices that require minimal operator training. Targeted AED therapy among high-risk patients, however, has not emerged as an effective treatment strategy for SCA. A recent trial

This work was supported by National Institutes of Health Grant U01HL089458.
Drs Lee and Olgin have received research support from Zoll Lifecor.
[a] Division of Cardiology, University of California, San Francisco, 505 Parnassus Avenue, San Francisco, CA 94143-0103, USA
[b] Electrophysiology and Arrhythmia Service, Division of Cardiology, University of California, San Francisco, 500 Parnassus Avenue, San Francisco, CA 94143-1354, USA
* Corresponding author. Electrophysiology and Arrhythmia Service, Division of Cardiology, University of California, San Francisco, 500 Parnassus Avenue, Box 1354, MU 429, San Francisco, CA 94143-1354.
E-mail address: leeb@medicine.ucsf.edu

Card Electrophysiol Clin 3 (2011) 339–347
doi:10.1016/j.ccep.2011.05.001

comparing home AED therapy to conventional cardiopulmonary resuscitation among patients with a history of prior anterior wall myocardial infarction failed to demonstrate an improvement in mortality among the device-treated cohort.[11] The notable disadvantage of an AED compared with implantable defibrillator therapy is the requirement of a bystander to witness the cardiac arrest and apply defibrillation pads. Delayed defibrillation is associated with reduced survival in multiple observational studies,[9,12,13] and only 36% of patients randomized to the treatment group in the previously mentioned trial suffered a witnessed cardiac arrest. Unstable arrhythmias that occur during sleep or when the patient is alone are likely to go untreated when AEDs are singularly used for sudden cardiac death prevention.

WEARABLE CARDIOVERTER-DEFIBRILLATOR

The wearable cardioverter-defibrillator (WCD) is an alternative device that combines the advantages of continuous cardiac monitoring with a noninvasive defibrillation system. The only WCD currently commercially available is the ZOLL LifeVest (ZOLL LifeCor, Pittsburgh, PA, USA). The United States Food and Drug Administration (FDA) initially approved the LifeVest for clinical use in October 2002. Now in its third generation, the device is composed of a vest assembly worn over the chest and a monitor unit carried in a holster at the waist (**Fig. 1**). The monitor unit includes the device battery, defibrillation capacitor, response buttons, signal processor, and a display. The entire system weighs approximately 1.3 kg. The vest is worn under the patient's clothing and holds 4 non-adhesive dry electrodes against the chest wall to facilitate the continuous collection of 2 electrocardiogram signals. In addition, 3 defibrillation electrodes are incorporated into the vest, allowing for defibrillation in the apex to posterior vector.

The LiveVest utilizes an advanced arrhythmia detection algorithm that uses heart rate, template matching, dual lead comparison, analog and digital signal filtering, rhythm stability analysis, and arrhythmia duration to guide therapy.[14] The treating physician can tailor the length of shock delay and rate thresholds for VT/VF in individual patients. When the device senses a treatable arrhythmia, a progressive alarm sequence consisting of a vibration alert, blinking light-emitting diode signals, and audible warnings is initiated. During this period, the patient has the ability to suspend therapy by pressing 2 buttons located on the alarm module, facilitating abortion of the defibrillation shock when consciousness is not impaired. If the warning sequence is not halted by response button activation, the device prepares to deliver therapy. While the WCD is charging, gel is extruded from the defibrillation electrodes to increase conduction to the skin using technology similar to that used by automobile airbags. An initial test pulse is delivered to measure thoracic impedance, resulting in automated adjustment of impulse duration. Therapy is delivered by means of up to 5 biphasic shocks at programmable energy levels between 75 and 150 J (**Fig. 2**). The device attempts to deliver each shock on a sensed R wave. If this is not possible after 3 seconds of monitoring, an unsynchronized shock is administered. The WCD vest assembly must be replaced after each treatment course. In addition to tachyarrhythmia treatment, the LifeVest also detects asystole and significant ventricular pauses. The device has the capacity to store and transmit electrocardiograms to facilitate analysis of alarmed events and overall signal quality.

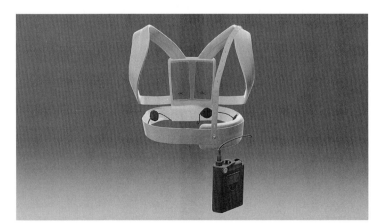

Fig. 1. WCD vest and monitor unit. (*Courtesy of* ZOLL Lifecor Corporation, Pittsburgh, PA, USA; with permission.)

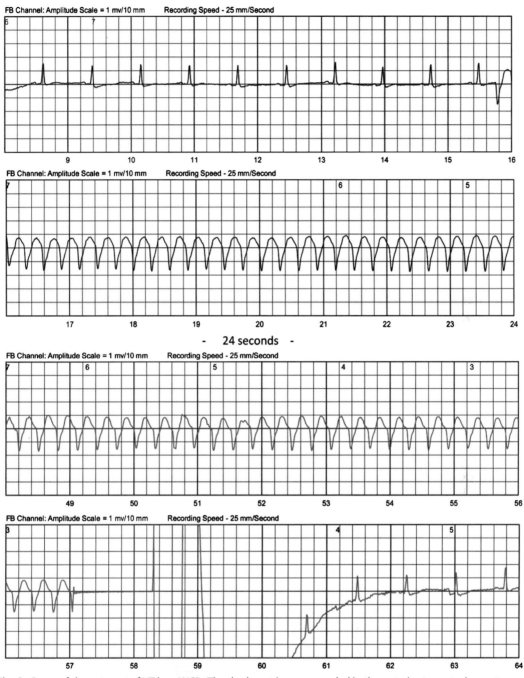

Fig. 2. Successful treatment of VT by a WCD. The rhythm strip was recorded in the anterior to posterior vector and saved by the device as the front-to-back (FB) channel. Between the second and third strips, 24 seconds of arrhythmia recording has been omitted. After arrhythmia identification, the device issued a progressive alarm sequence alerting the patient to the upcoming shock. Therapy was not suspended and a 150-J biphasic shock was delivered, resulting in restoration of sinus rhythm. (*Courtesy of* ZOLL Lifecor Corporation, Pittsburgh, PA, USA; with permission.)

EFFECTIVENESS OF WCD THERAPY

Efficacy of the WCD for the termination of ventricular arrhythmias was first reported in 1998. In this initial study, unstable VT/VF was induced in 10 survivors of SCA referred for electrophysiologic testing.[15] In all patients, a single monophasic 230-J shock delivered by a WCD successfully terminated the arrhythmia. A similarly designed follow-up study employing a next generation ICD using a biphasic shock again demonstrated the reliable termination of 22 episodes of induced VF among 12 patients.[16] In this follow-up investigation, both 70- and 100-J biphasic defibrillation energies were studied, providing assurance that the 150-J capacity of the current WCD model is sufficient for the treatment of clinical ventricular arrhythmias.

Data supporting the effectiveness of WCDs outside the electrophysiology laboratory are predominantly derived from multiple case series, including 2 large cohorts from the United States and Germany,[17,18] and a single prospective clinical trial.[19] Between 2002 and 2006, all of the nearly 3600 patients treated with the ZOLL LifeVest in the United States were enrolled in a clinical database maintained by the device manufacturer. A recent review of these data demonstrated that overall survival among patients enrolled in the registry was high (99.2%) and the first-shock success for the termination of VT/VF was 99%. Mean duration of therapy was 53 days.[17] Overall, the device was fairly well tolerated. Using duration of stored electrocardiogram data, investigators were able to quantify patient compliance. Of the patients who wore the LifeVest, the mean daily use was 19.9 ± 4.7 hours, and 52% of patients wore the device for longer than 90% of the day. Approximately 14% of patients prematurely discontinued WCD use, most commonly citing the size and weight of the device. Inappropriate shocks were experienced by 67 of the 3569 patients (1.9%) during a total of 4788 months of device use.

The WCD experience among a cohort of German patients has also been recently described.[18] Between 2000 and 2008, 354 patients were treated with a WCD for an average duration of 106 days. Mean daily use was 21.3 hours.[18] More than 70% of the patients in this study wore the device for greater than 22 hours a day. In 20 of the 21 VT/VF events, the first discharge was successful. The remaining VF event required 2 device-initiated defibrillation attempts to successfully treat the rhythm.

The Wearable Defibrillator Investigative Trial (WEARIT) and the Bridge to ICD in Patients at Risk of Sudden Arrhythmic Death (BIROAD) trial were 2 prospective, multicenter, nonrandomized clinical investigations designed to assess the safety and efficacy of WCD use in high-risk patient populations.[19] Patients were excluded from either study if they were candidates for ICD therapy but could be enrolled if a significant delay in device implantation was anticipated. These studies notably began recruitment before publication of the landmark primary-prevention ICD trials, including the MADIT II (Multicenter Autonomic Defibrillator Implantation Trial II) and the SCD-HeFT (Sudden Cardiac Death in Heart Failure Trial).[4,5] The WEARIT study enrolled outpatients with New York Heart Association class III or VI symptoms and an EF less than 30%. The BIROAD study was undertaken to evaluate the use of a WCD as a bridge to ICD decision in patients at elevated risk for ventricular arrhythmias. This second trial enrolled a much more heterogeneous population, including individuals with a recent myocardial infarction or coronary artery bypass graft (CABG) surgery complicated by high-risk features and patients unable or unwilling to receive an ICD in a timely manner. At the request of the FDA, the studies were eventually combined and reported as the WEARIT/BIROAD trial.

A total of 289 patients had been enrolled when the study was stopped after reaching prespecified safety and efficacy thresholds.[19] Eight episodes of VT/VF were observed in the combined study population; 6 of these events were successfully terminated by the WCD. The 2 unsuccessfully treated episodes occurred in patients with improperly mounted defibrillation electrodes. Subsequent changes in device design have eliminated the potential for this complication. Notably, the WEARIT/BIROAD study used an earlier version of the WCD that delivered monophasic defibrillation waveforms; present models use biphasic shocks.

It should be emphasized that all the present evidence supporting WCD use is derived from uncontrolled studies, and most of the reported experience is in the form of registry data. The WCD has not been compared in a randomized manner to either non–device-based therapy or treatment with an ICD. Although it is clear that early defibrillation is beneficial and that the WCD can reliably provide such timely therapy, the tendency to consider WCD and ICD treatment as analogous should be avoided in the absence of studies directly comparing these 2 fundamentally different devices.

CLINICAL USE OF WCD THERAPY

As the WCD is a readily removable noninvasive device that is significantly less expensive than traditional ICD therapy, the threshold for prescribing a WCD is likely to be lower than that required for an ICD. This ease of device discontinuation heightens the importance of patient compliance to ensure effective treatment. Given these issues, WCD therapy is best suited for clinical scenarios in which the risk of arrhythmia is temporary or when the wearable device can be used to bridge the patient to a more definitive treatment (ie, ICD implantation or heart transplantation).

The WCD can also be considered in patients with a temporarily elevated risk of arrhythmia in the absence of a validated ICD indication. The use of the WCD as an alternative to an implanted device should be discouraged and only considered in rare circumstances.

Current ICD implantation guidelines stress the importance of avoiding implantable defibrillator therapy in patients with reversible arrhythmic disorders or risk factors.[20] Accordingly, the WCD has been proposed for short-term use in patients with multiple conditions associated with VT/VF, including myocarditis,[21] newly diagnosed nonischemic cardiomyopathy,[22] proarrhythmic drug intoxication, recent CABG surgery complicated by a low EF,[23] or severe coronary disease before revascularization. The WCD is well suited to these clinical scenarios because the VT/VF risk factors associated with such conditions may diminish over time and with medical therapy. Using this strategy, the patient is not exposed to the immediate and long-term risks associated with surgical device implantation and can be adequately protected from arrhythmic death until the risk is diminished or a conventional indication for ICD therapy is identified.

The WCD should be considered for patients who have a conventional ICD indication but are not immediate candidates for surgical implantation. This situation is most commonly encountered in the setting of defibrillator generator or lead infection. The WCD may offer suitable protection for patients after device removal and throughout the course of antibiotic therapy, facilitating infection clearance and avoiding the risk of repeat hardware infection caused by premature reimplantation. Furthermore, this treatment strategy can potentially facilitate hospital discharge in an otherwise stable patient who is able to receive outpatient antibiotics. Approximately 10% and 23% of the patients in the German and United States WCD registries, respectively, were treated for this indication.[17,18]

Patients who develop an indication for an ICD but are being actively treated for a systemic infection or another reversible medical comorbidity precluding surgery (including ventricular thrombus or venous obstruction) can also be considered for WCD therapy as a bridge to eventual ICD insertion. In addition, individuals considered temporarily too unstable to endure a device implantation procedure and the attendant anesthesia may be appropriate for a WCD. In this instance, the desire to prevent an arrhythmic death must be framed by overall prognosis. Analogous to the concerns raised by ICD use in patients with end-stage disease, the WCD has the potential to transform a painless death into an uncomfortable and potentially traumatic experience heralded by a high-energy shock without promise of significant improvement in duration or quality of life.

Patients actively listed for cardiac transplantation are another high-risk population in which ICD implantation may be delayed. The yearly mortality among such patients approaches 25%, with sudden death (presumably because of ventricular arrhythmias) accounting for most of these fatalities. ICD therapy has been associated with improved survival among cardiac patients awaiting transplant.[24] However, an ICD is likely not required after transplantation, necessitates an implantation procedure with potentially lethal complications, and is costly. The WCD is an attractive alternative to bridge patients with severe systolic dysfunction to transplant when the wait for organ allocation is anticipated to be brief.

Temporary prophylaxis against arrhythmic death may also be warranted in patients who are suspected of having a congenital arrhythmia disorder, including the Brugada syndrome, long QT syndrome, and arrhythmogenic right ventricular cardiomyopathy. It is not uncommon to encounter patients in whom the clinical suspicion for such a condition has been raised after a family member suffers SCA or when other concerning features are incidentally found on an electrocardiogram, echocardiogram, or magnetic resonance image. The WCD can then be prescribed during the ensuing genetic and electrophysiologic workup, allowing the diagnosis to be confirmed before committing the patient to lifelong ICD treatment. Similarly, patients who have suffered a prior syncopal event caused by a suspected but yet unproven ventricular arrhythmia can be considered for WCD treatment while further testing is pending. WCD prescription is particularly advantageous over standard noninvasive event monitors in this setting because the device can provide potentially lifesaving therapy in addition to long-term rhythm monitoring. It is also reasonable to prescribe a WCD after an ICD indication is established in situations in which the patient requests more time to consider implantable therapy.

An additional broad category of WCD candidates encompasses those patients who were not included in the large primary-prevention ICD trials but are still believed to be at an increased risk for SCA. As previously mentioned, these trials predominantly used low EF as the criteria for enrollment. However, population-based studies indicate that significant proportions of SCA survivors do not have marked reductions in systolic function at the time of their arrest, suggesting other risk factors for SCA remain to be identified and studied in a prospective manner.[25,26] The WCD is a potentially appealing therapy in such situations in which the benefit of defibrillator therapy is less well established, especially when the heightened risk of ventricular arrhythmia is considered temporary.

Although patients with systolic dysfunction are at a significantly elevated risk of SCA in the period immediately after myocardial infarction,[27] ICD use does not have an established benefit in this setting. The Defibrillator in Acute Myocardial Infarction Trial examined ICD implantation in patients 6 to 40 days after a myocardial infarction complicated by a reduced EF ($\leq$35%) and impaired cardiac autonomic function.[28] Follow-up at a mean of 30 months failed to identify an improvement in mortality with this treatment strategy. Although defibrillator therapy reduced the incidence of arrhythmic death, this benefit was offset by an increase in non–sudden cardiac death. Explanation for this overall lack of benefit remains elusive. It is possible that successful defibrillation of an unstable arrhythmia shifted mortality from arrhythmic death to one by progressive heart failure. Alternatively, some aspect of ICD implantation and subsequent therapy, including the operative procedure, defibrillator threshold testing, or ventricular pacing, may have contributed to the observed increase in cardiac death. Treatment with a WCD has been proposed as a mechanism to deliver the benefits of ICD therapy in the immediate postinfarction period without exposing the patient to the potentially destabilizing side effects of device implantation.[29] The VEST (Vest prevention of Early Sudden death Trial) is an ongoing large-scale randomized trial to determine if WCD therapy reduces sudden death in the first 90 days after myocardial infarction. The findings of this trial have the potential to drastically affect care in the immediate postinfarction period and are expected in 2013.

Other novel indications for WCD continue to be identified and studied. For instance, the initiation of certain antiarrhythmic medications known to prolong the QT interval currently requires inpatient admission and telemetry monitoring to assess for proarrhythmic side effects. WCD use could potentially obviate hospitalization, making such therapy initiation more convenient and potentially more cost-effective.[18] Current indications for WCD therapy are likely to evolve as device technology progresses and further studies are published.

The WCD is a possible but problematic alternative treatment for patients with a guideline-based indication for ICD therapy who have declined device implantation. The average studied duration of WCD therapy is of the order of months, and the efficacy of a WCD treatment strategy over the years to decades during which an implantable device is expected to remain in place is unknown. Benefit of the WCD in this setting is undoubtedly less than that of an ICD given the substantial commitment required by the patient to ensure near-constant device use. Because of these issues, the WCD should not be considered a long-term alternative to ICD implantation.

COMPLICATIONS OF WCD USE

WCD therapy is overall well tolerated and is not associated with significant morbidity or mortality. Inappropriate therapy remains the most common complication associated with this treatment strategy. Among the 289 patients enrolled in the WEARIT/BIROAD study, 6 inappropriate shocks occurred in 6 patients. With 901 total months of patient follow-up, these shocks represented an inappropriate shock rate of 0.67% per month of WCD use.[19] In the German WCD cohort, only 3 inappropriate shocks were delivered among the 354 patients studied.[18] An analysis of roughly 9000 patients treated with a WCD for more than 18,000 aggregate months revealed 265 inappropriate shocks, suggesting an even lower inappropriate therapy rate of 0.009 episodes per month.[30] In all reports, the most common cause of an inappropriate shock was signal artifact.

One of the most compelling features of the WCD is the ability of the patient to abort therapy if consciousness is maintained, allowing for significant reductions in inappropriate treatment. The rate of incorrect identification of VT/VF by the device may be as high as 1 episode per 13.4 days.[18] Inability of the patient to prevent therapy in this setting has been attributed to multiple factors, including engagement in an activity that prohibits device deactivation, sleep, or failure to repetitively deactivate the device in the setting of recurrent inappropriate sensing.

Device usage was discontinued before reaching a study end point in 68 of the 289 patients (25%) enrolled in the WEARIT/BIOROAD trial.[19] The most commonly cited reason for self-discontinuation of WCD treatment was discomfort caused by the size and weight of the monitor. A small number of patients (6%) complained of a skin rash or itching associated with the device. Among the previously mentioned US LifeVest cohort, 307 of the 2169 patients (14.2%) self-discontinued the WCD because of discomfort or adverse reactions.[17]

GUIDELINE RECOMMENDATIONS FOR WCD USE

The *Guidelines for Device-Based Therapy of Cardiac Rhythm Abnormalities*, jointly published by the American College of Cardiology, American Heart Association, and the Heart Rhythm Society in 2008, does not specifically mention WCD therapy.[20] The International Society for Heart and Lung Transplantation gives a Class IC recommendation to the use of either an ICD or WCD in outpatients listed Status 1B for cardiac transplantation.[31]

The Centers for Medicare and Medicaid Services (CMS) approved WCD coverage in July 2005. WCD therapy is currently reimbursable by CMS when prescribed for patients with a prior ICD requiring explantation or in situations in which an ICD would be indicated (ie, a documented episode of sustained VT or VF in the absence of a reversible cause and more than 48 hours after myocardial infarction, in familial or inherited conditions associated with unstable ventricular arrhythmias, and as primary prevention in patients with an EF≤35%) but cannot be implanted because of other clinical factors.

CONTRAINDICATIONS TO WCD THERAPY

Contraindications to WCD use are few. A high-voltage pacing artifact produced by an implanted pacemaker may lead to either oversensing and inappropriate tachyarrhythmia treatment or pacing artifact misclassification resulting in shock inhibition.[32] As such, patients who are paced using a unipolar atrial or ventricular lead are not candidates for current WCD therapy. The WCD alerts the patient to an upcoming shock through audible, visual, and tactile alarms. Caution should be exercised when prescribing this device to individuals with significant hearing or other sensory difficulties. Furthermore, patients who are unable to abort therapy through response button activation secondary to either motor or cognitive impairment should not be treated with such a device. The FDA has only approved the WCD for adult patients at least 18 years of age, although a small case series documents its use in a pediatric population.[33] WCD treatment is not advised in patients who are pregnant or are exposed to excessive electromagnetic interference.

In contrast to ICDs, wearable defibrillators do not presently have pacing capabilities. This property may be most relevant in the immediate postdefibrillation period, during which asystole of variable duration of may be encountered. Retrospective analysis of 142 shocks delivered by the LifeVest to treat VT/VF identified 4 episodes of postshock asystole longer than 10 seconds.[34] Of the 4 patients, 3 survived. If a significant bradycardia is sensed by the WCD, the device issues an audible alarm to bystanders to contact emergency medical services. Patients with a concomitant need for bradycardia therapies should not be solely treated with a WCD.

SUMMARY

The WCD is an antiarrhythmic device that provides continuous cardiac monitoring and defibrillation capabilities through a noninvasive electrode-based system. WCD therapy has been shown to be highly effective at restoration of sinus rhythm in patients with ventricular tachyarrhythmia, and multiple clinical case series document its use in the treatment of patients who are either unable to undergo ICD implantation or are without an accepted indication for such invasive therapy. Because of variable patient adherence and lack of long-term follow-up, the WCD should not be considered a replacement for ICD therapy. Randomized trials using the WCD in patient populations at elevated risk of arrhythmic death have not been reported. Clinical indications for WCD use are varied and continue to evolve as further experience with this relatively new technology emerges.

REFERENCES

1. Zoll PM, Linenthal AJ, Gibson W, et al. Termination of ventricular fibrillation in man by externally applied electric countershock. N Engl J Med 1956;254(16): 727–32.
2. Rosamond W, Flegal K, Furie K, et al. Heart disease and stroke statistics—2008 update: a report from the American Heart Association Statistics Committee and Stroke Statistics Subcommittee. Circulation 2008;117(4):e25–146.
3. Moss AJ, Hall WJ, Cannom DS, et al. Improved survival with an implanted defibrillator in patients with coronary disease at high risk for ventricular arrhythmia. Multicenter Automatic Defibrillator Implantation Trial Investigators. N Engl J Med 1996;335(26):1933–40.
4. Bardy GH, Lee KL, Mark DB, et al. Amiodarone or an implantable cardioverter-defibrillator for congestive heart failure. N Engl J Med 2005; 352(3):225–37.
5. Moss AJ, Zareba W, Hall WJ, et al. Prophylactic implantation of a defibrillator in patients with myocardial infarction and reduced ejection fraction. N Engl J Med 2002;346(12):877–83.
6. A comparison of antiarrhythmic-drug therapy with implantable defibrillators in patients resuscitated from near-fatal ventricular arrhythmias. The Antiarrhythmics versus Implantable Defibrillators (AVID) Investigators. N Engl J Med 1997; 337(22):1576–83.

7. Caffrey SL, Willoughby PJ, Pepe PE, et al. Public use of automated external defibrillators. N Engl J Med 2002;347(16):1242–7.

8. Page RL, Joglar JA, Kowal RC, et al. Use of automated external defibrillators by a U.S. airline. N Engl J Med 2000;343(17):1210–6.

9. Valenzuela TD, Roe DJ, Nichol G, et al. Outcomes of rapid defibrillation by security officers after cardiac arrest in casinos. N Engl J Med 2000;343(17):1206–9.

10. Sanna T, La Torre G, de Waure C, et al. Cardiopulmonary resuscitation alone vs. cardiopulmonary resuscitation plus automated external defibrillator use by non-healthcare professionals: a meta-analysis on 1583 cases of out-of-hospital cardiac arrest. Resuscitation 2008;76(2):226–32.

11. Bardy GH, Lee KL, Mark DB, et al. Home use of automated external defibrillators for sudden cardiac arrest. N Engl J Med 2008;358(17):1793–804.

12. Chan PS, Krumholz HM, Nichol G, et al. Delayed time to defibrillation after in-hospital cardiac arrest. N Engl J Med 2008;358(1):9–17.

13. Peberdy MA, Kaye W, Ornato JP, et al. Cardiopulmonary resuscitation of adults in the hospital: a report of 14720 cardiac arrests from the National Registry of Cardiopulmonary Resuscitation. Resuscitation 2003;58(3):297–308.

14. Dillon KA, Szymkiewicz SJ, Kaib TE. Evaluation of the effectiveness of a wearable cardioverter defibrillator detection algorithm. J Electrocardiol 2010;43(1):63–7.

15. Auricchio A, Klein H, Geller CJ, et al. Clinical efficacy of the wearable cardioverter-defibrillator in acutely terminating episodes of ventricular fibrillation. Am J Cardiol 1998;81(10):1253–6.

16. Reek S, Geller JC, Meltendorf U, et al. Clinical efficacy of a wearable defibrillator in acutely terminating episodes of ventricular fibrillation using biphasic shocks. Pacing Clin Electrophysiol 2003;26(10):2016–22.

17. Chung MK, Szymkiewicz SJ, Shao M, et al. Aggregate national experience with the wearable cardioverter-defibrillator: event rates, compliance, and survival. J Am Coll Cardiol 2010;56(3):194–203.

18. Klein HU, Meltendorf U, Reek S, et al. Bridging a temporary high risk of sudden arrhythmic death. Experience with the wearable cardioverter defibrillator (WCD). Pacing Clin Electrophysiol 2009;33(3):353–67.

19. Feldman AM, Klein H, Tchou P, et al. Use of a wearable defibrillator in terminating tachyarrhythmias in patients at high risk for sudden death: results of the WEARIT/BIROAD. Pacing Clin Electrophysiol 2004;27(1):4–9.

20. Epstein AE, DiMarco JP, Ellenbogen KA, et al. ACC/AHA/HRS 2008 Guidelines for Device-Based Therapy of Cardiac Rhythm Abnormalities: a report of the American College of Cardiology/American Heart Association Task Force on Practice Guidelines (Writing Committee to Revise the ACC/AHA/NASPE 2002 Guideline Update for Implantation of Cardiac Pacemakers and Antiarrhythmia Devices): developed in collaboration with the American Association for Thoracic Surgery and Society of Thoracic Surgeons. Circulation 2008;117(21):e350–408.

21. Prochnau D, Surber R, Kuehnert H, et al. Successful use of a wearable cardioverter-defibrillator in myocarditis with normal ejection fraction. Clin Res Cardiol 2009;99(2):129–31.

22. Traub D, Alpert B, Donahue B, et al. Sudden cardiac arrest aborted by a wearable cardioverter-defibrillator in newly diagnosed non-ischemic cardiomyopathy. Heart Rhythm 2007;4(5):S101.

23. Meltendorf U, Reek S, Buhtz F, et al. Using the wearable cardioverter defibrillator—a strategy for bridging high risk patients after CABG. Heart Rhythm 2005;2(5):S32.

24. Sandner SE, Wieselthaler G, Zuckermann A, et al. Survival benefit of the implantable cardioverter-defibrillator in patients on the waiting list for cardiac transplantation. Circulation 2001;104(12 Suppl 1):I171–6.

25. Gorgels AP, Gijsbers C, de Vreede-Swagemakers J, et al. Out-of-hospital cardiac arrest—the relevance of heart failure. The Maastricht Circulatory Arrest Registry. Eur Heart J 2003;24(13):1204–9.

26. Stecker EC, Vickers C, Waltz J, et al. Population-based analysis of sudden cardiac death with and without left ventricular systolic dysfunction: two-year findings from the Oregon Sudden Unexpected Death Study. J Am Coll Cardiol 2006;47(6):1161–6.

27. Solomon SD, Zelenkofske S, McMurray JJV, et al. Sudden death in patients with myocardial infarction and left ventricular dysfunction, heart failure, or both. N Engl J Med 2005;352(25):2581–8.

28. Hohnloser SH, Kuck KH, Dorian P, et al. Prophylactic use of an implantable cardioverter-defibrillator after acute myocardial infarction. N Engl J Med 2004;351(24):2481–8.

29. Choudhuri I, Tverskaya R, Kazanikova G, et al. Arrhythmic events during the 40/90 days "cooling off" period: clinical utility of the wearable defibrillator. Circulation 2007;116(16):II 348.

30. Szymkiewicz S. Incidence and causes of inappropriate defibrillation during wearable defibrillator use. Heart Rhythm 2009;6(5):S74.

31. Gronda E, Bourge RC, Costanzo MR, et al. Heart rhythm considerations in heart transplant candidates and considerations for ventricular assist devices: International Society for Heart and Lung Transplantation guidelines for the care of cardiac

transplant candidates—2006. J Heart Lung Transplant 2006;25(9):1043–56.

32. LaPage MJ, Canter CE, Rhee EK. A fatal device-device interaction between a wearable automated defibrillator and a unipolar ventricular pacemaker. Pacing Clin Electrophysiol 2008; 31(7):912–5.

33. Everitt MD, Saarel EV. Use of the wearable external cardiac defibrillator in children. Pacing Clin Electrophysiol 2010;33(6):742–6.

34. Freeman G, Quan W, Szymkiewicz S. Is severe post-shock bradyarrhythmia in patients using wearable defibrillators common or serious? Circulation 2007; 116(16):II 931.

Implantable Cardioverter–Defibrillator Therapy in Pediatric Patients and Congenital Heart Disease

Allison C. Hill, MD[a], Anne M. Dubin, MD[a,b],*

KEYWORDS

- Implantable cardioverter–defibrillator • Pediatric
- Congenital heart disease • Sudden cardiac death

Sudden cardiac death (SCD) in children is rare, but the frequency has increased in recent years.[1,2] The disease processes underlying SCD are heterogeneous, although arrhythmias cause the majority of SCDs in children.[3] One important and growing high-risk group is congenital heart disease patients. Children who have had surgical repair or palliation for congenital heart disease have a 25 to 100 times greater risk of SCD than those without underlying heart disease.[3] The small but growing group of adults with congenital heart disease is also at risk for fatal arrhythmias.[4]

Regardless of cause, SCD has devastating consequences, as only 8% of children who suffer out of hospital arrests survive to hospital discharge.[5] SCD and resuscitated death in adults and children represent significant morbidity and mortality. Multiple large population-based trials of adults with ischemic and idiopathic cardiomyopathy have established the superiority of implantable cardioverter–defibrillators (ICDs) to medical treatment in preventing sudden arrhythmic death.[6–8] This overwhelming evidence was extrapolated to children at risk for SCD. The first ICDs were placed in children in the 1980s, and since then, the number has

grown consistently. In 2006, 396 children received ICDs, and they tended to be younger at time of ICD placement than in previous decades.[9]

Although experience with ICDs in children is growing, there are still significant and unique challenges. Technical difficulties exist due to the design of ICDs. Since less than 1% of all ICDs are placed in children, ICDs are designed for adults.[10] The long-term management of ICDs in children also presents challenges. Children have a longer life expectancy compared with adults, which means appropriate ICD therapy can prolong life significantly at the cost of multiple procedures for generator replacements and lead revisions and extractions.

ICD INDICATIONS

The indications for ICDs in children have evolved significantly over the past 30 years. Because there have been no large prospective trials in pediatric patients, the American College of Cardiology and the American Heart Association suggest using similar indications to those for adults despite the inherent differences between adult coronary artery disease and various diseases that put children at

No external sources of funding were used. Dr Dubin receives fellowship support from Medtronic.
a Department of Pediatrics, MC MSO/LPCH Stanford Hospitals & Clinics, 300 Pasteur Drive, Stanford, CA 94305, USA
b Division of Cardiology, Stanford University, 750 Welch Road, MC 5912, Palo Alto, CA, USA
* Corresponding author.
E-mail address: amdubin@stanford.edu

Card Electrophysiol Clin 3 (2011) 349–357
doi:10.1016/j.ccep.2011.05.002

risk for SCD.[11] Recommendations regarding ICD implantation for primary prevention of sudden death in children are based on limited clinical experience and small retrospective studies. Indications for both adult and pediatric ICD implantation have transitioned from secondary to primary prevention of SCD. Berul and colleagues conducted a large retrospective study of 443 pediatric and young adult patients in which 52% of patients had ICDs placed for primary prevention and 48% for secondary prevention.[12] Underlying diseases in this study are shown in **Fig. 1**.

Pediatric Conditions Associated with SCD

Hypertrophic cardiomyopathy
Hypertrophic cardiomyopathy (HCM) is the most common cause of SCD in young people in the United States. Approximately 1 to 2 per 1000 Americans have HCM, and the mortality is 4% to 6%.[13] At present there are several possible therapies that have been proposed for HCM. However, the 1 therapy that has been shown to improve survival has been the ICD.[14] ICDs were traditionally placed for secondary prevention, but there has been a trend toward placement for primary prevention.

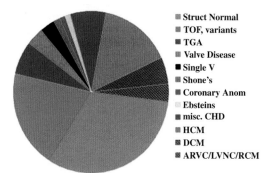

Fig. 1. Anatomic diagnoses of pediatric and congenital implantable cardioverter–defibrillator recipients. Congenital heart disease (CHD) accounts for 46% of total, cardiomyopathies (CM) 23%, and structurally normal hearts with primary electrical diseases 31% of all patients. Among CHD patients, diagnoses included tetralogy of Fallot (TOF), transposition of great arteries (TGA), atrial or ventricular septal defects, valve abnormalities, single ventricle, Shone complex, coronary artery congenital anomalies, Ebstein anomaly of tricuspid valve, and others. Cardiomyopathies included hypertrophic cardiomyopathy (HCM), dilated cardiomyopathy (DCM), arrhythmogenic right ventricular dysplasia/cardiomyopathy (ARVC), left ventricular noncompaction (LVNC), and restrictive cardiomyopathy (RCM). (*From* Berul CI, Van Hare GF, Kertesz NJ, et al. Results of a multicenter retrospective implantable cardioverter–defibrillator registry of pediatric and congenital heart disease patients. J Am Col Cardiol 2008; 51(17):1687; with permission.)

Although ICDs placed for secondary prevention have more discharges (10% per year), those placed for primary prevention have a significant number of discharges as well (3.6% per year).[15] Survival is equivalent for patients who have ICDs placed for primary and secondary prevention.[16] ICDs have also been placed in patients with fewer risk factors than in the past. Maron and colleagues found that 35% of patients with HCM who had ICDs placed for primary prevention had only 1 risk factor at the time of implantation. There was no significant difference in the likelihood of appropriate therapy if patients had 1, 2, or 3 risk factors at the time of ICD implantation.

Long QT syndrome
Long QT syndrome is caused by a variety of genetic mutations that transcribe myocardial sodium and potassium channels. The result is prolonged ventricular repolarization, which predisposes patients to polymorphic ventricular tachycardia (VT). Risk of sudden death is directly related to type of LQT, with LQT3 being the most lethal of the 3 major types of LQTS.[17]

Despite the widespread use of beta-blockers, up to 14% of patients with LQTS still have syncope or SCD.[18] Thus, ICDs are indicated in many patients with LQTS. In a large review of the LQTS registry, Zareba and colleagues found that only 1 out of 73 patients with ICDs died, compared with 26 of the 161 matched patients without ICDs.[19]

Congenital heart disease
Select patients with congenital heart disease are at risk for SCD from arrhythmias. In fact, 25% of patients with structural heart disease had inducible sustained VT on electrophysiological testing and had an increased risk of clinical arrhythmia and death.[20] Thus many of these patients could benefit from ICD placement. In Silka and colleagues' large retrospective study of 3589 patients with congenital heart disease, 41 had late SCD mostly related to aortic stenosis, aortic coarctation, and tetralogy of Fallot.[3] Subsequent studies have confirmed the risk of SCD in patients with tetralogy of Fallot in particular; thus most patients with congenital heart disease and an ICD have tetralogy of Fallot.[4,21]

Safety and Efficacy

Safety
ICDs are generally a safe therapeutic option for patients at risk for life-threatening arrhythmias. No implant-related deaths occurred in Berul and colleagues' study of 443 pediatric and young adult patients with ICDs.[12] There is an overall higher complication rate for ICDs in children compared

with adults.[22–24] As advances have been made, complication rates in children have trended down from 16% in 2000 to 10% in 2006.[9] The most common complications in children are infection and lead-related problems such as dislodgement and failure (**Fig. 2**).[12,25] Children remain more active than adults after ICD placement, and their physical activity puts stressors on the ICD leads. Other potential complications include hematoma, pneumothorax, stroke, or cardiac perforation at implantation and tricuspid regurgitation if a lead is positioned across the valve.[26]

When a patient experiences infection or a lead fracture, the lead must be extracted. Lead extraction can be particularly difficult if it has adhered to the endocardium or vascular structures. This process usually occurs after the lead has been in place for over 6 months, thus recently placed leads can be extracted with less difficulty.[27] Other indications that lead extraction may be challenging depend on how the lead was placed. Passive fixation can cause leads to adhere to the endocardium. Dual-coil defibrillation leads may have adherence between the proximal coil and the surrounding veins.[28] The most significant lead adherence sites are at the lead entry, lead tip, and high-voltage shocking coils.

Despite the challenges of lead adherence, extraction can be done successfully in children with a low complication rate by experienced providers.[18] Appropriate techniques of lead extraction, such as with use of interlocking sheaths and laser cutting sheaths, have been associated with a 95% to 98% success rate, which is similar to rates reported in adults.[28–30]

A major concern for patients and physicians is the risk of inappropriate ICD discharges. The rate is higher for pediatric patients than adults (21%–25% vs 14%).[12,31,32] Within all pediatric patients, those with primary electrical disease or congenital heart disease are at higher risk for inappropriate ICD discharge than those with cardiomyopathy.[12] Multiple factors contribute to these discrepancies. Children have higher sinus tachycardia rates, which can be misinterpreted as VT or ventricular fibrillation. Also, patients with congenital heart disease frequently have atrial arrhythmias. As many as 30% of patients with congenital heart disease and ICDs develop supraventricular tachycardia.[33,34] These atrial arrhythmias can cause an ICD to discharge. Patients with LQTS have prolonged repolarization, which can make an ICD double count the ventricular rate. In these cases, the ICD sensing electrode must be placed such that T-wave sensing can be blanked and still allow for reliable arrhythmia detection.

Efficacy

A large range of appropriate and inappropriate discharge rates has been reported.[35–41] In 1993, Silka and colleagues noted 59% of 125 pediatric patients with ICDs had appropriate discharges.[42] Fifteen years later, Berul and colleagues found that 26% of 443 patients with ICDs had appropriate discharges.[12] The decreased rate of appropriate discharge is likely due to the trend from placing ICDs for secondary prevention to primary prevention, since ICDs placed for secondary prevention have more appropriate discharges than those placed for primary prevention (32% vs 18%). Other factors associated with appropriate discharges are older patients and a longer time elapsed between ICD placement and time of the study. Even though there are significant numbers of life-saving discharges from ICDs placed in children, there is still a small (1%) risk of sudden cardiac death in children with ICDs.[12]

CONSIDERATIONS FOR ICD PLACEMENT IN CHILDREN
Pulse Generator

An inevitable obstacle in ICD placement in children is the size of the components, since ICDs were developed for adults and there are no specially designed pediatric ICDs.[42] As technology has advanced, pulse generators have become smaller, but size is limited by high-energy capacitors and battery life. A shorter battery life means more generator changes, especially since children have a longer lifetime ahead of them than adults when ICDs are placed.

There are various location options for pulse generator placement, based mostly on the size of the patient. Traditionally, pulse generators are placed

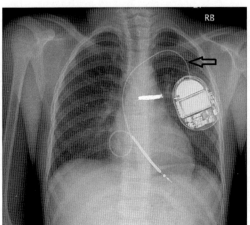

Fig. 2. Lead fracture (*arrow*) in a single-coil transvenous implantable cardioverter-defibrillators (ICD).

in the prepectoral location. In children with thin chest walls and a paucity of fat, the pulse generator can be placed subpectorally. In addition to an improved cosmetic appearance, the subpectoral location has been associated with a decreased risk of superficial erosion, but does require increased time for placement and revision.[43–45] There have been reports of inappropriate ICD discharge from the stress of local musculoskeletal activity.[43]

In children who are too small for a prepectoral or subpectoral placement, the pulse generator can also be placed abdominally (**Fig. 3**). In general, infants and young children less than 25 kg require an abdominal pulse generator. In these cases, the pacing and sensing leads can be placed on the epicardial surface, or a transvenous system can be tunneled subcutaneously to the heart. Tunneled leads are at risk for fracture due to movement at the inferior costal margin. Various hybrid systems have been used for patients at the border between requiring abdominal placement and tolerating subpectoral or prepectoral placement.

Leads

There is a variety of anatomic challenges with transvenous lead placement in the pediatric and congenital heart disease patient. Infants and young children may have systemic veins that are too small for 1 or more leads. In patients with an intracardiac shunt or single ventricle, intracardiac leads could cause thrombosis and stroke. Venous anomalies of the upper extremity such as persistent left superior vena cava without bridging vein can also make transvenous lead placement difficult. Cardiac surgery can preclude transvenous lead placement if there is no access to the ventricles due to cavopulmonary anastamosis with

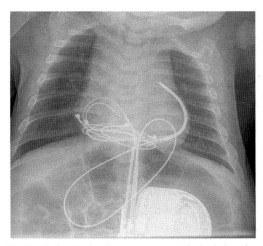

Fig. 3. Abdominal pulse generator with dual chamber leads in an infant.

a Glenn or Fontan procedure or if extensive atrial reconstruction has led to venous stenosis. During cardiopulmonary bypass, the right atrial appendage may be amputated during cannulation, which makes atrial lead placement difficult and requires active fixation. Ventricular inversion or atrial baffle for d-transposition of the great arteries can change the location of the ventricular shock in relation to the myocardium.

In these cases, epicardial leads have been placed. However, there are risks associated with epicardial leads. Surgical placement via thoracotomy is required, which carries a higher mortality rate than transvenous lead placement (t2% vs 5%).[46] Long-term risks include lead failure, ventricular stricture, or strangulation.[42,47]

Various newer configurations have been reported.[48–54] Subcutaneous array was initially used as an adjunct to transvenous defibrillator leads to improve higher defibrillation thresholds. It has several fingers of unipolar coil leads in the subcutaneous fascia of the lateral ribcage. The aim of this configuration is to provide a defibrillation discharge wavefront that covers a greater area of myocardium with less energy.[55] Berul successfully defibrillated animal models as well as a 2 year old child with a circuit between an 'active-can' pulse generator and a subcutaneous array.[48] A single-finger lead with an abdominal pulse generator has also been successful, even in small infants.[49,56–59] Although subcutaneous placement is most commonly used, a coil in the pericardial or pleural space has been reported.[49] Even fully subcutaneous ICDs have recently been reported.[60] However, nontransvenous ICDs, excluding epicardial shocking patches, have shorter survival than transvenous ICDs.[61]

In addition to choosing optimal placement of leads, leads can also be fixed to the ventricle actively or passively. Ninety-seven percent of pediatric ICDs use active fixation leads, which have a helical screw that is deployed into the myocardium at the time of placement.[12] Passive fixation leads have tines meant to secure themselves into the ventricular trabeculae, but are more susceptible to getting tangled in the heavily trabeculated right ventricle in children. Active fixation leads are also more easily removed, which must always be a consideration in children who will potentially need several system revisions throughout their lifetimes.

Dual-coil systems, commonly used in adults receiving ICDs to ensure adequate defibrillation thresholds, must be used with caution in children. The dual-coil system can be less ideal in small children in whom the proximal coil would not be positioned in the superior vena cava, and more likely would be found in the right subclavian vein, or at times even in the pocket. The proximal coil segment of the lead often causes fibrosis at the venous contact site, which makes it a prime target for lead breaks that require revision or extraction. Dual-coil systems are also associated with more late complications in children due to growth.[28]

Arrhythmia detection

Children are at a higher risk of receiving inappropriate shocks than adults due to differences in sinus tachycardia rates and atrial arrhythmias in congenital heart disease patients. In an attempt to improve arrhythmia detection, the dual-chamber ICD has been used in children, as this configuration is better able to discriminate between atrial and ventricular rhythms. Some have reported fewer inappropriate ICD discharges with the dual-chamber ICD, while others have shown no significant difference in the rate of inappropriate discharges.[33,62] Here again, size may be a limiting factor for many children whose venous anatomy is inadequate for 2 cardiac leads.

In adults, arrhythmia detection has also been improved by the use of algorithms to identify a 1:1 atrial ventricular relationship, PR and RP ratios.[63] These algorithms have not been tested in children with higher atrial rates and shorter refractory periods.

Growth considerations

Placement of an ICD in young children requires special consideration of growth. A change in body surface area has the highest hazard ratio for lead failure.[31] Both epicardial and transvenous systems are associated with high rates of complications such as lead dislodgement or fracture, which can be directly related to patient growth.[25] Epicardial leads have higher failure rates than transvenous leads, and require additional thoracotomies.[46] Even in older children whose veins are large enough for leads, growth carries the risk of lead fracture.

Systemic venous stenosis can be a major issue in a child with a small subclavian vein. These stenoses can preclude placement of any subsequent leads through the vessel, which can significantly complicate future lead revisions or extractions. Studies of upper extremity venography in adult patients undergoing defibrillator revision find a venous stenosis rate as high as 50% to 67%.[64,65]

Defibrillator lead extraction can be performed in children with or without congenital heart disease with a low incidence of complications.[18,66] Active fixation leads tend to be more easily removed than passive fixation, and thus should be preferentially considered in the small child who has a higher likelihood of requiring lead extraction within his or her lifetime. Avoiding a dual-coil defibrillator system in a small patient is also preferred, as binding of the proximal coil to the vasculature is commonly seen when attempting extraction of these leads in children.[28]

It is important to try and allow for some redundancy of the ventricular lead in the small child who is undergoing ICD placement to allow for growth. As the heart grows, the apex moves away from the base. A lead with the tip at the apex can be stretched or dislodged as the heart grows. Thus, children whose venous anatomy allows transvenous lead placement, but who still have years of growth ahead of them must have ICD leads placed with redundancy to allow growth. Lead redundancy is most commonly left in the atrium, and less commonly in the inferior vena cava.[67,68] Some authors have suggested the use of absorbable anchor sutures to permit inward migration of the ventricular lead with growth.[69] Another option to decrease the complications related to growth is placement of the right ventricular lead on the ventricular septum. This lessens the stress of the lead with growth, but may create a suboptimal shock vector.

A significant difference between pediatric and adult patients with defibrillators is the functional capacity of the patient. Children tend to have a better left ventricular (LV) ejection fraction when compared with adult recipients (54 ± 14% vs 33 ± 13%).[25] These children are likely to have a higher activity level and thus may subject leads to repeated stresses over a longer period to time. These stresses may result in damage to chronically implanted leads. They may also place the leads under unique stressors such as roller coasters or trampolines.

Quality of life

Children can have a long life expectancy after ICD placement, making quality-of-life considerations particularly important. Children with ICDs have adjustment issues such as decreased social interactions, less physical activity including sexual activity, and concerns of body image due to the ICD appearance.[70] However, they tend to have less clinical depression compared with adults. Still, anxiety about shocks and fear of device failure are common. These factors must be carefully considered, anticipated, and recognized, and support groups can be encouraged to improve patient acceptance and understanding.[71–74]

FUTURE DIRECTIONS

There are 2 major areas of potential advancement when contemplating ICD therapy in the pediatric and congenital heart disease patient: a better understanding of indications and improvement in the technical aspects of ICDs.

At present the pediatric and congenital heart disease population requiring an ICD is quite limited and heterogeneous, which makes prospective multicenter studies impossible. However, the national ICD registry American College of Cardiology National Cardiovascular Data Registry began in 2006 with enrollment of adult patients. Phase 2 of this registry, with pediatric- and congenital heart disease-specific enrollment started earlier this year. Further studies from this registry will expand knowledge on ICD indications, outcomes, lead survival, and other issues regarding pediatric ICDs.[75]

There is also a need for improvements in the technical aspects of ICDs. As the number of children necessitating ICDs increases, the need for models designed for pediatric patients expands. Miniaturization of ICD components will allow for more options as to where ICDs can be implanted. Improved computer programming will allow safer and more effective ICD care. Upgrading previously placed ICDs with a software download has been shown to reduce inappropriate shocks due to lead fractures, and may be further developed to help combat other lead complications.[76] Complicated computer modeling studies predict energy requirements for defibrillation in patients with complex anatomy and differing configurations.[77,78] These models will potentially be extremely useful in patients with nontraditional lead placement, and may indeed help plan for patient growth. Smaller-sized parts and even leadless ICDs may be on the horizon. Once available, this device could obviate the need for additional hardware and potentially eliminate a cause of late complications for patients with a defibrillator.

SUMMARY

ICDs in children are safe and effective. The indications are expanding from mostly secondary to primary prevention of SCD. Several technical limitations exist due to the lack of ICDs specifically designed for children, the small size of children, and the variety of underlying pathology and anatomy of children requiring ICDs. Given the long life expectancy of children, considerations for long-term durability and growth of ICDs are crucial.

REFERENCES

1. Maron BJ, Doerer JJ, Haas TS, et al. Sudden deaths in young competitive athletes: analysis of 1866 deaths in the United States, 1980–2006. Circulation 2009; 119(8):1085–92.

2. Liberthson RR. Sudden death from cardiac causes in children and young adults. N Engl J Med 1996; 334(16):1039–44.

3. Silka MJ, Hardy BG, Menashe VD, et al. A population-based prospective evaluation of risk of sudden cardiac death after operation for common congenital heart defects. J Am Coll Cardiol 1998; 32(1):245–51.

4. Oechslin EN, Harrison DA, Connelly MS, et al. Mode of death in adults with congenital heart disease. Am J Cardiol 2000;86(10):1111–6.

5. Nadkarni VM, Larkin GL, Peberdy MA, et al. First documented rhythm and clinical outcome from in-hospital cardiac arrest among children and adults. JAMA 2006;295(1):50–7.

6. A comparison of antiarrhythmic drug therapy with implantable defibrillators in patients resuscitated from near-fatal ventricular arrhythmias. The Antiarrhythmics versus Implantable Defibrillators (AVID) Investigators. N Engl J Med 1997;337(22): 1576–83.

7. Moss AJ, Zareba W, Hall WJ, et al. Prophylactic implantation of a defibrillator in patients with myocardial infarction and reduced ejection fraction. N Engl J Med 2002;346(12):877–83.

8. Bardy GH, Lee KL, Mark DB, et al. Amiodarone or an implantable cardioverter–defibrillator for congestive heart failure. N Engl J Med 2005;352(3):225–37.

9. Burns KM, Evans F, Kaltman J. Pediatric ICD Utilization in the United States from 1997–2006. Heart Rhythm 2010. Available at: http://www.ncbi.nlm.nih.gov.laneproxy.stanford.edu/pubmed/20887811. Accessed October 24, 2010.

10. Epstein AE, DiMarco JP, Ellenbogen KA, et al. ACC/AHA/HRS 2008 Guidelines for device-based therapy of cardiac rhythm abnormalities: a report of the American College of Cardiology/American Heart Association Task Force on Practice Guidelines (Writing Committee to Revise the ACC/AHA/NASPE 2002 Guideline Update for Implantation of Cardiac Pacemakers and Antiarrhythmia Devices): developed in collaboration with the American Association for Thoracic Surgery and Society of Thoracic Surgeons. Circulation 2008;117(21):e350–408.

11. Gregoratos G, Abrams J, Epstein AE, et al. ACC/AHA/NASPE 2002 guideline update for implantation of cardiac pacemakers and antiarrhythmia devices–summary article: a report of the American College of Cardiology/American Heart Association Task Force on Practice Guidelines (ACC/AHA/NASPE Committee to Update the 1998 Pacemaker Guidelines). J Am Coll Cardiol 2002;40(9):1703–19.

12. Berul CI, Van Hare GF, Kertesz NJ, et al. Results of a multicenter retrospective implantable cardioverter–defibrillator registry of pediatric and congenital heart disease patients. J Am Coll Cardiol 2008;51(17): 1685–91.

13. Maron BJ. Risk stratification and prevention of sudden death in hypertrophic cardiomyopathy. Cardiol Rev 2002;10(3):173–81.

14. Maron BJ, Shen WK, Link MS, et al. Efficacy of implantable cardioverter–defibrillators for the prevention of sudden death in patients with hypertrophic cardiomyopathy. N Engl J Med 2000;342(6): 365–73.

15. Maron BJ, Spirito P, Shen W, et al. Implantable cardioverter–defibrillators and prevention of sudden cardiac death in hypertrophic cardiomyopathy. JAMA 2007;298(4):405–12.

16. Begley DA, Mohiddin SA, Tripodi D, et al. Efficacy of implantable cardioverter–defibrillator therapy for primary and secondary prevention of sudden cardiac death in hypertrophic cardiomyopathy. Pacing Clin Electrophysiol 2003;26(9):1887–96.

17. Zareba W, Moss AJ, Schwartz PJ, et al. Influence of genotype on the clinical course of the long-QT syndrome. International Long-QT Syndrome Registry Research Group. N Engl J Med 1998;339(14):960–5.

18. Friedman RA, Van Zandt H, Collins E, et al. Lead extraction in young patients with and without congenital heart disease using the subclavian approach. Pacing Clin Electrophysiol 1996;19(5):778–83.

19. Zareba W, Moss AJ, Daubert JP, et al. Implantable cardioverter–defibrillator in high-risk long QT syndrome patients. J Cardiovasc Electrophysiol 2003; 14(4):337–41.

20. Alexander ME, Walsh EP, Saul JP, et al. Value of programmed ventricular stimulation in patients with congenital heart disease. J Cardiovasc Electrophysiol 1999;10(8):1033–44.

21. Nollert GD, Däbritz SH, Schmoeckel M, et al. Risk factors for sudden death after repair of tetralogy of Fallot. Ann Thorac Surg 2003;76(6):1901–5.

22. Chatrath R, Porter CJ, Ackerman MJ. Role of transvenous implantable cardioverter–defibrillators in preventing sudden cardiac death in children, adolescents, and young adults. Mayo Clin Proc 2002;77(3):226–31.

23. Stefanelli CB, Bradley DJ, Leroy S, et al. Implantable cardioverter–defibrillator therapy for life-threatening arrhythmias in young patients. J Interv Card Electrophysiol 2002;6(3):235–44.

24. Wilson WR, Greer GE, Grubb BP. Implantable cardioverter–defibrillators in children: a single-institutional experience. Ann Thorac Surg 1998;65(3):775–8.

25. Link MS, Hill SL, Cliff DL, et al. Comparison of frequency of complications of implantable cardioverter–defibrillators in children versus adults. Am J Cardiol 1999;83(2):263–6.

26. Sherrid MV, Daubert JP. Risks and challenges of implantable cardioverter–defibrillators in young adults. Prog Cardiovasc Dis 2008;51(3):237–63.

27. Bracke F, Meijer A, Van Gelder B. Extraction of pacemaker and implantable cardioverter defibrillator leads: patient and lead characteristics in relation to the requirement of extraction tools. Pacing Clin Electrophysiol 2002;25(7):1037–40.

28. Cooper JM, Stephenson EA, Berul CI, et al. Implantable cardioverter–defibrillator lead complications and laser extraction in children and young adults with congenital heart disease: implications for implantation and management. J Cardiovasc Electrophysiol 2003;14(4):344–9.

29. Saad EB, Saliba WI, Schweikert RA, et al. Nonthoracotomy implantable defibrillator lead extraction: results and comparison with extraction of pacemaker leads. Pacing Clin Electrophysiol 2003;26(10):1944–50.

30. Epstein LM, Byrd CL, Wilkoff BL, et al. Initial experience with larger laser sheaths for the removal of transvenous pacemaker and implantable defibrillator leads. Circulation 1999;100(5):516–25.

31. Alexander ME, Cecchin F, Walsh EP, et al. Implications of implantable cardioverter–defibrillator therapy in congenital heart disease and pediatrics. J Cardiovasc Electrophysiol 2004;15(1):72–6.

32. Rinaldi CA, Simon RD, Baszko A, et al. A 17-year experience of inappropriate shock therapy in patients with implantable cardioverter–defibrillators: are we getting any better? Heart 2004;90(3):330–1.

33. Love BA, Barrett KS, Alexander ME, et al. Supraventricular arrhythmias in children and young adults with implantable cardioverter–defibrillators. J Cardiovasc Electrophysiol 2001;12(10):1097–101.

34. Korte T, Köditz H, Niehaus M, et al. High incidence of appropriate and inappropriate ICD therapies in children and adolescents with implantable cardioverter–defibrillator. Pacing Clin Electrophysiol 2004; 27(7):924–32.

35. Goel AK, Berger S, Pelech A, et al. Implantable cardioverter–defibrillator therapy in children with long QT syndrome. Pediatr Cardiol 2004;25(4):370–8.

36. Botsch MP, Franzbach B, Opgen-Rhein B, et al. ICD therapy in children and young adults: low incidence of inappropriate shock delivery. Pacing Clin Electrophysiol 2010;33(6):734–41.

37. Werner B, Przybylski A, Kucińska B, et al. Implantable cardioverter–defibrillators in children. Kardiol Pol 2004;60(3):239–46.

38. Eicken A, Kolb C, Lange S, et al. Implantable cardioverter–defibrillator (ICD) in children. Int J Cardiol 2006;107(1):30–5.

39. Pablo Kaski J, Tomé Esteban MT, Lowe M, et al. Outcomes after implantable cardioverter–defibrillator treatment in children with hypertrophic cardiomyopathy. Heart 2007;93(3):372–4.

40. Celiker A, Olgun H, Karagoz T, et al. Midterm experience with implantable cardioverter–defibrillators in children and young adults. Europace 2010;12(12): 1732–8.

41. Heersche JHM, Blom NA, van de Heuvel F, et al. Implantable cardioverter–defibrillator therapy for

prevention of sudden cardiac death in children in the Netherlands. Pacing Clin Electrophysiol 2010; 33(2):179–85.

42. Silka MJ, Kron J, Dunnigan A, et al. Sudden cardiac death and the use of implantable cardioverter–defibrillators in pediatric patients. The Pediatric Electrophysiology Society. Circulation 1993;87(3): 800–7.

43. Kistler PM, Fynn SP, Mond HG, et al. The subpectoral pacemaker implant: it isn't what it seems! Pacing Clin Electrophysiol 2004;27(3):361–4.

44. Lee JCR, Shannon K, Boyle NG, et al. Evaluation of safety and efficacy of pacemaker and defibrillator implantation by axillary incision in pediatric patients. Pacing Clin Electrophysiol 2004;27(3):304–7.

45. Gold MR, Peters RW, Johnson JW, et al. Complications associated with pectoral cardioverter–defibrillator implantation: comparison of subcutaneous and submuscular approaches. Worldwide Jewel Investigators. J Am Coll Cardiol 1996;28(5):1278–82.

46. Trappe HJ. The modern implantable cardioverter–defibrillator: comparing it to those of the late 1980s. Am J Cardiol 1996;78(5A):3–8.

47. Chevalier P, Moncada E, Canu G, et al. Symptomatic pericardial disease associated with patch electrodes of the automatic implantable cardioverter–defibrillator: an underestimated complication? Pacing Clin Electrophysiol 1996;19:2150–2.

48. Berul CI, Triedman JK, Forbess J, et al. Minimally invasive cardioverter–defibrillator implantation for children: an animal model and pediatric case report. Pacing Clin Electrophysiol 2001;24(12):1789–94.

49. Stephenson EA, Batra AS, Knilans TK, et al. A multicenter experience with novel implantable cardioverter–defibrillator configurations in the pediatric and congenital heart disease population. J Cardiovasc Electrophysiol 2006;17(1):41–6.

50. Cannon BC, Friedman RA, Fenrich AL, et al. Innovative techniques for placement of implantable cardioverter–defibrillator leads in patients with limited venous access to the heart. Pacing Clin Electrophysiol 2006;29(2):181–7.

51. Tomaske M, Prêtre R, Rahn M, et al. Epicardial and pleural lead ICD systems in children and adolescents maintain functionality over 5 years. Europace 2008;10(10):1152–6.

52. Hsia T, Bradley SM, LaPage MJ, et al. Novel minimally invasive, intrapericardial implantable cardioverter–defibrillator coil system: a useful approach to arrhythmia therapy in children. Ann Thorac Surg 2009;87(4):1234–8 [discussion 1238–39].

53. Kaltman JR, Gaynor JW, Rhodes LA, et al. Subcutaneous array with active can implantable cardioverter–defibrillator configuration: a follow-up study. Congenit Heart Dis 2007;2(2):125–9.

54. Kriebel T, Ruschewski W, Gonzalez y Gonzalez M, et al. ICD Implantation in infants and small children:

the extracardiac technique. Pacing Clin Electrophysiol 2006;29(12):1319–25.

55. Gradaus R, Hammel D, Kotthoff S, et al. Nonthoracotomy implantable cardioverter–defibrillator placement in children: use of subcutaneous array leads and abdominally placed implantable cardioverter defibrillators in children. J Cardiovasc Electrophysiol 2001;12(3):356–60.

56. Luedemann M, Hund K, Stertmann W, et al. Implantable cardioverter defibrillator in a child using a single subcutaneous array lead and an abdominal active can. Pacing Clin Electrophysiol 2004;27(1):117–9.

57. Madan N, Gaynor JW, Tanel R, et al. Single-finger subcutaneous defibrillation lead and active can: a novel minimally invasive defibrillation configuration for implantable cardioverter–defibrillator implantation in a young child. J Thorac Cardiovasc Surg 2003;126(5):1657–9.

58. Watanabe H, Hayashi J, Haga M, et al. Successful implantation of a cardioverter–defibrillator in an infant. Ann Thorac Surg 2001;72(6):2125–7.

59. Greene AE, Berger JT, Heshmat Y, et al. Transcutaneous implantation of an internal cardioverter–defibrillator in a small infant with recurrent myocardial ischemia and cardiac arrest simulating sudden infant death syndrome. Pacing Clin Electrophysiol 2004;27(1):112–6.

60. McLeod KA, McLean A. Implantation of a fully subcutaneous ICD in Children. Pacing Clin Electrophysiol 2010. [Epub ahead of print].

61. Radbill AE, Triedman JK, Berul CI, et al. System survival of nontransvenous implantable cardioverter–defibrillators compared to transvenous implantable cardioverter–defibrillators in pediatric and congenital heart disease patients. Heart Rhythm 2010;7(2):193–8.

62. Lawrence D, Von Bergen N, Law IH, et al. Inappropriate ICD discharges in single-chamber versus dual-chamber devices in the pediatric and young adult population. J Cardiovasc Electrophysiol 2009; 20(3):287–90.

63. Wilkoff BL, Kühlkamp V, Volosin K, et al. Critical analysis of dual-chamber implantable cardioverter–defibrillator arrhythmia detection: results and technical considerations. Circulation 2001;103(3):381–6.

64. Lickfett L, Bitzen A, Arepally A, et al. Incidence of venous obstruction following insertion of an implantable cardioverter–defibrillator. A study of systematic contrast venography on patients presenting for their first elective ICD generator replacement. Europace 2004;6(1):25–31.

65. Sticherling C, Chough SP, Baker RL, et al. Prevalence of central venous occlusion in patients with chronic defibrillator leads. Am Heart J 2001;141(5):813–6.

66. Cecchin F, Atallah J, Walsh EP, et al. Lead extraction in pediatric and congenital heart disease patients. Circ Arrhythm Electrophysiol 2010;3(5):437–44.

67. Gasparini M, Mantica M, Galimberti P, et al. Inferior vena cava loop of the implantable cardioverter–defibrillator endocardial lead: a possible solution of the growth problem in pediatric implantation. Pacing Clin Electrophysiol 2000;23(12):2108–12.

68. Antretter H, Hangler H, Colvin J, et al. Inferior vena caval loop of an endocardial pacing lead did not solve the growth problem in a child. Pacing Clin Electrophysiol 2001;24(11):1706–8 [discussion: 1709].

69. Stojanov P, Velimirović D, Hrnjak V, et al. Absorbable suture technique: solution to the growth problem in pediatric pacing with endocardial leads. Pacing Clin Electrophysiol 1998;21:65–8.

70. Dubin AM, Batsford WP, Lewis RJ, et al. Quality-of-life in patients receiving implantable cardioverter–defibrillators at or before age 40. Pacing Clin Electrophysiol 1996;19:1555–9.

71. Sears SF, Conti JB. Implantable cardioverter–defibrillators for children and young adolescents: mortality benefit confirmed—what's next? Heart 2004;90(3):241–2.

72. Sears SF, Burns JL, Handberg E, et al. Young at heart: understanding the unique psychosocial adjustment of young implantable cardioverter–defibrillator recipients. Pacing Clin Electrophysiol 2001;24(7):1113–7.

73. Sears SF, St Amant JB, Zeigler V. Psychosocial considerations for children and young adolescents with implantable cardioverter–defibrillators: an update. Pacing Clin Electrophysiol 2009;32(Suppl 2):S80–2.

74. DeMaso DR, Lauretti A, Spieth L, et al. Psychosocial factors and quality of life in children and adolescents with implantable cardioverter–defibrillators. Am J Cardiol 2004;93(5):582–7.

75. Hammill SC, Kremers MS, Stevenson LW, et al. Review of the registry's fourth year, incorporating lead data and pediatric ICD procedures, and use as a national performance measure. Heart Rhythm 2010;7(9):1340–5.

76. Swerdlow CD, Gunderson BD, Ousdigian KT, et al. Downloadable software algorithm reduces inappropriate shocks caused by implantable cardioverter–defibrillator lead fractures: a prospective study. Circulation 2010;122(15):1449–55.

77. Jolley M, Stinstra J, Pieper S, et al. A computer modeling tool for comparing novel ICD electrode orientations in children and adults. Heart Rhythm 2008;5(4):565–72.

78. Vadakkumpadan F, Rantner LJ, Tice B, et al. Image-based models of cardiac structure with applications in arrhythmia and defibrillation studies. J Electrocardiol 2009;42(2):157, e1–10.

ICD Lead Extraction

Melanie Maytin, MD*, Laurence M. Epstein, MD

KEYWORDS

• ICD • Transvenous lead extraction • ICD lead

Implantable cardioverter-defibrillator (ICD) technology has been lifesaving for many patients. Original devices required a sternotomy or thoracotomy for implantation, thereby limiting their applicability to secondary prevention patients. The advent of the transvenous ICD lead was a major breakthrough and allowed for current expanded indications. Unfortunately, benefits usually come with a cost. Eliminating the need for major surgery was crucial to expanded usage, but it created the problem of having to manage chronic transvenous ICD leads. Beyond the issues related to chronic transvenous pacing leads, ICD leads pose their own unique challenges. ICD leads are significantly more complex than traditional pacemaker leads. Most pacing leads are unipolar or bipolar whereas most ICD leads are tripolar or quadripolar. This complexity has created leads with multiple lumens and conductors that are less resistant to chronic wear, yielding a significantly higher failure rate. In addition, ICD leads are larger and older models often are nonisodiametric, making removal more challenging. Lastly, integral to ICD leads is one or more high voltage "shocking" coil electrode. These coils are susceptible to in-growth of fibrotic tissue, again increasing the difficulty of lead removal. Given these considerations, the management of chronic transvenous leads is significantly different from that of standard pacing leads.

PATHOLOGY OF THE HUMAN-LEAD INTERACTION

The challenges and risks of transvenous lead extraction (TLE) are principally related to the body's foreign body response to the cardiovascular implantable electronic device (CIED). This response begins at implantation with thrombus development along the lead. Fibrosis of the thrombus occurs next with near-complete encapsulation of the leads with a fibrin sheath within 4 to 5 days of implant.[1,2] Robust fibrosis develops in areas of direct contact between the lead and the vasculature and endocardium (**Fig. 1**). The most common adhesion sites include the venous entry site, the superior vena cava (SVC), and the electrode-myocardial interface with multiple areas of scar tissue found in the majority of patients.[3] The exposed defibrillator coils of ICD leads enable fibrous tissue in-growth, resulting in dense vascular and myocardial adhesions and adding to the challenge of extraction.[4,5] Aggressive fibrosis of an SVC coil, which lies in an area at high risk for vascular injury, presents additional problems. Calcification of the fibrotic lesions can occur over time, further cementing the adhesion site and increasing the difficulties and risks of the extraction. Although predictors of severe scar formation have not been clearly identified, it seems that younger patients develop more vigorous fibrotic responses and more frequently develop progressive calcification.[6] In addition to human-lead interaction, lead-lead binding can significantly increase the difficulty of lead extraction. Thus, lead type, the presence of multiple leads, and implant duration are important factors impacting the safety and efficacy of TLE.

Think Before You Choose

As described previously, the high-voltage coils of ICD leads pose a particular challenge to extraction. Most current ICD leads come in two versions, a dual coil and single coil. The majority of ICD leads implanted worldwide are dual coil leads.

Dr Maytin has no disclosures. Dr Epstein has received research grants from and is a consultant for Boston Scientific, Medtronic, Spectranetics, and St Jude Medical and has equity in and served as a board member for Carrot Medical.
Cardiovascular Division, Brigham and Women's Hospital, 75 Francis Street, Boston, MA 02215, USA
* Corresponding author.
E-mail address: mmaytin@partners.org

Card Electrophysiol Clin 3 (2011) 359–372
doi:10.1016/j.ccep.2011.05.003

cardiacEP.theclinics.com

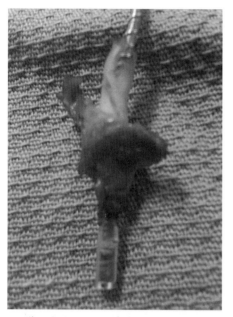

Fig. 1. Fibrosis in areas of direct contact. Vigorous fibrosis develops in areas of direct contact between the lead and the vasculature and myocardium. Extracted defibrillator lead found to have a large amount of organized fibrosis at the electrode tip-myocardial interface.

Those who extract leads more often choose single coil leads to reduce the need to deal with the SVC coil during future extractions. The authors believe the preference of dual coil leads is purely habit in most cases. Early transvenous ICD lead systems required both a right ventricular (RV) and an SVC coil for an adequate shocking vector because the device was implanted in the abdomen. The first of these systems consisted of separate RV and SVC defibrillator leads. A major advance was the development of a dual coil lead that allowed for the implantation of a single lead. Since these early systems, the ICD has continued to evolve. Devices now deliver a biphasic waveform, dramatically reducing defibrillation thresholds. In addition, devices are now small enough for pectoral implant and have active cans, thus eliminating the need for a second high-voltage electrode. Studies have demonstrated no difference in defibrillation thresholds with dual coil and single coil leads with current ICD systems. The authors, therefore, suggest that implanters consider the potential need for extraction when choosing a lead.

TLE INDICATIONS

As advances in extraction techniques have made the procedure safer and more successful, TLE indications have expanded to include more clinical situations.[7] The 2009 Heart Rhythm Society Expert Consensus Statement on Transvenous Lead Extraction has extended class I indications to include patients with CIED pocket infection, occult gram-positive infection, and functional leads that, due to design or failure, may pose an immediate threat if left in place (**Table 1**). Additionally, the class II indications for TLE are divided into IIa (reasonable to perform the procedure) and IIb (may consider performing the procedure) indications. CIED patients with occult gram-negative bacteremia, severe chronic pain, ipsilateral venous occlusion with contraindication to contralateral implantation, nonfunctional leads, need for MRI with no other imaging alternatives, and in whom implantation would result in more than 4 leads on one side or more than 5 leads through the SVC represent class IIa indications for TLE. Class IIb indications for TLE include CIED patients with superfluous functional or nonfunctional leads and with functional leads that pose risk of device interference or that due to design or failure pose potential future risk.

In assessing an individual's indication for TLE, a comparison of the risks of extraction with the risks of lead abandonment is mandated (**Fig. 2**). The consideration of patient and lead characteristics and, importantly, operator experience must be factored into the risk assessment of extraction. Specifically, the risk assessment evaluation must include specific attention to the number of leads, implant duration, defibrillator versus pacing electrodes, and patient age.

It cannot be emphasized enough that decisions regarding lead extraction must be made on a case-by-case basis integrating various patient and lead characteristics and operator-related variables. In patients with a poor prognosis or where the risks of intervention clearly outweigh the risks of lead abandonment, lead extraction with its potential for significant morbidity and mortality may not be warranted. Moreover, those inexperienced in the procedure should not perform lead extractions nor should those without the necessary tools available to attain complete success or in a setting not prepared and committed to the complete and safe performance of the procedure.[7]

TLE TECHNIQUES AND TOOLS
Preprocedure and Patient Preparation

TLE, like any surgical procedure, requires a team approach with anticipation of and planning for all potential situations. At minimum, the required personnel of the extraction team include the physician performing the extraction, a cardiothoracic surgeon, anesthesia support, an x-ray technician or other person to operate the fluoroscopy, and both scrubbed and nonscrubbed assistants. Although complications occur, the single most important factor in preventing a major complication from becoming a death is the time to definitive intervention. Thus, the procedure location (ie, operating room or catheterization/electrophysiology laboratory) is less important than the immediate availability of cardiothoracic surgical intervention. This mandates that a surgeon proficient at managing the potential complications is on site during the extraction procedure and that the equipment necessary for cardiopulmonary bypass is readily available. Additional emergency equipment that should be present in the room or immediately available includes transthoracic and/or transesophageal echocardiography, pericardiocentesis tray, vacuum containers for chest tube drainage, temporary pacing equipment, and an anesthesia cart for general anesthesia as well as vasopressors and other emergency medications. The authors have fashioned a mobile extraction cart that contains all the aforementioned emergency equipment in addition to extraction tools (locking stylets, nonpowered and powered sheaths, femoral workstations, extraction snares, and so forth) and CIED implant tools (stylets, wrenches, fixation tools, introducer sheaths, intravenous contrast, repair kits, and so forth).

Recognizing the potential need for emergent surgical intervention (**Table 2**), the authors' patients are prepared for the procedure in such a way so as to eliminate delays. Patients are prepped with a chlorhexadine solution and draped to allow access for contralateral implant or emergent pericardiocentesis, thoracentesis, thoracotomy, sternotomy, or cardiopulmonary bypass. It is the authors' practice that all patients have bilateral peripheral venous access with large bore catheters, femoral venous access, invasive hemodynamic monitoring with a radial arterial line, general endotracheal anesthesia, and 4 units of packed red blood cells immediately available. In addition, the entire team performing the procedure is aware and prepared to act in the event of any potential complications, from asystole due to a dislodged temporary wire to cardiac or SVC tear requiring immediate intervention.

Techniques

The authors use a stepwise approach to lead extraction in every case with the goal of complete success using the fewest number of tools (**Fig. 3**). Because TLE is routinely performed by superior approach via the implant vein, the initial step in the extraction procedure is an appropriately positioned incision that permits easy access to the venous entry site in a plane parallel to the leads. It is the authors' practice to attempt to use the existing incision whenever possible and perform an elliptical incision excising the existing incisional scar. Occasionally, two incisions are necessary—one over the venous entry site of the leads and a second over the pocket or area of skin erosion or adherence. Once the pocket is entered, microbial cultures of pocket tissue are obtained in all cases of CIED infection. Then, the device is removed and the leads are dissected free back to their venous entry site. Dissection around the venous entry site is important to allow easy passage of any devices that may be necessary for lead extraction but aggressive dissection can result in transient issues with hemostasis secondary to back bleeding. The anchor sleeves are then removed and all extraneous material, including suture material, is eliminated from the pocket. Complete removal of infected tissue and foreign material is mandatory in cases of CIED infection. Additionally, it is the authors' routine practice to perform a capsulectomy whenever ipsilateral reimplantation is planned.

If ipsilateral reimplantation is planned (never in the setting of infection), ipsilateral venous access is attempted under fluoroscopic guidance with or without the aid of intravenous contrast. In the authors' experience, stenotic lesions and even total occlusions can often be crossed with a use of a 5-French dilator and Terumo Glidewire (Terumo Medical Corporation, Somerset, New Jersey). If the vein is successfully cannulated and a wire could be passed into the inferior vena cava or if ipsilateral reimplantation is not planned, lead removal with simple traction is attempted after extraction of the active fixation screw, if present. If this proves unsuccessful, the lead is cut and a locking stylet is introduced, a #5 silk is tied around the lead body, and traction reattempted. The #5 silk is used to reinforce the lead and to prevent the insulation from bunching up or snow plowing under the force of counterpressure. In the case of multipolar ICD leads, the individual cables can be tied together and then another suture applied to the joined cables to provide additional traction. If lead removal still proves unsuccessful, a nonpowered or powered sheath is used. Sheath selection is determined by the clinical situation and the operator's preference and experience. If the lead is not retrievable from the implant vein or lead disruption occurs, transfemoral retrieval is performed.

Counterpressure, traction, and countertraction
Counterpressure is the force applied by the nonpowered or powered sheath as it is advanced

Table 1
Indications for transvenous lead extraction

Indication	Class I Procedure *SHOULD* be Performed	Class IIa *REASONABLE* to Perform Procedure	Class IIb Procedure *MAY BE CONSIDERED*	Class III Procedure Should *NOT* be Performed
Infection	1. Definite CIED infection (eg, valvular endocarditis, DRE, or sepsis) *(LOE: B)* 2. CIED pocket infection (eg, abscess, erosion, or chronic draining sinus) *(LOE: B)* 3. Valvular endocarditis w/o definite lead and/or device involvement *(LOE: B)* 4. Occult gram-positive bacteremia *(LOE: B)*	1. Persistent occult gram-negative bacteremia *(LOE: B)*		1. Superficial or incisional infection w/o involvement of device/leads *(LOE: C)* 2. Chronic bacteremia due to a source other than CIED when long-term suppressive antibiotics are required *(LOE: C)*
Thrombosis or Venous Stenosis	1. Clinically significant TE events associated w/ thrombus on lead or fragment *(LOE: C)* 2. Bilateral SCV or SVC occlusion precluding implant of needed TV lead *(LOE: C)* 3. Planned stent deployment in vein w/ TV lead already to avoid entrapment *(LOE: C)* 4. Symptomatic SVC stenosis/occlusion *(LOE: C)* 5. Ipsilateral venous occlusion precluding implant of additional lead when contralateral implant contraindicated (AVF, shunt or vascular access port, mastectomy) *(LOE: C)*	1. Ipsilateral venous occlusion precluding ipsilateral implant of additional lead w/o contraindication to contralateral implant *(LOE: C)*		

	Class I	Class IIa	Class IIb
Functional Leads	1. Life-threatening arrhythmias due to retained leads (LOE: B) 2. Leads, due to design or failure, may pose immediate threat if left in place (LOE: B) 3. Leads that interfere w/ CIED function (LOE: B) 4. Leads that interfere w/ treatment of malignancy (radiation, surgery) (LOE: C)	1. Leads w/ potential interference w/ CIED function (LOE: C) 2. Leads, due to design or failure, w/ potential threat if left in place (LOE: C) 3. Abandoned leads (LOE: C) 4. Need for MRI imaging w/o alternative (LOE: C) 5. Need for MRI conditional CIED system (LOE: C)	1. Redundant leads with <1 y life expectancy (LOE: C) 2. Known anomalous lead placement (SCA, Ao, pleura, etc.) or through a systemic atrium or ventricle* (LOE: C) * Can be considered w/ surgical backup
Non Functional Leads	1. Leads, due to design or failure, w/ potential threat if left in place (LOE: C) 2. CIED implant would yield >4 leads on 1 side or >5 leads through SVC (LOE: C) 3. Need for MRI imaging w/o alternative (LOE: C)	1. At time of indicated CIED procedure w/o contraindication to TLE (LOE: C) 2. Need for MRI conditional CIED system (LOE: C)	1. Redundant leads with <1 y life expectancy (LOE: C) 2. Known anomalous lead placement (SCA, Ao, pleura, etc.) or through a systemic atrium or ventricle* (LOE: C) * Can be considered w/ surgical backup
Chronic Pain	1. Severe chronic pain at device or lead insertion site w/ significant discomfort not manageable by medical or surgical techniques and w/o acceptable alternative (LOE: C)		

Abbreviations: Ao, aorta; AVF, arteriovenous fistula; DRE, device-related endocarditis; LOE, level of evidence; SCA, subclavian artery; SCV, subclavian vein; TE, thromboembolic; TV, transvenous; w/, with; w/o, without.

Adapted from Wilkoff BL, Love CJ, Byrd CL, et al. Transvenous lead extraction: Heart Rhythm Society Expert consensus on facilities, training, indications, and patient management: this document was endorsed by the American Heart Association (AHA). Heart Rhythm 2009;6:1085; with permission.

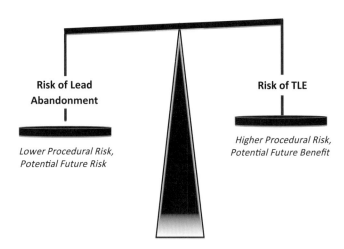

Risk vs. Risk

Fig. 2. Risk versus risk. The decision regarding lead extraction or abandonment requires comparison of the current risks of lead extraction with the future risks of both lead abandonment and potential lead extraction.

over the lead, interrupting areas of adherent scar tissue. Sufficient traction must be applied to the lead and locking stylet so that the lead acts as a rail. This allows the sheath to follow the lead body and not damage the vasculature as the leads curves within the vein. This is especially true when passing the sheath from the brachiocephalic vein through the SVC to the right atrium. By exerting significantly more pull than push, the lateral force on the SVC can be reduced. Countertraction is a technique used once the sheath has been advanced to the lead tip-myocardium interface. Applying countertraction limits the traction forces on an entrapped electrode to the circumference of the sheath at the lead tip-myocardium interface. Once the lead is released from the fibrous tissue, the myocardium falls away from the sheath, reducing the risk of myocardial invagination and injury (**Fig. 4**).[8–10]

Approaches
Leads are typically extracted by a superior approach via the implant vein although alternative approaches are used in certain situations. For example, when the free lead tip cannot be reached from the implant vein, an inferior approach via the

Table 2	
Potential complications of TLE	

Major Complications	Minor Complications
Death	Pericardial effusion not requiring intervention
Cardiac avulsion requiring intervention (percutaneous or surgical)	Hemothorax not requiring intervention
Vascular injury requiring intervention (percutaneous or surgical)	Pocket hematoma requiring reoperation
Pulmonary embolism requiring surgical intervention	Upper extremity thrombosis resulting in medical treatment
Respiratory arrest/anesthesia-related complication prolonging hospitalization stroke	Vascular repair near implant site or venous entry site
CIED infection at previously noninfected site	Hemodynamically significant air embolism migrated lead fragment without sequelae Blood transfusion as a result of intraoperative blood loss Pneumothorax requiring a chest tube Pulmonary embolism not requiring surgical intervention

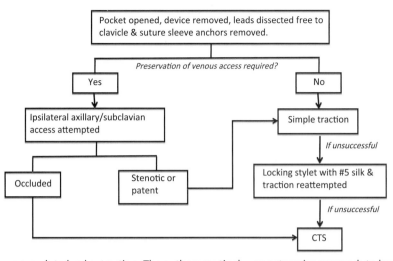

Fig. 3. Stepwise approach to lead extraction. The authors routinely use a stepwise approach to lead extraction so as to achieve the highest rate of complete success using the least amount of tools. CTS, countertraction sheath, including mechanical dilating sheaths, laser sheaths, or mechanical cutting sheaths.

femoral vein is necessary. Occasionally, hybrid or alternative venous approaches are used. The success of a combined approach via the femoral and internal jugular veins for free-floating leads and leads with dense SVC adhesions has been reported by Bongiorni and colleagues.[11] Lead stabilization by femoral snaring via an inferior approach provides a straighter rail for extraction approach from the right internal jugular vein, decreasing the likelihood of SVC avulsion. Recently, Fischer and colleagues[12] described a hybrid superior and inferior approach with femoral snaring of the lead to provide stability from below while counterpressure and traction were applied from above.

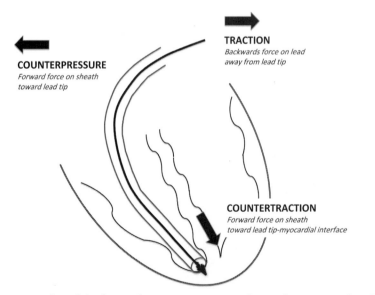

Fig. 4. Schematic representation of the forces of counterpressure, traction, and countertraction. Counterpressure is the force applied by the nonpowered or powered sheath as it is advanced forward over the lead interrupting areas of adherent scar tissue. Traction is the pulling force on the lead to provide a straight "rail" so as to allow the sheath to follow the lead. Countertraction is the forward force applied by the sheath at the myocardium to limit the traction forces on an entrapped electrode to the circumference of the sheath at the lead tip-myocardium interface. Once the lead is released from the fibrous tissue, the myocardium falls away from the sheath reducing the risk of myocardial invagination and injury.

They demonstrated this as a safe and effective technique for lead extraction with maintenance of venous access.

Tools

Locking stylets

The ability to successfully extract a lead with traction is directly dependent on the lead construction and its tensile strength.[6] Locking stylets were developed to reinforce the lead, transmit the extraction force to the tip of the lead, reduce the risk of lead disruption, and increase the likelihood of complete lead removal.[8,13,14] The authors believe the ability to place a locking stylet to the distal portion of the lead dramatically increases the chance of the complete extraction. Several types of locking stylets have been designed. Although the original locking stylets had to be sized to the luminal diameter of the conductor coil, the most commonly used locking stylets today are designed to accommodate a range of conductor coil diameters. The Liberator (Cook Medical, Bloomington, Indiana) and Lead Locking Device (LLD) EZ (Spectranetics, Colorado Springs, CO, USA) stylets offer similar support but differ in their locking mechanism design. The locking mechanism of the Liberator is at the distal tip of the stylet providing focal traction at the tip of the lead whereas the LLD EZ stylet grabs the lead in multiple areas and exerts force along the length of the lead (**Fig. 5**). In a lead that cannot receive a locking stylet, either due to extensive damage, inner conductor fracture, or a solid core design, applying sufficient traction can prove challenging. The Bulldog Lead Extender (Cook Medical) is a tool that can be useful in this situation (**Fig. 6**).

It consists of a wire with a threadable handle through which the lead is passed and secured, thereby locking the insulation and conductor to the extender. The advent of locking stylets has permitted safer and more successful TLE via the implant vein, stimulating the development of new techniques and technologies.

Telescoping sheaths

Telescoping sheaths are nonpowered sheaths available in a range of sizes from 7 to 16 French and made of different materials with varying properties, including stainless steel, Teflon, and polypropylene (**Fig. 7**). Teflon is soft and flexible but is unable to cut through dense scar tissue whereas polypropylene is stiffer and better at disrupting encapsulating scar but must be used with caution to avoid vascular injury. Stainless steel sheaths are used only for disrupting dense and calcified fibrosis as the central venous circulation is entered. The inner and outer sheath pair is advanced along the lead with alternating counterclockwise and clockwise motions with moderate pressure. The soft inner sheath is used as a guide whereas the more rigid outer sheath serves to disrupt and dilate the encapsulating fibrous tissue. Sufficient traction is essential to insure that the sheaths track the path of the lead and remain within the confines of the vasculature under fluoroscopic guidance. Utilizing telescoping TLE success rates via a superior (ie, implant vein) approach range from 71% to 97%.[8,9,13,15]

Powered sheaths

Powered sheaths use a source of energy to make the dissection of encapsulating fibrous tissue easier and more efficient, thus enabling the

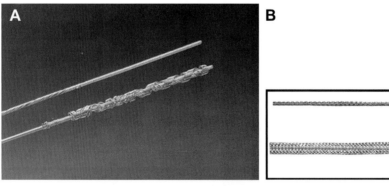

Fig. 5. Locking stylets. (*A*) The Liberator Locking Stylet (Cook Medical) fits leads with lumen diameters of 0.016 to 0.032 in. An undeployed Liberator locking stylet is shown above a deployed Liberator locking stylet. When deployed, the wound spring at the end of the stylet opens up, locking into place. (*Courtesy of* Cook Medical, Inc; with permission.) (*B*) LLD EZ (Spectranetics) has a radiopaque tip and accommodates inner coil diameters of 0.015 to 0.026 in (undepolyed stylet) (*top image*). In contrast to the Liberator locking stylet, the LLD locking stylet has a braided mesh over the entire length of a solid lead that expands when deployed (*bottom image*). (*Courtesy of* The Spectranetics Corporation, Inc; with permission.)

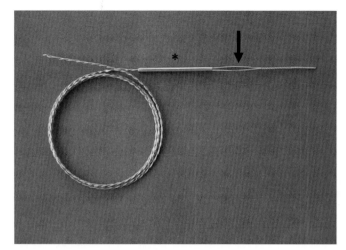

Fig. 6. Bulldog Lead Extender (Cook Medical). The Bulldog Lead Extender is a useful tool for leads that cannot receive a locking stylet, either due to extensive damage or a solid core design. The exposed end of the lead is passed through the loop of the Bulldog (*arrow*) and the metal sleeve (*asterisk*) is advanced over the loop grasping the lead. (*Courtesy of* Cook Medical, Inc; with permission.)

advancement of the sheath along the lead with reduced countertraction and counterpressure forces.[6,16] One such powered sheath is the Excimer Laser System (Spectranetics), a "cool," pulsed ultraviolet laser at a wavelength of 308 nm available in 12, 14, and 16 French sizes. The laser sheath applies circumferential pulses of energy at its distal end dissolving tissue in contact with the tip of the sheath by photochemical destruction of molecular bonds and photothermal ablation that vaporizes water and ruptures cells with resultant photomechanical creation of kinetic energy (**Fig. 8**).[17] The sheath is advanced over the lead body using the standard techniques of counterpressure and countertraction, and laser energy is delivered when encapsulating fibrous tissue halts sheath advancement. Tissue in direct contact with the sheath tip is ablated to a depth of 50 μm until the distal electrode is reached; countertraction is still necessary to dislocate the lead tip. In comparison with mechanical telescoping sheaths,

laser-assisted extraction resulted in more frequent complete lead removal and shortened extraction times without an increase in procedural risk.[18–20] The introduction of laser extraction changed the landscape of transvenous extraction, providing a highly effective and low morbidity technique with broad applications.[19–21]

The Perfecta Electrosurgical Dissection Sheath (Cook Medical) represents another type of powered sheath. The electrosurgical dissection sheath consists of an inner polytetrafluoroethylene sheath with bipolar tungsten electrodes exposed at the distal tip and an outer sheath for counterpressure and countertraction. Radiofrequency energy is delivered between the bipoles to dissect through fibrous binding sites, much like a surgical cautery tool, although the lead tip must be liberated with countertraction. In contrast to the Excimer Laser Sheath, the Electrosurgical Dissection Sheath permits a localized application of radiofrequency energy with linear rather than circumferential

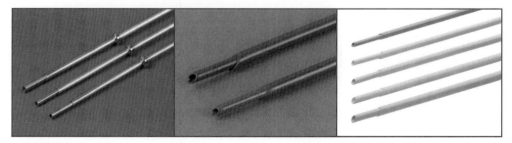

Fig. 7. Telescoping nonpowered countertraction sheaths. Telescoping sheaths are available in a range of sizes from 7 to 16 French and made of different materials with varying properties, including stainless steel, Teflon, and polypropylene (from left to right). (*Courtesy of* Cook Medical, Inc; with permission.)

A

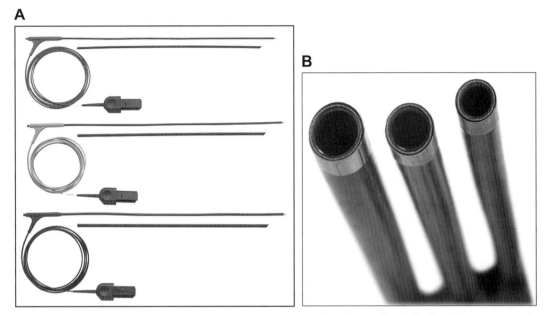

B

Fig. 8. Excimer laser sheaths (Spectranetics). (*A*) The Excimer laser sheath uses ultraviolet laser energy to vaporize tissue in contact with the tip of the sheath where the optical fibers terminate. The sheath available in a range of sizes (12 French, 14 French, and 16 French) displayed from top to bottom. (*B*) End-on view of the laser sheath demonstrating the distal end where the optical fibers terminate. (*Courtesy of* The Spectranetics Corporation, Inc; with permission.)

dissection of the encapsulating fibrous tissue. The focused and steerable dissection plane offers the potential advantages of improved precision however the sheath may have to be repositioned repeatedly as a result.

Despite the improved success rates of lead extraction with powered sheath technologies, disruption of calcified binding sites remains difficult with either system. The most recent addition to the armamentarium of lead extraction tools provides a solution. The Evolution Mechanical Dilator Sheath and Evolution Shortie Mechanical Dilator Sheath (Cook Medical) are hand-powered mechanical sheaths that consist of a flexible, braided stainless steel sheath with a stainless steel spiral cut dissection tip. The sheath is attached to a trigger activation handle that rotates the sheath and allows the threaded metal end to bore through calcified and dense adhesions (**Fig. 9**).[22] The authors' experience have found the Evolution sheath useful for

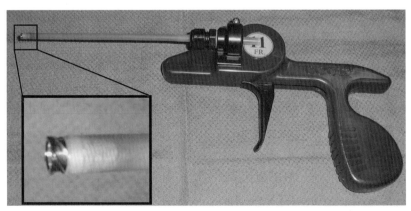

Fig. 9. The Evolution device. The Evolution Mechanical Dilator Sheath and Evolution Shortie Mechanical Dilator Sheath (Cook Medical) are hand-powered mechanical sheaths that consist of a flexible, braided stainless steel sheath with a stainless steel spiral cut dissection tip (*inset*). The sheath is attached to a trigger handle that rotates the sheath and allows the threaded metal end to agar out the scar tissue.

disrupting sites of calcified fibrosis but often at the expense of functional leads that were attempt to be preserved. Specifically, care must be taken to prevent nontargeted leads from becoming entwined by the Evolution sheath. Regardless, this technology has provided an effective alternative for dealing with the challenges densely scarred venous entry sites and heavily calcified adhesions.[23]

Femoral tools

Transfemoral lead retrieval with the Byrd Workstation (Cook Medical) is a necessary skill for successful lead extraction, particularly in cases when the lead is not accessible from the implant vein either as a result of previously cut leads that have retracted into the vasculature (**Fig. 10**) or lead disruption that occurs during the extraction procedure. The Byrd Workstation consists of a 16-French outer sheath with one-way valve that is advanced over a wire into the femoral vein and a 12-French inner sheath through which a number of retrieval snares can be advanced. The Workstation package contains a Needle's Eye Snare but several other snares can be used, including Mini-ENSnare (Angiotech, Gainesville, Florida) and Amplatz GooseNeck (ev3 Endovascular, Plymouth, Minnesota) snares. If lead retrieval with a Needle's Eye Snare proves unsuccessful, the combination of a gooseneck snare and bioptome forceps has been successful. The authors preload the gooseneck snare on the bioptome, advance the two together to the lead fragment, grasp the free lead tail with the bioptome, and then advance the GooseNeck snare over the bioptome to the ensnare the lead. The challenge of femoral retrieval remains manipulating the tools

and snaring the lead in 3-D using 2-D fluoroscopic imaging. The recent description of a novel technology to facilitate extraction and the maintenance of vascular access proposed a hybrid superior and inferior approach with femoral snaring of the lead to stabilize the lead while countertraction and counterpressure are used to free the lead reiterates the clinical importance of femoral retrieval[12] as does the internal jugular approach described by Bongiorni and colleagues.[11]

OUTCOMES

Early studies of TLE action of pacemaker leads with a laser sheath, such as the Pacemaker Lead Extraction with the Excimer Sheath (PLEXES) trial, demonstrated a marked improvement in extraction efficacy from 64% with traditional extraction techniques to 94% with laser-assisted extraction without a significant difference in complications, although significant crossover between groups occurred.[20] Similar success was observed with the use of larger laser sheaths for the removal of large diameter and ICD leads.[19] Coincident with the growth of the discipline of TLE, the authors have witnessed a marked decline in the incidence of procedure-related morbidity and mortality with several high-volume single centers reporting morbidity and mortality rates less than 1.0% and 0.3%, respectively, with ICD lead extraction experience ranging from approximately 5% to 50%.[11,24,25] A recent multicenter study of transvenous laser lead extraction of 2405 leads (29.2% ICD leads) demonstrated similarly low morbidity and mortality complication rates of 1.1% and 0.28%, respectively, with a higher clinical success

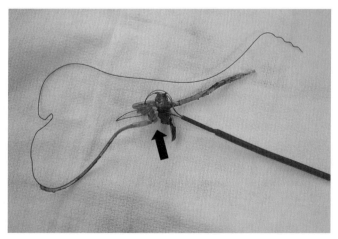

Fig. 10. Transfemoral snaring of lead. Transfemoral lead retrieval with the Byrd Workstation (Cook Medical) is a necessary skill for successful lead extraction, particularly in cases when the lead is not accessible from the implant vein as in a cut or fractured lead. The lead has been snared and wound up by the Needle's Eye Snare (*arrow*), allowing successful removal of the lead.

rate of 98.8%. Although data are limited, the success and complication rates for TLE of ICD as compared with pacemaker leads seem similar.[26–28] Newer ICD lead coil treatments, such as expanded polytetrafluoroethylene-coated and medical adhesive backfilled coils, have been demonstrated to facilitate ICD lead extraction albeit without an improvement in success rate or a reduction in complications.[5,29]

Complication rates with TLE directly parallel operator experience. Major and minor complications are reduced by approximately 50% with increased operator experience from 20 to 120 cases to more than 300 cases performed.[30] Large-scale multicenter randomized trials have confirmed the effect of experience on outcomes.[3,19–21,30] Likewise, observational registries of experienced, high-volume extractionists have consistently demonstrated even higher success rates (>99%) with exceedingly low major complication (<1.0%) and mortality rates (<0.3%).[11,24,25] Consequently, the 2009 Heart Rhythm Society Expert Consensus Statement on Transvenous Lead Extraction recommended that physicians being trained in TLE extract a minimum of 40 leads as primary operators under the direct supervision of a qualified physician and extract a minimum of 20 leads annually to maintain their skills.[7] This is a minimum recommendation; there are many experts who believe that the best outcomes come with additional experience. The ability for trainees and those post training to gain this experience is limited. Recently, Spectranetics and others have begun the development of a realistic simulator to allow for those interested in performing extractions to practice, gain experience, and confront emergencies in a safe and controlled environment.

LEAD MANAGEMENT

CIED use has increased exponentially over the past decade[31–33] with more than 4.5 million active devices and more than 1 million new leads implanted annually.[34,35] With expanded CIED use and indications for device therapy, observed complications have increased in parallel.[36–44] The occurrence of more frequent device system revisions for complications,[36,38,44] system upgrade,[45–47] and/or lead malfunction[37,39–42] and longer patient life expectancies have mandated a paradigm shift toward premeditated lead management strategies from implant to removal or replacement. Proactive lead management requires both forethought and conscious decisions at the time of CIED implantation with respect to hardware selection (eg, single coil versus dual coil defibrillator leads), implant vein access, and lead abandonment versus extraction, if necessary.

SUMMARY

TLE has evolved dramatically over the past 30 years and exponentially throughout the past decade. Despite these advances, the basic tenants of counterpressure, traction, and countertraction remain critical to insuring successful and safe outcomes regardless of lead type. As indications for device therapy expand and younger patients receive devices, it is likely that the number of lead extractions performed will increase and similarly the pressure on the field to continue to evolve not only as a technique but also as a discipline and a science. Future developments in ICD lead extraction are likely to focus on comprehensive device management, alternative systems for extraction training, and the design of new leads conceived to facilitate future extraction. Regardless of the field's future directions, the decision to extract a lead in any patient must involve an individualized process considering all patient variables and the experience and outcomes of the extraction program.

REFERENCES

1. Huang TY, Baba N. Cardiac pathology of transvenous pacemakers. Am Heart J 1972;83:469.
2. Robboy SJ, Harthorne JW, Leinbach RC, et al. Autopsy findings with permanent pervenous pacemakers. Circulation 1969;39:495.
3. Smith HJ, Fearnot NE, Byrd CL, et al. Five-years experience with intravascular lead extraction. U.S. lead extraction database. Pacing Clin Electrophysiol 1994;17:2016.
4. Epstein AE, Kay GN, Plumb VJ, et al. Gross and microscopic pathological changes associated with nonthoracotomy implantable defibrillator leads. Circulation 1998;98:1517.
5. Hackler JW, Sun Z, Lindsay BD, et al. Effectiveness of implantable cardioverter defibrillator lead coil treatments in facilitating ease of extraction. Heart Rhythm 2010;7(7):890–7.
6. Smith MC, Love CJ. Extraction of transvenous pacing and ICD leads. Pacing Clin Electrophysiol 2008;31:736.
7. Wilkoff BL, Love CJ, Byrd CL, et al. Transvenous lead extraction: Heart Rhythm Society Expert consensus on facilities, training, indications, and patient management: this document was endorsed by the American Heart Association (AHA). Heart Rhythm 2009;6: 1085.
8. Byrd CL, Schwartz SJ. Transatrial implantation of transvenous pacing leads as an alternative to implantation of epicardial leads. Pacing Clin Electrophysiol 1856;13:1990.

9. Byrd CL, Schwartz SJ, Hedin N. Intravascular techniques for extraction of permanent pacemaker leads. J Thorac Cardiovasc Surg 1991;101:989.

10. Byrd CL, Schwartz SJ, Hedin N. Lead extraction. Indications and techniques. Cardiol Clin 1992;10:735.

11. Bongiorni MG, Soldati E, Zucchelli G, et al. Transvenous removal of pacing and implantable cardiac defibrillating leads using single sheath mechanical dilatation and multiple venous approaches: high success rate and safety in more than 2000 leads. Eur Heart J 2008;29:2886.

12. Fischer A, Love B, Hansalia R, et al. Transfemoral snaring and stabilization of pacemaker and defibrillator leads to maintain vascular access during lead extraction. Pacing Clin Electrophysiol 2009;32:336.

13. Fearnot NE, Smith HJ, Goode LB, et al. Intravascular lead extraction using locking stylets, sheaths, and other techniques. Pacing Clin Electrophysiol 1864;13:1990.

14. Goode LB, Byrd CL, Wilkoff BL, et al. Development of a new technique for explantation of chronic transvenous pacemaker leads: five initial case studies. Biomed Instrum Technol 1991;25:50.

15. Brodell GK, Castle LW, Maloney JD, et al. Chronic transvenous pacemaker lead removal using a unique, sequential transvenous system. Am J Cardiol 1990;66:964.

16. Bongiorni MG, Giannola G, Arena G, et al. Pacing and implantable cardioverter-defibrillator transvenous lead extraction. Ital Heart J 2005;6:261.

17. Gijsbers GH, van den Broecke DG, Sprangers RL, et al. Effect of force on ablation depth for a XeCl excimer laser beam delivered by an optical fiber in contact with arterial tissue under saline. Lasers Surg Med 1992;12:576.

18. Byrd CL, Wilkoff BL, Love CJ, et al. Clinical study of the laser sheath for lead extraction: the total experience in the United States. Pacing Clin Electrophysiol 2002;25:804.

19. Epstein LM, Byrd CL, Wilkoff BL, et al. Initial experience with larger laser sheaths for the removal of transvenous pacemaker and implantable defibrillator leads. Circulation 1999;100:516.

20. Wilkoff BL, Byrd CL, Love CJ, et al. Pacemaker lead extraction with the laser sheath: results of the pacing lead extraction with the excimer sheath (PLEXES) trial. J Am Coll Cardiol 1999;33:1671.

21. Wazni O, Epstein LM, Carrillo RG, et al. Lead extraction in the contemporary setting: the LExICon study an observational retrospective study of consecutive laser lead extractions. J Am Coll Cardiol 2010;55:579.

22. Dello Russo A, Biddau R, Pelargonio G, et al. Lead extraction: a new effective tool to overcome fibrous binding sites. J Interv Card Electrophysiol 2009;24:147.

23. Hussein AA, Wilkoff BL, Martin DO, et al. Initial experience with the Evolution mechanical dilator sheath for lead extraction: Safety and efficacy. Heart Rhythm 2010;7(7):870-3.

24. Jones SO, Eckart RE, Albert CM, et al. Large, single-center, single-operator experience with transvenous lead extraction: outcomes and changing indications. Heart Rhythm 2008;5:520.

25. Kennergren C, Bjurman C, Wiklund R, et al. A single-centre experience of over one thousand lead extractions. Europace 2009;11:612.

26. Bracke F, Meijer A, Van Gelder B. Extraction of pacemaker and implantable cardioverter defibrillator leads: patient and lead characteristics in relation to the requirement of extraction tools. Pacing Clin Electrophysiol 2002;25:1037.

27. Malecka B, Kutarski A, Grabowski M. Is the transvenous extraction of cardioverter-defibrillator leads more hazardous than that of pacemaker leads? Kardiol Pol 2010;68:884.

28. Saad EB, Saliba WI, Schweikert RA, et al. Nonthoracotomy implantable defibrillator lead extraction: results and comparison with extraction of pacemaker leads. Pacing Clin Electrophysiol 2003;26:1944.

29. Di Cori A, Bongiorni MG, Zucchelli G, et al. Transvenous extraction performance of expanded polytetrafluoroethylene covered ICD leads in comparison to traditional ICD leads in humans. Pacing Clin Electrophysiol 2010;33:1376.

30. Byrd CL, Wilkoff BL, Love CJ, et al. Intravascular extraction of problematic or infected permanent pacemaker leads: 1994-1996. U.S. Extraction Database, MED Institute. Pacing Clin Electrophysiol 1999;22:1348.

31. DeFrances CJ, Lucas CA, Buie VC, et al. 2006 National hospital discharge survey. Natl Health Stat Report 2008;(5):1–20.

32. Hammill SC, Kremers MS, Kadish AH, et al. Review of the ICD Registry's third year, expansion to include lead data and pediatric ICD procedures, and role for measuring performance. Heart Rhythm 2009;6:1397.

33. Maisel WH, Moynahan M, Zuckerman BD, et al. Pacemaker and ICD generator malfunctions: analysis of Food and Drug Administration annual reports. JAMA 2006;295:1901.

34. Agarwal SK, Kamireddy S, Nemec J, et al. Predictors of complications of endovascular chronic lead extractions from pacemakers and defibrillators: a single-operator experience. J Cardiovasc Electrophysiol 2009;20:171.

35. Borek PP, Wilkoff BL. Pacemaker and ICD leads: strategies for long-term management. J Interv Card Electrophysiol 2008;23:59.

36. Cabell CH, Heidenreich PA, Chu VH, et al. Increasing rates of cardiac device infections among

Medicare beneficiaries: 1990–1999. Am Heart J 2004;147:582.

37. Dorwarth U, Frey B, Dugas M, et al. Transvenous defibrillation leads: high incidence of failure during long-term follow-up. J Cardiovasc Electrophysiol 2003;14:38.

38. Eckstein J, Koller MT, Zabel M, et al. Necessity for surgical revision of defibrillator leads implanted long-term: causes and management. Circulation 2008;117:2727.

39. Ellenbogen KA, Wood MA, Shepard RK, et al. Detection and management of an implantable cardioverter defibrillator lead failure: incidence and clinical implications. J Am Coll Cardiol 2003;41:73.

40. Haqqani HM, Mond HG. The implantable cardioverter-defibrillator lead: principles, progress, and promises. Pacing Clin Electrophysiol 2009;32:1336.

41. Kleemann T, Becker T, Doenges K, et al. Annual rate of transvenous defibrillation lead defects in implantable cardioverter-defibrillators over a period of >10 years. Circulation 2007;115:2474.

42. Luria D, Glikson M, Brady PA, et al. Predictors and mode of detection of transvenous lead malfunction in implantable defibrillators. Am J Cardiol 2001;87: 901.

43. Pakarinen S, Oikarinen L, Toivonen L. Short-term implantation-related complications of cardiac rhythm management device therapy: a retrospective single-centre 1-year survey. Europace 2010;12:103.

44. Voigt A, Shalaby A, Saba S. Continued rise in rates of cardiovascular implantable electronic device infections in the united states: temporal trends and causative insights. Pacing Clin Electrophysiol 2010;33:414.

45. Foley PW, Muhyaldeen SA, Chalil S, et al. Long-term effects of upgrading from right ventricular pacing to cardiac resynchronization therapy in patients with heart failure. Europace 2009;11:495.

46. Sweeney MO, Shea JB, Ellison KE. Upgrade of permanent pacemakers and single chamber implantable cardioverter defibrillators to pectoral dual chamber implantable cardioverter defibrillators: indications, surgical approach, and long-term clinical results. Pacing Clin Electrophysiol 2002;25: 1715.

47. Vatankulu MA, Goktekin O, Kaya MG, et al. Effect of long-term resynchronization therapy on left ventricular remodeling in pacemaker patients upgraded to biventricular devices. Am J Cardiol 2009;103: 1280.

Strategies to Reduce ICD Shocks: The Role of Supraventricular Tachycardia–Ventricular Tachycardia Discriminators

Joseph J. Gard, MD, Paul A. Friedman, MD*

KEYWORDS

- Cardioverter defibrillator • Supraventricular tachycardia
- Inappropriate therapy

Implantable cardioverter defibrillators (ICDs) are designed to offer survival benefit by treating life-threatening tachyarrhythmias such as ventricular tachycardia (VT) and ventricular fibrillation (VF).[1–5] In isolation, ICDs do not provide symptomatic improvement, although therapy may abort pending syncope caused by bradyarrhythmias or tachyarrhythmias. However, cardiac resynchronization therapy-defibrillators (CRT-D) improve symptoms of heart failure, exercise tolerance, and longevity, and prevent heart failure hospitalizations by means of left ventricular pacing and resynchronization.[6,7] Despite their benefits, ICDs are a potential cause of significant morbidity because of inappropriate shocks, which are common and occur in roughly a quarter of patients with ICDs.[8–10] Shocks may cause patients physical pain, psychological trauma, and reduce their quality of life.[11] Inappropriate and appropriate shocks may also be associated with increased mortality.[12,13]

Because inappropriate shocks are a potential source of harm to the patient, the potential life-saving benefit of an ICD must be balanced against the physician's responsibility to do no harm (primum non nocere). Thus, means to reduce inappropriate shocks must be considered. Traditional causes of inappropriate shocks include electrical noise classified as external (electromagnetic interference) or internal, occurring within the circuit because of a conductor defect, loose set-screw, or air in the header; oversensing of cardiac or extracardiac physiologic signals; and inappropriate detection of supraventricular tachycardia (SVT) as VT.[14,15] Detection of self-terminating arrhythmias, although often classified as appropriate because the arrhythmia before therapy delivery is ventricular, leads to unnecessary battery depletion and shocks.[16] A comprehensive programming strategy can reduce the risk of inappropriate and appropriate shocks.

Disclosures: Joseph J. Gard, MD: none. Paul A. Friedman, MD, research support from Medtronic (grant administered by Mayo Clinic for investigator initiated study) and Pfizer. Intellectual property rights: Bard EP, Hewlett Packard, Medical Positioning, Inc, Aegis Medical, NeoChord. Speaker or Consultant: Medtronic, Boston Scientific, St Jude, Bard.
Division of Cardiovascular Disease, Mayo Clinic, Rochester, MN, USA
* Corresponding author. Division of Cardiovascular Diseases, Mayo Clinic, 200 1st Street SW, Rochester, MN 55905.
E-mail address: friedman.paul@mayo.edu

Card Electrophysiol Clin 3 (2011) 373–387
doi:10.1016/j.ccep.2011.05.004
1877-9182/11/$ – see front matter © 2011 Elsevier Inc. All rights reserved.

cardiacEP.theclinics.com

THE CASCADE OF EVENTS LEADING TO AN ICD SHOCK

Once a tachycardia occurs, a cascade of events transpires before ICD shock delivery (**Fig. 1**). Thoughtful programming at each step of the cascade offers an opportunity for shock prevention. There are some fundamental concepts in minimizing ICD morbidity:

- Avoid treatment of slower tachycardias
- Avoid treatment of nonsustained tachycardias
- Use SVT-VT discriminators to avoid shocking SVT
- Apply antitachycardia pacing (ATP) before shock delivery
- Deliver shocks of sufficient energy to ensure that the first shock succeeds
- Minimize ventricular pacing in non-CRT devices to avoid congestive heart failure (CHF) exacerbation and atrial fibrillation (AF).[17–20]

The risk of inappropriate therapy increases with the number of tachycardias to which an ICD is exposed.[21] In the Detect SVT study, in which a cutoff rate of 150 beats per minute (bpm) was used, 52% or 400 subjects had an ICD tachycardia detection of any kind at 6 months.[21] In contrast, the PREPARE study used a detection rate of 182, and approximately 25% of subjects experienced events at 1 year. Because of differences in populations and other detection parameters (including duration), a direct comparison cannot be made. Nonetheless, it is clear that an ICD cannot treat a tachycardia it does not detect, and that

withholding therapy for tachycardias slower than 182 bpm in a large primary prevention population does not seem to increase mortality or syncope.[22]

Rapid delivery of ICD shocks results in overtreatment of self-terminating arrhythmias, and accelerated battery depletion.[16] Increasing the number of intervals required to detect VF from 12 to 18 reduces the episode rate by 22% with a clinically insignificant added shock delay of less than 2 seconds.[16] In a large primary prevention study, setting VF detection to 30 out of 40 intervals (approximately 9 seconds delay from arrhythmia onset to detection), was associated with significantly fewer shocks without increased syncope risk compared with historical controls.[22] Increasing the required duration to therapy prevents treatment of nonsustained supraventricular and ventricular episodes. Because most noise caused by lead fracture is brief and occurs during less than 10% of the cardiac cycle, with extending detection the risk of noise-related inappropriate shock is also reduced.[14,15,23]

Once a tachycardia meets rate and duration thresholds, SVT-VT discriminators are applied to avoid therapy delivery for SVT; these are reviewed in greater detail later. If the tachycardia is not rejected as SVT, ATP terminates 72% of fast monomorphic VTs without the need for a shock.[17,18] ATP also terminates atrioventricular (AV) node-dependent SVTs, provides additional time for spontaneous arrhythmia termination, and may transiently slow the ventricular response during AF via concealed conduction into the AV node. The investigators' suggested programming to address all of the major steps in the cascade to shock are summarized at the end of this article.

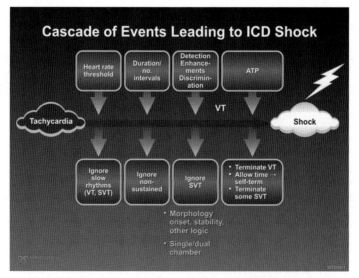

Fig. 1. Cascade of events leading to ICD shock. A sequence of events occurs before an ICD delivers a shock. Each offers an opportunity from programming to minimize appropriate and inappropriate shock delivery. Full details in text.

The Big Picture

Use of upstream therapies prevents tachycardias from occurring, and is an important part of comprehensive care for the arrhythmia patient. Inflammation,[24] sleep apnea,[25] hypercatecholaminergic states,[26] alcohol ingestion,[27] ischemia,[28] progressive heart failure,[5] and obesity[29] may contribute to arrhythmogenesis. Retrospective studies and post hoc analysis of prospective randomized trials have found that, in patients with ICDs, statin use is associated with reduced inappropriate shocks caused by AF,[30] fewer ventricular tachyarrhythmia episodes,[31,32] and improved survival (**Table 1**).[33] These findings were present in patients with ischemic and nonischemic cardiomyopathy, suggesting that among the pleiotropic effects of statins, their antiinflammatory properties may be contributatory.[34] Patients with ICDs similarly benefit from angiotensin-converting enzyme (ACE) inhibitor and β-blocker therapy with fewer VT/VF episodes and a survival benefit.[35,36] The role of upstream therapies has been reviewed elsewhere.[37]

SVT DISCRIMINATORS AND THEIR APPLICATION

SVT-VT discriminators are algorithms that analyze ventricular and atrial intervals and/or morphologic features to distinguish SVT from VT. In order for discriminators to be applied, a tachycardia must exceed the VT detection rate, discriminators must be programmed on, and the tachycardia must be slower than the VF detection rate or an explicitly programmed SVT upper detection limit, depending on the manufacturer. In St Jude devices, the SVT discriminators can be programmed in either or both VT zones but not the VF zone. Similarly, Boston Scientific devices, since the introduction of Vitality in 2004, have allowed SVT discriminators to be programmed in either or both VT zones. However, Boston Scientific devices in generations before Vitality only allowed for SVT discriminators within the slow VT zone. Medtronic devices allow an SVT limit to be programmed irrespective of ranges set for the VT and VF zones. However, discriminator function is modified in the VF zone; SVT with AV dissociation (ie, AF) is not classified as SVT when its rate is within the VF zone[14] because both are irregular. Approximately 25% of SVTs receive ventricular therapy because their cycle length falls within a zone for which discriminators are not applied; appropriate programming is critical to ensure that SVT-VT discriminators are applied.[38] SVT-VT discriminators available in single-chamber ICDs include stability, onset, and morphology.

SVT DISCRIMINATORS IN SINGLE-CHAMBER DEVICES
Stability

Interval stability distinguishes AF, characterized by irregular R-R intervals, from VT, which is regular.[39–42] In published studies, the sensitivity and specificity of stability algorithms has varied depending on the stability value programmed and the heart rate it is applied to; with a stability of 30 milliseconds applied to heart rates of 150 to 169 bpm, a sensitivity of 94.5% and specificity of 76.5% has been reported.[40,42–44] When used in dual-chamber ICDs, confirmation of a rapid

Table 1						
Role of statin therapy in ICD recipients						
Trial	No.	On Statin (%)	Follow-up Duration	Population	HR for Mortality with Statin (95% CI)	HR for VT/VF Occurrence with Statin (95% CI)
AVID	362	21[a]	28	Secondary prevention	0.36 (0.15–0.68)	0.40 (0.15–0.58)
DEFINITE	458	24	29	Primary prevention: nonischemic cardiomyopathy	0.22 (0.09–0.55)	0.78 (0.34–1.82)
MADIT-II	654[b]	77[c]	17	Primary prevention: ischemic cardiomyopathy	NG	0.72 (0.52–0.99)
SCD-HeFT	2512	47	46	Primary prevention: ischemic + nonischemic cardiomyopathy	0.70 (0.58–0.83)	N/A

Abbreviations: CI, confidence interval; HR, heart rate; N/A, not available.
  [a] Denotes that AVID evaluated lipid therapy involving statins.
  [b] Denotes that, in MADIT-II, only the ICD subpopulation was included in the nested cohort study.
  [c] Denotes that MADIT-II compared patients with greater than 90% use of statins versus less than or equal to 10% usage.

atrial rate in association with ventricular irregularity enhances algorithmic function (discussed later). Unlike onset, which only makes a determination of SVT versus VT as the rate crosses the VT cutoff, stability continually assesses an ongoing tachycardia, lowering the risk of underdetection of significant VT to less than 0.5%.[45] Sinus tachycardia with ectopy, or ventricular tachycardia made irregular in the setting of antiarrhythmic drugs (amiodarone or Class 1C agents) can lead to classification errors.[46,47] AF at rates greater than approximately 170 bpm becomes more regular, limiting SVT-VT discrimination based on interval stability alone.[41]

Onset

The sudden onset detection enhancement analyzes the rate at which a tachycardia begins to distinguish sinus tachycardia, which starts with a gradual heart rate increase, from VT, which begins abruptly.[41,42] The use of the onset discriminator has been shown to reduce shocks caused by sinus tachycardia.[42] Misclassification can occur when VT begins at less than the VT detection rate, and then gradually increases across the sinus-VT rate boundary, or when ectopy during sinus tachycardia produces abrupt interval changes.[44] A limitation of the onset discriminator is that is assesses a tachyarrhythmia only at its onset so that it cannot correct misclassifications. Underdetection of significant VT occurs in 0.5% to 5% of episodes.[41,44] Sudden onset is not used during redetection. An example of the use of sudden onset (in a dual-chamber ICD) is shown in **Fig. 2.**

Morphology

Morphology algorithms compare a stored sinus or baseline rhythm template with a template acquired during a tachycardia. With VT, the morphology of the ventricular electrogram differs from the reference; during SVT the acquired morphology matches the baseline template. This finding has been shown as an effective SVT-VT discriminator when used in conjunction with other discriminators.[48–51]

The general steps within an morphology discrimination algorithm are to (1) obtain a representative ventricular electrogram template during baseline rhythm; (2) generate a quantitative representation of this template that is stored for future comparison; (3) obtain a ventricular electrogram during an unknown tachycardia and translate it into a quantitative representation; (4) time align the ventricular electrograms for comparison; (5) compare the degree of similarity between the quantitative representation of the unknown tachycardia with that of the reference template during baseline rhythm; (6) classify the unknown tachycardia either as VT, if the morphology is significantly different from the baseline, or as SVT if the morphologies are similar.[14] Because the morphology of an electrogram may change during lead maturation after being newly implanted,[52] algorithms automatically acquire and update the templates periodically. Defibrillation alters the surface electrocardiograph (ECG) and electrogram morphology for minutes after shock delivery,[53] so morphology algorithms are not used during redetection. There are differences in how the device manufacturers implement each of the steps of morphology detection enhancements, but all have common failure modes.

An inaccurate template will lead to inappropriate classification of SVT as VT. Ectopy and intermittent bundle branch block that occur during template acquisition can lead to its inaccuracy. Because the morphology of the ventricular electrogram can also change as the lead matures following implant, the inability to acquire updated templates because of frequent ectopy or absence of an intrinsic rhythm may lead to inaccuracies. If periodic templates cannot be acquired, morphology should not be used until lead maturation is complete, typically around 3 months after implantation.

An electrogram is truncated when its amplitude exceeds the sensing amplifier's dynamic range. Truncation can affect feature extraction by altering the electrogram waveform and, in Medtronic ICDs, affect alignment, because the electrogram peak is used to align baseline with tachycardia templates (**Fig. 3**).[14] In Medtronic and St Jude ICDs, the electrogram amplitude scale is manually adjustable, and should be sized so that the electrogram uses 25% to 75% of the dynamic range.

Alignment errors lead to misclassification of similar electrograms as different because of improper alignment. St Jude ICDs use the onset of the electrogram as the point of reference for alignment. Because ICD sensing is dynamic and affected by heart rate, the electrogram onset point may vary based on the rate at the time of acquisition, leading to misalignment (see **Fig. 3**B and C).[14] In Medtronic ICDs, the tallest peak of the electrogram is for alignment; peak distortion caused by truncation or rate-related changes may lead to misalignment.[14,54,55] Boston Scientific ICDs assess morphology by a vector timing and correlation algorithm that uses the near-field electrogram, which is generally sharper (greater slew) for alignment, and then following alignment compares features of the far-field electrogram.[14,56] Alignment errors can occur if there are changes in the near-field electrogram (see **Fig. 3**B).

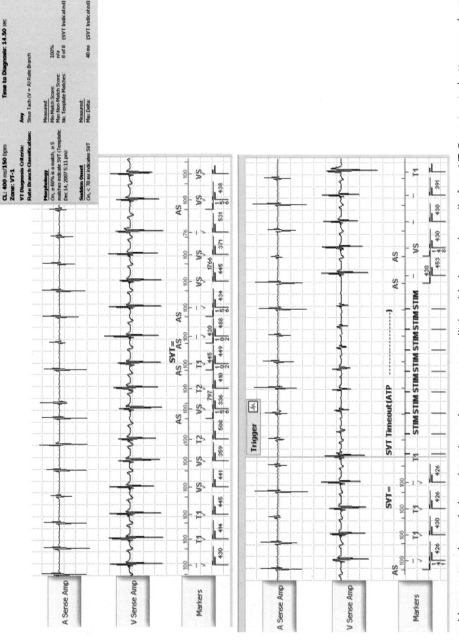

Fig. 2. Use of the sudden onset and morphology detection enhancements to distinguish sinus tachycardia from VT. From top to bottom are shown the atrial channel, ventricular channel, and markers. In the top panel the rhythm is sinus tachycardia with occasional premature atrial complexes (PACs; fourth and eighth complexes). Note that the PACs advance the next ventricular event, consistent with an atrially driven rhythm. The tachycardia is detected in the VT-1 zone (box, inset above right). SVT indicates the V = A rate branch classification. Sudden onset indicates SVT, as does morphology (match scores of 100, and check marks to indicate template match). The third from last complex has a lower match score (76) and a PR interval shorter than other complexes, suggesting a PVC fused with the sinus complex. Because the logic used in the V = A rate branch is ANY if either morphology or sudden onset had indicated VT, therapy would have been delivered. In the bottom panel, the duration timer expires, and SVT-VT discriminators are overridden, so therapy is delivered.

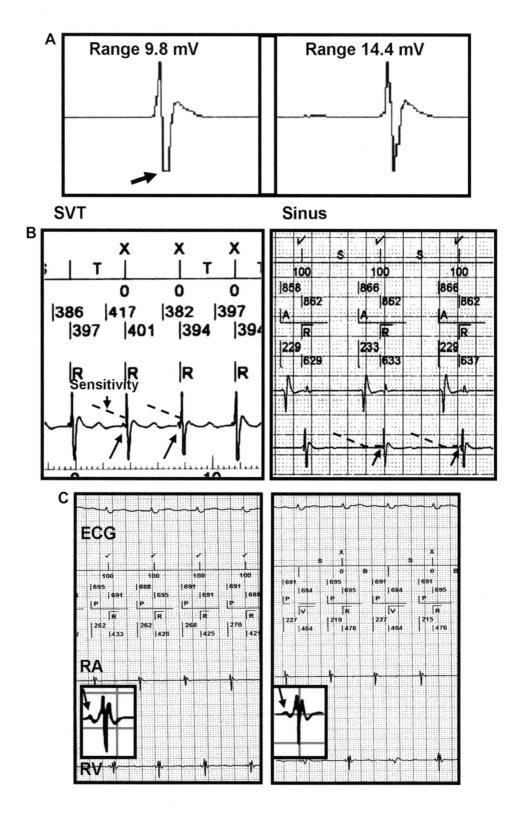

Rate-related aberrancy may result in misclassification of SVT as VT. If it occurs reproducibly, automatic template updating should be turned off and a template acquired while pacing in the AAI mode at a rate sufficient to acquire the aberrancy. Because the degree of aberrancy may be variable during irregular SVTs such as AF, reducing the fraction of electrogram required to exceed the match threshold (from 5 of 8 to 4 of 8 in St Jude ICDs) may ameliorate the problem without impairment of VT detection.[14]

SVT soon after shocks may lead to misclassification because of postshock electrogram distortion. Although morphology is not used during redetection, if an episode during which a shock is delivered is terminated and a new episode develops within several minutes, residual electrogram distortion may be present during detection.

Pectoral myopotentials do not result in shocks in the absence of tachycardia, because the pulse generator is not used as a sensing electrode in the rate detecting channel. However, pectoral myopotentials can lead to inappropriate detection of SVT as VT by distorting the far-field electrogram during SVT, leading to mismatch, which may be seen during sinus tachycardia caused by exercise. Medtronic (nominally) and Boston Scientific ICDs use the far-field electrogram during morphology discrimination, whereas St Jude ICDs use the near-field electrogram, and thus are not susceptible to pectoral myopotential oversensing.

Sustained-rate Timers

Sustained-duration timers override SVT-VT discriminators and deliver therapy once the timer expires. The underlying hypothesis is that an SVT is unlikely to remain rapid for the duration of the timer, whereas VT will. Because all detection enhancements necessarily increase VT specificity at the cost of sensitivity, the timers are designed to prevent prolonged VT episodes. In patients with known VT, extending timers to 2 to 5 minutes is reasonable. Several large trials with mostly patients receiving primary prevention have turned timers off, and it is reasonable to do so when detection enhancements are limited to heart rates less than 200 bpm. Timers can lead to inappropriate shocks despite correct rhythm discrimination.

SVT DISCRIMINATORS IN DUAL-CHAMBER DEVICES

Dual-chamber devices use substantial additional information from the atrial electrogram for rhythm determination. Accurate atrial sensing is essential for proper rhythm classification. To prevent far-field R wave oversensing, major manufacturers use dynamic blanking following ventricular events (St Jude and Boston Scientific) or algorithmic assessment of atrial events that occur around the time of ventricular events to distinguish atrial and ventricular events recorded on the atrial channel (Medtronic). Avoidance of large R waves (more than one-quarter the size of the P wave) on the atrial channel at the time of lead insertion is critical. Atrial sensing errors accounted for 41% to 75% of inappropriately treated SVTs in early studies.[57–59] However, in a study of 400 patients in which far-field R waves were avoided at the time of implant, only 5% of misclassifications resulted from far-field R wave oversensing. Atrial lead dislodgment, oversensing, and

---

Fig. 3. Inappropriate detection of SVT by St Jude MD morphology algorithm. (*A*) Electrogram truncation: template electrogram is truncated (*arrow*) with amplifier range of 9.8 mV. Truncation was corrected by increasing range to 14.4 mV. Inconsistent truncation may prevent SVT morphology from matching template. (*B*) Interaction of automatic sensitivity control and morphology analysis. Left panel shows stored electrogram of SVT inappropriately detected as VT. Right panel shows programmer strip of validated template in sinus rhythm. Despite identical ventricular electrograms, morphology match scores are 0% in SVT and 100% in sinus rhythm. Slanted line denotes slope of automatic sensitivity control. In sinus rhythm, automatic sensitivity control reaches minimum value before the next ventricular electrogram so that the small peak at onset of electrogram (*arrow*) is used for alignment. In SVT, automatic sensitivity control does not reach minimum, and small peak is not used for alignment. (*C*) Programmer strip showing ECG, marker, and atrial and ventricular electrograms in sinus rhythm at left and intermittent atrial-sensed ventricular paced rhythm at right. Insert shows identical ventricular electrogram morphology in 2 panels recorded seconds apart in time. Morphology match is 100% for consistently conducted sinus beats and 0% for sinus beats following ventricular paced beats. The most likely explanation for this discrepancy is an alignment error: automatic sensitivity control is more sensitive after paced beats than during consistently conducted sinus rhythm. Thus the small peak at the onset of the ventricular electrogram is used for alignment only after paced beats. Failure of morphology match only on postpaced beats does not degrade algorithm performance during tachycardia. S denotes intervals interval the sinus zone longer than the VT detection interval. T denotes intervals in VT zone. (*From* Swerdlow CD, Friedman PA. Advanced ICD troubleshooting: part I. Pacing Clin Electrophysiol 2005;28(12):1322–46; with permission.)

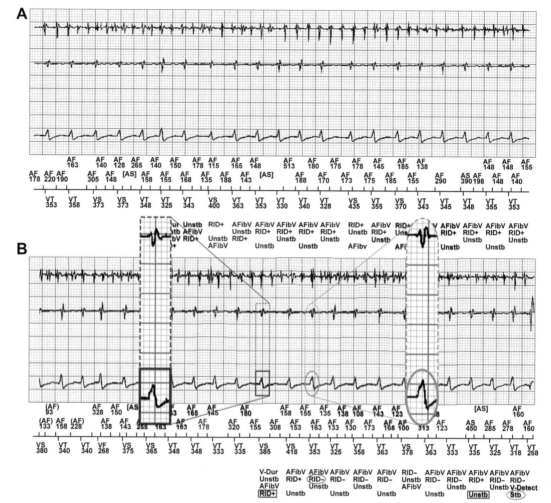

Fig. 4. An example of correct and incorrect classification via Rhythm ID dual-chamber algorithm. From top to bottom are shown the atrial channel (top), ventricular near-field (middle), and ventricular far-field (lower) electrograms, with the device markers shown at the bottom. (*A*) Appropriate withholding of therapy for AF. AF is evident on the atrial electrogram. The device correctly identifies the rhythm as AF via Rhythm ID. Once 8 out of 10 ventricular events exceed the VT detection rate, a duration timer is started. Once the duration timer is met (nominally 2.5 seconds in the VT zone), the device proceeds to therapy delivery unless Rhythm ID indicates SVT. In the top panel, the morphology of the far-field ventricular electrogram during tachycardia matches the baseline template (RID+) so therapy is withheld. In addition, interval stability indicates an unstable (Unstb) rhythm, consistent with AF. (*B*) Inappropriate therapy delivery. Note that duration is met with the occurrence of the complex in the red box, with the marker V-Dur underneath. Initially, the Unstb marker indicates QRS interval variability consistent with AF. The RID+ marker indicates that the morphology analysis indicates supra-ventricular tachycardia as well. With the blue-circled complex, the marker changes to RID-. This indicates that the morphology is now considered different than the baseline template, and suggests VT base on morphology. However, because Rhythm ID also assesses interval stability, and the overall rhythm remains unstable (Unstb), therapy is withheld at this point. Note that the change in the morphology of the complexes in the rectangle and circle is small. During AF, small morphology changes can often occur because of longitudinal dissociation (activation of different fibers in the His-Purkinje system). These morphologic changes are usually much smaller than the gross distortions seen with rate-related bundle branch block (aberrancy). The algorithm in this device uses both the near-field and far-field electrograms to assess morphology, and changes in either could lead to misclassification. When the ventricular response during AF regularizes, the classification changes from Unstb to Stb (last blue circle) and therapy is delivered.

undersensing can all lead to inappropriate classifications with dual-chamber SVT discrimination.[14]

In general, preclassification of the relative atrial and ventricular rates or patterns enhances the sensitivity and specificity of onset, stability, and morphology algorithms. Thus, stability is only applied when the atrial lead confirms AF, or onset when atrial and ventricular rates match. Accurate preclassification of relative atrial and ventricular rates also eliminates many arrhythmias from additional analysis, eliminated possible error. A ventricular rate greater than the atrial rate was

Table 2
Disease-specific programming considerations

	Programming	Rationale
Sensing	Screen for far-field R wave oversensing and program to eliminate it if present	Ensure appropriate detection enhancement operation
	Screen for T-wave oversensing and program to eliminate it if present	Avoid double counting and inappropriate detection
Detection	Use detection enhancements in all patients with intact AV nodal conduction and VT zone with HR cutoff <200 bpm	Minimize the risk of inappropriate detection
	Prolong number of intervals to detect or detection time in patients with frequent self-terminating arrhythmias (up to 30 out of 40 in Medtronic VF zone)	Prevent unnecessary capacitor charging and shocks
Bradycardia therapy	Minimize RV pacing in all non-CRT systems	RV apical pacing promotes AF and CHF
	Promote atrial pacing in patients with sinus node dysfunction	Reduce the risk of AF
Tachycardia therapy	Program liberal ATP in VT zones <200 bpm and 1–2 ATP sequences in faster detection zones	Minimize the risk of inappropriate and appropriate shocks
	Program first shock strength for VT or VF based on DFT or ULV testing or to maximum output. Program all subsequent shocks at maximum output	DFT of ULV-based shock output not likely to transform VT to VF. Maximum output shocks more likely to be effective and lower risk of repetitive shocks; longer charge time may allow spontaneous termination
Device function/surveillance	Check for device-specific recalls at routine follow-up and reprogram accordingly	Some device malfunction can be corrected by specific manufacturer-recommended programming. Example include software errors (such as latching) eliminated by turning off certain features
	Enable patient alerts	These generate audible tones or vibratory alerts, advising the patient to seek care
	Enable remote monitoring	Automated monitoring generates Web-based or other forms of physician notification when parameters (eg, lead impedance) are out of range suggesting incipient malfunction

Abbreviations: DFT, defibrillation threshold; RV, right ventricle; ULV, upper limit of vulnerability.
From Hayes DL, Swerdlow CD, Friedman PA. Programming. In Hayes DL, Friedman PA. Cardiac Pacing, Defibrillation, and Resynchronization: A Clinical Approach. 2nd edition. Wiley-Blackwell, Chichester, West Sussex, UK; 2009; 372; with permission.

present in more than 80% of arrhythmias in one study, and accurately identified VT in 100%.[60] Implementation of dual-chamber information varies among major device manufactures.

The Boston Scientific Rhythm ID is simply programmed on or off. When active, it first compares the ventricular and atrial rates. If ventricular rate is greater than the atrial rate plus 10 bpm, VT is identified. Otherwise, a morphology analysis is performed (unless redetection is underway). If the tachycardia matches the template, SVT is diagnosed. Otherwise, if the atrial rate is less than 200 bpm (indicating AF is absent) or the ventricular intervals vary by 20 ms or less, the rhythm is treated as VT.[61] An example of correct and incorrect classification via Rhythm ID is shown in **Fig. 4**.

St Jude's rate branch algorithm initially sorts tachycardia into 3 arms: V greater than A, A equal to V, or A greater than V.[62] If V greater than A is true, VT is diagnosed. In the other 2 rate branch arms, the individual detection enhancements (stability, morphology for A>V; onset, morphology for A = V) are individually programmed and combined using ANY or ALL logic (indicating how many of the SVT-VT discriminators must indicate VT for the episode to be classified as VT).[60] Based on the sensitivity and specificity of these combinations when applied to stored electrograms from spontaneous tachycardias in a clinical cohort, we use morphology in the A equals V branch, and morphology or stability (ANY logic) in the A greater than V branch.[14,60] St Jude dual-chamber ICDs also analyze AV association in conjunction with stability to test for N:1 flutters.

Medtronic's PR Logic contains 3 rules that are independently programmed on or off.: AF/AT, sinus tachycardia, and other 1:1 SVT. The logic then analyzes the pattern of AA, VV, AV, and VA intervals hierarchically to classify the arrhythmia. An SVT limit criterion defines the fastest ventricular rate that the algorithm can classify as VT. The other 1:1 SVT rule is programmed off during the first month after implantation in case of lead dislodgement, which could result in misclassification of VT as SVT.

In nonresynchronization patients who are not in permanent AF and who do not have a bradycardia indication for dual-chamber pacing, the choice between a single and dual chamber remains controversial. A meta-analysis of trials randomizing patients to dual-chamber versus single-chamber ICDs showed no reduction in the risk of inappropriate shocks for an individual with dual-chamber ICDs, although the number of individual shocks an individual might get was significantly reduced.[63] A subsequent study did show a reduction in a composite morbidity index with use of dual-chamber ICDs, predominantly because of a reduction

---

Table 3
Company-specific program parameters to minimize shock risk in primary prevention

Manufacturer	Detection	Rate	Beats to Detection/ Duration	Enhancement	Therapy
Medtronic	VT (monitor)	167 bpm	32 intervals	AF/AFL on	Off
	FVT via VF	182 bpm	30 of 40 intervals	ST (1:1 VT/ST = 66%) on wavelet (match = 70%) SVT limit = 300 ms	Burst × 1, 30–35 J × 5
	VF	250 bpm	30 of 40 intervals	—	30–35 J × 6
Boston Scientific	VT-1 (monitor)	165 bpm	9.0 s	Monitor only	Off
	VT	180 bpm	7.0 s	Rhythm ID on	Burst ×1, 41 J × 6
	VF	200 bpm	7.0 s	Not applicable	41 J shocks × 8[a]
St Jude	VT-1 (monitor)	166 bpm	30 intervals	—	Off (monitor)
	VT-2	181 bpm	30 intervals	V<A: if ALL[b] morphology internal stability V = A if ANY morphology SVT limit = 300 ms	ATP, 30 J, 40 J × 3
	VF	240 bpm	30 intervals	—	30 J, 40 J × 5[a]

(1) Extended duration timers turned off; (2) ATP burst = 8 intervals, at 88% cycle length; (3) these have only been validated for Medtronic devices in the PREPARE study. Other manufacturers' settings are an approximation of the Medtronic settings and have not been prospectively tested.
   [a] While not used in PREPARE, it is reasonable to program ATP during or before charge ON.
   [b] Based on unpublished analysis of detect SVT data.

Table 4
Patient-independent programming optimization

Disease State	Arrhythmia Characteristic	Programming Considerations	Rationale
Channelopathies	Rapid polymorphic VT/VF	Single detection zone for HR >200 bpm	Clinical arrhythmia is rapid (so that a high cutoff rate is unlikely to underdetect significant arrhythmias; young patients can achieve rapid HRs with exercise, increasing the risk of inappropriate detection of rhythms with HR<200 bpm
		Detection enhancements off / Avoid ATP	Enhancements are generally not effective in VF zone at rapid rates / Role in polymorphic VT/VF not established; possibility of proarrhythmia
	Frequent, nonsustained episodes	Prolong detection (to 30 of 40 beats has been used in one clinical trial; analogous programming for other manufacturers' ICDs exist)	Prevent inappropriate charging and shocks
	Long QT during sinus episodes	Screen for T-wave oversensing and reprogram as necessary	Avoid inappropriate shocks
Primary prevention (CAD or DCM)	Fast VT/VF is often monomorphic, HR >200	Use 2 detection zones, VT cutoff 180–190 / ATP: use 1–2 sequences for HR<250	Minimize risk for inappropriate detections by not exposing detection algorithms to slower rates; 2 zones permit increased ATP use in the lower HR zone / Reduce risk of inappropriate and appropriate shock
Secondary prevention (CAD, DCM)	Monomorphic VT with HRs 120–200	Use 3 detection zones / Program detection enhancements on; use dual-chamber enhancements if available	Permit increased detection enhancements and ATP for slower VT and tiered therapies / Decrease risk of inappropriate shock
	Fast VT/VF is often monomorphic, HR>200	Multiple sequence of ATP in slower zones; 1–2 sequences for 200<HR<250	Terminate SVT and VT; reduce risk of appropriate and inappropriate shock
CHF	Bradycardias	Avoid RV pacing in non-CRT systems. Use RV pacing avoidance algorithms if available	Chronic RV apical pacing desynchronizes the ventricles, increasing the risk of CHF
	VT/VF	Program as for primary and secondary prevention	
PAF	AF and sinus bradycardia	Promote atrial pacing and minimize RV apical pacing / Atrial prevention and termination algorithms (if available)	Increased atrial pacing modestly reduces AF RV apical pacing increases risk of AF / Atrial termination algorithms (ATP,HFB) reduce arrhythmia burden, but clinical significance is uncertain / May be particularly useful in patients with atrial flutter, incisional atrial reentrant circuits / Avoid use in first month (possible lead dislodgment) / Avoid shocks for atrial arrhythmias

Abbreviations: CAD, coronary artery disease; DCM, dilated cardiomyopathy.
From Hayes DL, Swerdlow CD, Friedman PA. Programming. In Hayes DL, Friedman PA. Cardiac Pacing, Defibrillation, and Resynchronization: A Clinical Approach. 2nd edition. Wiley-Blackwell, Chichester, West Sussex, UK; 2009; 371; with permission.

in the number of shock episodes and in the frequency of sustained symptomatic atrial tachycarrhythmias.[64] Ongoing studies (The RAPTURE Study; ClinicalTrials.gov identifier: NCT00787800) may further define the role of dual-chamber versus single-chamber ICDs. In patients with complete AV block, there is no role for the use of discriminators.

STRATEGIES TO AVOID INAPPROPRIATE SHOCKS CAUSED BY SVT

ICDs have hundreds of programmable parameters. Clinical trials have shown that carefully selected empiric settings perform as well as clinician-tailored individualized settings.[22,65] Population-specific parameters (eg, primary prevention), when specifically selected to follow the principals discussed earlier, seem to reduce all-cause shocks by 50%.[22] General considerations for programming parameters based on disease condition are summarized in **Table 2**. Company-specific recommended parameters to minimize shocks in patients receiving primary prevention is shown in **Table 3**. **Table 4** summarizes patient-independent and general programming optimization steps.

In addition to programming considerations, steps taken at implantation may reduce the risk of shocks during follow-up. These steps include ventricular lead placement to ensure a suitably sized R wave (generally ≥ 5 mV) and a small T wave relative to the R wave (R/T ratio >4:1) that is not sensed. As noted earlier, if an atrial lead is used, the lead should be positioned to minimized far-field R waves. Use of leads with closer tip-ring distances minimize far-field R waves because the lead's antenna is smaller.[66] Novel leads in which both sensing electrodes are intramyocardial hold promise for superior far-field R wave rejection, and enhanced rhythm discrimination.[67,68] Specific programming details to further reduce oversensing has been previously reviewed.[14]

Pharmacologic therapy may reduce the frequency of appropriate and inappropriate shocks by preventing VT/VF episodes, slowing sinus tachycardia, slowing the ventricular rate during atrial arrhythmias, or suppressing them.[69] The authors favor aggressive use of guideline directed β-blockers, ACE inhibitors, and statins, which have been shown to reduce mortality in populations with heart disease; membrane-active drugs are routinely reserved for patients with difficult to control arrhythmias. Catheter ablation is useful in reducing the frequency of ventricular[70] and atrial arrhythmias,[71] and is used adjunctively. New advances in automated remote monitoring permit the generation Internet-based automated alerts

to warn of impending lead failure, battery depletion, asymptomatic atrial arrhythmias, and hemodynamic changes. An ICD is no longer an isolated device, but is now part of a connected, proactive ecosystem that can further manage health and minimize shock risk. The role of drugs, ablation, and remote monitoring is beyond the scope of this review.

SUMMARY

ICDs can offer lifesaving therapy for patients at risk for VT and VF. ICDs detect tachyarrhythmias when the cycle lengths are within the programmed VT and VF zones. Because SVTs, oversensing, component failure, and nonsustained VT may also result in sensed ventricular events within the detection zones, these may lead to unnecessary shocks. Thoughtful programming minimizes shock risk and enhances the patient's wellbeing.

REFERENCES

1. Kuck KH, Cappato R, Siebels J, et al. Randomized comparison of antiarrhythmic drug therapy with implantable defibrillators in patients resuscitated from cardiac arrest: the Cardiac Arrest Study Hamburg (CASH). Circulation 2000;102(7):748–54.
2. Writing Committee M, Epstein AE, DiMarco JP, et al. ACC/AHA/HRS 2008 Guidelines for Device-Based Therapy of Cardiac Rhythm Abnormalities: a report of the American College of Cardiology/American Heart Association Task Force on Practice Guidelines (Writing Committee to Revise the ACC/AHA/NASPE 2002 Guideline Update for Implantation of Cardiac Pacemakers and Antiarrhythmia Devices): developed in collaboration with the American Association for Thoracic Surgery and Society of Thoracic Surgeons. Circulation 2008;117(21):e350–408.
3. A comparison of antiarrhythmic-drug therapy with implantable defibrillators in patients resuscitated from near-fatal. ventricular arrhythmias. N Engl J Med 1997;337(22):1576–84.
4. Connolly SJ, Gent M, Roberts RS, et al. Canadian Implantable Defibrillator Study (CIDS): a randomized trial of the implantable cardioverter defibrillator against amiodarone. Circulation 2000;101(11):1297–302.
5. Bardy GH, Lee KL, Mark DB, et al. Amiodarone or an implantable cardioverter-defibrillator for congestive heart failure. N Engl J Med 2005;352(3):225–37.
6. Cleland JGF, Daubert J-C, Erdmann E, et al. The effect of cardiac resynchronization on morbidity and mortality in heart failure. N Engl J Med 2005; 352(15):1539–49.
7. Young JB, Abraham WT, Smith AL, et al. Combined cardiac resynchronization and implantable cardioversion defibrillation in advanced chronic heart

failure: the MIRACLE ICD Trial. JAMA 2003;289(20):2685–94.

8. Wood MA, Stambler BS, Damiano RJ, et al. Lessons learned from data logging in a multicenter clinical trial using a late-generation implantable cardioverter-defibrillator. J Am Coll Cardiol 1994;24(7):1692–9.

9. Schmitt C, Montero M, Melichercik J. Significance of supraventricular tachyarrhythmias in patients with implanted pacing cardioverter defibrillators. Pacing Clin Electrophysiol 1994;17(3 Pt 1):295–302.

10. Grimm W, Flores BF, Marchlinski FE. Electrocardiographically documented unnecessary, spontaneous shocks in 241 patients with implantable cardioverter defibrillators. Pacing Clin Electrophysiol 1992;15(11 Pt 1):1667–73.

11. Ahmad M, Bloomstein L, Roelke M, et al. Patients' attitudes toward implanted defibrillator shocks. Pacing Clin Electrophysiol 2000;23(6):934–8.

12. Poole JE, Johnson GW, Hellkamp AS, et al. Prognostic importance of defibrillator shocks in patients with heart failure. N Engl J Med 2008;359(10):1009–17.

13. Sweeney MO, Sherfesee L, DeGroot PJ, et al. Differences in effects of electrical therapy type for ventricular arrhythmias on mortality in implantable cardioverter-defibrillator patients. Heart Rhythm 2010;7(3):353–60.

14. Swerdlow CD, Friedman PA. Advanced ICD troubleshooting: part I. Pacing Clin Electrophysiol 2005;28(12):1322–46.

15. Swerdlow CD, Friedman PA. Advanced ICD troubleshooting: part II. Pacing Clin Electrophysiol 2006;29(1):70–96.

16. Gunderson BD, Abeyratne AI, Olson WH, et al. Effect of programmed number of intervals to detect ventricular fibrillation on implantable cardioverter-defibrillator aborted and unnecessary shocks. Pacing Clin Electrophysiol 2007;30(2):157–65.

17. Wathen MS, Sweeney MO, DeGroot PJ, et al. Shock reduction using antitachycardia pacing for spontaneous rapid ventricular tachycardia in patients with coronary artery disease. Circulation 2001;104(7):796–801.

18. Wathen MS, DeGroot PJ, Sweeney MO, et al. Prospective randomized multicenter trial of empirical antitachycardia pacing versus shocks for spontaneous rapid ventricular tachycardia in patients with implantable cardioverter-defibrillators: Pacing Fast Ventricular Tachycardia Reduces Shock Therapies (PainFREE Rx II) trial results. Circulation 2004;110(17):2591–6.

19. The DAVID Trial Investigators. Dual-chamber pacing or ventricular backup pacing in patients with an implantable defibrillator: the Dual Chamber and VVI Implantable Defibrillator (DAVID) Trial. JAMA 2002;288(24):3115–23.

20. Sweeney MO, Bank AJ, Nsah E, et al. Minimizing ventricular pacing to reduce atrial fibrillation in sinus-node disease. N Engl J Med 2007;357(10):1000–8.

21. Friedman PA, McClelland RL, Bamlet WR, et al. Dual-chamber versus single-chamber detection enhancements for implantable defibrillator rhythm diagnosis: the Detect Supraventricular Tachycardia study. Circulation 2006;113(25):2871–9.

22. Wilkoff BL, Williamson BD, Stern RS, et al. Strategic programming of detection and therapy parameters in implantable cardioverter-defibrillators reduces shocks in primary prevention patients: results from the PREPARE (Primary Prevention Parameters Evaluation) study. J Am Coll Cardiol 2008;52(7):541–50.

23. Swerdlow CD, Gunderson BD, Ousdigian KT, et al. Downloadable software algorithm reduces inappropriate shocks caused by implantable cardioverter-defibrillator lead fractures: a prospective study. Circulation 2010;122(15):1449–55.

24. Patel P, Dokainish H, Tsai P, et al. Update on the Association of inflammation and atrial fibrillation. J Cardiovasc Electrophysiol 2010;21(9):1064–70.

25. Gami AS, Hodge DO, Herges RM, et al. Obstructive sleep apnea, obesity, and the risk of incident atrial fibrillation. J Am Coll Cardiol 2007;49(5):565–71.

26. Napolitano C, Priori SG. Diagnosis and treatment of catecholaminergic polymorphic ventricular tachycardia. Heart Rhythm 2007;4(5):675–8.

27. Krishnamoorthy S, Lip GYH, Lane DA. Alcohol and illicit drug use as precipitants of atrial fibrillation in young adults: a case series and literature review. Am J Med 2009;122(9):851–6, e853.

28. Furukawa T, Moroe K, Mayrovitz H, et al. Arrhythmogenic effects of graded coronary blood flow reductions superimposed on prior myocardial infarction in dogs. Circulation 1991;84(1):368–77.

29. Pietrasik G, Goldenberg I, McNitt S, et al. Obesity as a risk factor for sustained ventricular tachyarrhythmias in MADIT II patients. J Cardiovasc Electrophysiol 2007;18(2):181–4.

30. Bhavnani SP, Coleman CI, White CM, et al. Association between statin therapy and reductions in atrial fibrillation or flutter and inappropriate shock therapy. Europace 2008;10(7):854–9.

31. Vyas AK, Guo H, Moss AJ, et al. Reduction in ventricular tachyarrhythmias with statins in the Multicenter Automatic Defibrillator Implantation Trial (MADIT)-II. J Am Coll Cardiol 2006;47(4):769–73.

32. Chiu JH, Abdelhadi RH, Chung MK, et al. Effect of statin therapy on risk of ventricular arrhythmia among patients with coronary artery disease and an implantable cardioverter-defibrillator. Am J Cardiol 2005;95(4):490–1.

33. Dickinson MG, Ip JH, Olshansky B, et al. Statin use was associated with reduced mortality in both ischemic and nonischemic cardiomyopathy and in patients with implantable defibrillators: mortality data and mechanistic insights from the Sudden

Cardiac Death in Heart Failure Trial (SCD-HeFT). Am Heart J 2007;153(4):573–8.

34. Goldberger JJ, Subacius H, Schaechter A, et al. Effects of statin therapy on arrhythmic events and survival in patients with nonischemic dilated cardiomyopathy. J Am Coll Cardiol 2006;48(6): 1228–33.

35. Brodine WN, Tung RT, Lee JK, et al. Effects of beta-blockers on implantable cardioverter defibrillator therapy and survival in the patients with ischemic cardiomyopathy (from the Multicenter Automatic Defibrillator Implantation Trial-II). Am J Cardiol 2005;96(5):691–5.

36. Tandri H, Griffith LS, Tang T, et al. Clinical course and long-term follow-up of patients receiving implantable cardioverter-defibrillators. Heart Rhythm 2006;3(7):762–8.

37. Nattel S, Carlsson L. Innovative approaches to anti-arrhythmic drug therapy. Nat Rev Drug Discov 2006; 5(12):1034–49.

38. Wilkoff BL, Kuhlkamp V, Volosin K, et al. Critical analysis of dual-chamber implantable cardioverter-defibrillator arrhythmia detection: results and technical considerations. Circulation 2001;103(3):381–6.

39. Daubert JP, Zareba W, Cannom DS, et al. Inappropriate implantable cardioverter-defibrillator shocks in MADIT II: frequency, mechanisms, predictors, and survival impact. J Am Coll Cardiol 2008; 51(14):1357–65.

40. Higgins SL, Lee RS, Kramer RL. Stability: an ICD detection criterion for discriminating atrial fibrillation from ventricular tachycardia. J Cardiovasc Electrophysiol 1995;6(12):1081–8.

41. Swerdlow CD, Chen PS, Kass RM, et al. Discrimination of ventricular tachycardia from sinus tachycardia and atrial fibrillation in a tiered-therapy cardioverter-defibrillator. J Am Coll Cardiol 1994; 23(6):1342–55.

42. Weber M, Böcker D, Bänsch D, et al. Efficacy and safety of the initial use of stability and onset criteria in implantable cardioverter defibrillators. J Cardiovasc Electrophysiol 1999;10(2):145–53.

43. Kettering K, Dornberger V, Lang R, et al. Enhanced detection criteria in implantable cardioverter defibrillators: sensitivity and specificity of the stability algorithm at different heart rates. Pacing Clin Electrophysiol 2001;24(9 Pt 1):1325–33.

44. Brugada J, Mont L, Figueiredo M, et al. Enhanced detection criteria in implantable defibrillators. J Cardiovasc Electrophysiol 1998;9(3):261–8.

45. Swerdlow CD. Supraventricular tachycardia-ventricular tachycardia discrimination algorithms in implantable cardioverter defibrillators: state-of-the-art review. J Cardiovasc Electrophysiol 2001;12(5): 606–12.

46. Le Franc P, Kus T, Vinet A, et al. Underdetection of ventricular tachycardia using a 40 ms stability criterion: effect of antiarrhythmic therapy. Pacing Clin Electrophysiol 1997;20(12 Pt 1):2882–92.

47. Garcia-Alberola A, Yli-Mayry S, Block M, et al. RR interval variability in irregular monomorphic ventricular tachycardia and atrial fibrillation. Circulation 1996;93(2):295–300.

48. Boriani G, Biffi M, Frabetti L, et al. Clinical evaluation of morphology discrimination: an algorithm for rhythm discrimination in cardioverter defibrillators. Pacing Clin Electrophysiol 2001;24(6):994–1001.

49. Grönefeld GC, Schulte B, Hohnloser SH, et al. Morphology discrimination: a beat-to-beat algorithm for the discrimination of ventricular from supraventricular tachycardia by implantable cardioverter defibrillators. Pacing Clin Electrophysiol 2001;24(10): 1519–24.

50. Klingenheben T, Sticherling C, Skupin M, et al. Intracardiac QRS electrogram width—an arrhythmia detection feature for implantable cardioverter defibrillators: exercise induced variation as a base for device programming. Pacing Clin Electrophysiol 1998;21(8):1609–17.

51. Lüthje L, Vollmann D, Rosenfeld M, et al. Electrogram configuration and detection of supraventricular tachycardias by a morphology discrimination algorithm in single chamber ICDs. Pacing Clin Electrophysiol 2005;28(6):555–60.

52. Barold HS, Newby KH, Tomassoni G, et al. Prospective evaluation of new and old criteria to discriminate between supraventricular and ventricular tachycardia in implantable defibrillators. Pacing Clin Electrophysiol 1998;21(7):1347–55.

53. Jung W, Manz M, Moosdorf R, et al. Changes in the amplitude of endocardial electrograms following defibrillator discharge: comparison of two lead systems. Pacing Clin Electrophysiol 1995;18(12 Pt 1): 2163–72.

54. Toquero J, Alzueta J, Mont L, et al. Morphology discrimination criterion wavelet improves rhythm discrimination in single-chamber implantable cardioverter-defibrillators: Spanish Register of Morphology Discrimination criterion wavelet (REMEDIO). Europace 2009;11(6):727–33.

55. Medtronic SECURA VR D224VRC Clinician Manual ICD 2008.

56. Gold MR, Shorofsky SR, Thompson JA, et al. Advanced rhythm discrimination for implantable cardioverter defibrillators using electrogram vector timing and correlation. J Cardiovasc Electrophysiol 2002;13(11):1092–7.

57. Kulhlkamp V, Dörnberger V, Mewis C, et al. Clinical experience with the new detection algorithms for atrial fibrillation of a defibrillator with dual chamber sensing and pacing. J Cardiovasc Electrophysiol 1999;10(7):905–15.

58. Deisenhofer I, Kolb C, Ndrepepa G, et al. Do current dual chamber cardioverter defibrillators have

advantages over conventional single chamber cardioverter defibrillators in reducing inappropriate
therapies? A randomized, prospective study. J Cardiovasc Electrophysiol 2001;12(2):134–42.

59. Theuns DA, Klootwijk APJ, Simoons ML, et al. Clinical variables predicting inappropriate use of
implantable cardioverter-defibrillator in patients
with coronary heart disease or nonischemic dilated
cardiomyopathy. Am J Cardiol 2005;95(2):271–4.

60. Glikson M, Swerdlow CD, Gurevitz OT, et al. Optimal
combination of discriminators for differentiating
ventricular from supraventricular tachycardia by
dual-chamber defibrillators. J Cardiovasc Electrophysiol 2005;16(7):732–9.

61. Aliot E, Nitzsche R, Ripart A. Arrhythmia detection
by dual-chamber implantable cardioverter defibrillators. Europace 2004;6(4):273–86.

62. Boriani G, Biffi M, Dall'Acqua A, et al. Rhythm discrimination by rate branch and QRS morphology in dual
chamber implantable cardioverter defibrillators.
Pacing Clin Electrophysiol 2003;26(1 Pt 2):466–70.

63. Theuns DA, Rivero-Ayerza M, Boersma E, et al.
Prevention of inappropriate therapy in implantable
defibrillators: a meta-analysis of clinical trials
comparing single-chamber and dual-chamber
arrhythmia discrimination algorithms. Int J Cardiol
2008;125(3):352–7.

64. Almendral J, Arribas F, Wolpert C, et al. Dual-
chamber defibrillators reduce clinically significant
adverse events compared with single-chamber
devices: results from the DATAS (Dual chamber

and Atrial Tachyarrhythmias Adverse events Study)
trial. Europace 2008;10(5):528–35.

65. Wilkoff BL, Ousdigian KT, Sterns LD, et al.
A comparison of empiric to physician-tailored programming of implantable cardioverter-defibrillators:
results from the prospective randomized multicenter
EMPIRIC trial. J Am Coll Cardiol 2006;48(2):330–9.

66. de Voogt W, van Hemel N, Willems A, et al. Far-field
R-wave reduction with a novel lead design: experimental and human results. Pacing Clin Electrophysiol 2005;28(8):782–8.

67. Henz BD, Friedman PA, Bruce CJ, et al. Synchronous
ventricular pacing without crossing the tricuspid valve
or entering the coronary sinus—preliminary results.
J Cardiovasc Electrophysiol 2009;20(12):1391–7.

68. Asirvatham SJ, Bruce CJ, Danielsen A, et al. Intramyocardial pacing and sensing for the enhancement of
cardiac stimulation and sensing specificity. Pacing
Clin Electrophysiol 2007;30(6):748–54.

69. Connolly SJ, Dorian P, Roberts RS, et al. Comparison
of {beta}-blockers, amiodarone plus {beta}-blockers,
or sotalol for prevention of shocks from implantable
cardioverter defibrillators: the OPTIC Study: a randomized trial. JAMA 2006;295(2):165–71.

70. Reddy VY, Reynolds MR, Neuzil P, et al. Prophylactic
catheter ablation for the prevention of defibrillator
therapy. N Engl J Med 2007;357(26):2657–65.

71. Calkins H, Reynolds MR, Spector P, et al. Treatment
of atrial fibrillation with antiarrhythmic drugs or radiofrequency ablation/CLINICAL PERSPECTIVE. Circ
Arrhythm Electrophysiol 2009;2(4):349–61.

Complications of ICD Generator Change and Implantations

Jordan M. Prutkin, MD, MHS, Jeanne E. Poole, MD*

KEYWORDS

- ICD • Complications • ICD leads • Generator change
- Cardiac implantable electronic device infection

Although implantable cardioverter-defibrillator (ICD) therapy can be lifesaving, complications are a possibility with implantation and during long-term follow-up. Though early ICDs, placed via open thoracotomy, were associated with a significant risk, the modern era of transvenous ICD implantation has reduced the surgical risk substantially. The conclusion of several decades of randomized clinical trials supporting the use of ICDs and cardiac resynchronization therapy (CRT) in patients with moderate-to-advanced heart failure highlights an important paradox. Whereas nonthoracotomy ICD implantation can be performed with fewer complications than early devices, the patients now considered for this therapy are generally more ill and often with advanced heart failure. The impact of significant cardiac disease and associated comorbid medical illness on complication rates must also be considered. This article reviews the available data reporting complications associated with ICD procedures. Adverse events associated with both the acute procedural risk as well as those events that occur later are examined.

COMPLICATIONS ASSOCIATED WITH INITIAL ICD AND CRT IMPLANTATION

Most of the large randomized clinical trials of ICDs reported adverse events (**Table 1**). Comparison of these results is hindered by differences in patient populations, definitions of complications, and whether complications were prespecified for inclusion in the clinical data. The secondary prevention studies reported a complication rate for any adverse event at 8.0% to 22.2%[8–10] while the primary prevention studies reported rates from 2.4% to 22%.[1–7]

The largest randomized clinical trial of primary prevention ICD therapy is the Sudden Cardiac Death in Heart Failure Trial (SCD-HeFT).[6,20] It was unique in that the protocol included a large number of predefined complications to be reported over the course of the 5 years of follow-up. Overall, 13.1% of patients had any complication. There were no deaths due to the implant, though 2.3% had a major early complication and 5.7% had a minor early complication. While 51.9% of complications happened within 30 days of implant, 20.8% presented between 1 and 3 months and 27.4% presented after 3 months. This led to an estimated complication rate of 1% per month after the first 30 days.

The Multicenter Automatic Defibrillator Implantation Trial II (MADIT II) reported adverse events at 20 months of follow-up.[2] Only a selected group of complications was reported in this study. There were no perioperative deaths, and the investigators reported that 1.8% of patients had lead-related problems, and five patients had infections that required ICD removal.

Financial disclosures: Dr Prutkin has no financial disclosures. Dr Poole receives honoraria for speaking from Biotronik, Boston Scientific, Medtronic, and St Jude Medical, and honoraria for scientific board advisory with Boston Scientific and Medtronic. Dr Poole also reports NHLBI research grant support for CABANA and SCD-HeFT 10 year Follow Up.
Division of Cardiology, University of Washington, Box 356422, 1959 Northeast Pacific Street, Seattle, WA 98195, USA
* Corresponding author.
E-mail address: jpoole@cardiology.washington.edu

Table 1
Complication rates reported from randomized ICD and CRT clinical trials

Trial Name	Follow-up	Periprocedural Complications	Postprocedural Complications	Total Complications	Infection Rates
ICD-Primary Prevention					
MADIT I[1]	27 mo		7/95 (7.4%)		2/95 (2.1%)
MADIT II[2]	20 mo		18/742 (2.4%)		5/742 (0.7%)
CAT[3]	24 mo	0/50 (0%)		11/50 (22%)	2/50 (4%)
AMIOVIRT	2.0 y	Not reported	Not reported		Not reported
DEFINITE[4]	29 mo	3/229 (1.3%)		10/229 (4.4%)	1/229 (0.4%)
DINAMIT[5]	In-hospital		25/310 (8.1%)		Not reported
SCD-HeFT[6]	45.5 mo		106/811 (13.1%)		36/811 (4.4%)
IRIS[7]	37 mo		65/415 (15.7%)		Not reported
ICD-Secondary Prevention					
AVID[8]	18.2 mo		43/539 (8.0%)		14/539 (2.8%)
CIDS[9]	36 mo		48/328 (14.6%)		15/328 (4.6%)
CASH[10,a]	57 mo	6/99 (6.1%)		22/99 (22.2%)	3/99 (3.0%)
CRT-ICD or CRT-Pacemaker					
MIRACLE[11]	6 mo	56/571 (9.8%)		64/528 (12.1%)	7/528 (1.3%)
MUSTIC[12]	26 wk	Not reported		2/67 (3.0%)	0/67 (0%)
VENTAK CHF/CONTAK CD[13,b]	2.5 y	9/512 (1.8%)		80/443 (18.1%)	5/443 (1.1%)
INSYNC III[14]	6 mo	38/422 (9.0%)		35/397 (8.8%)	3/397 (0.8%)
MIRACLE ICD[14]	6 mo	207/1085 (19.0%)		121/978 (12.4%)	11/978 (1.1%)
MIRACLE II[15]	6 mo	6/210 (2.9%)		20/210 (9.5%)	Not reported
COMPANION[16]	15.7–16.2 mo	8% in CRT-ICD and 10% in CRT-P		Not reported	Not reported
CARE-HF[17]	19.4 mo		52/409 (12.7%)	101/621 (16.3%)	11/409 (2.7%)
REVERSE[18]	12 mo	26/642 (4.0%)			0/610 (0%)
MADIT-CRT[19]	30 d	21/1089 (1.9%) in CRT-D / 6/731 (0.8%) in ICD-only		92/1089 (8.5%) in CRT-D / 23/731 (3.1%) in ICD-only	12/1089 (1.1%) in CRT-D / 5/731 (0.7%) in ICD-only

Generator malfunction and complications from defibrillation threshold testing were excluded for this analysis, when identified. Complications are reported as the number of patient with the complication out of the total number of patients in the patient group examined (%).

Abbreviation: CRT-D, CRT combined with ICD.

a Includes 55 patients with epicardial systems.
b Includes 53 patients with epicardial leads.

Data from the randomized trials examining the use of CRT in advanced heart failure suggest that the overall complication rates are higher than with single-chamber or dual-chamber ICD implantation (see **Table 1**). This may be due to the more advanced heart failure status and the increased risk associated with transvenous left ventricular lead placement. CRT randomized trials have reported periimplant complication rates ranging from 4.0% to 16.0%, a periimplant mortality rate of 0.2% to 0.8%, and follow-up complication rates at 30 days to 1 year of 4.5% to 23.8%.[14,16–19,21,22]

The largest dataset reporting early complications comes from the ongoing National Cardiovascular Disease Registry (NCDR).[22,23] The NCDR ICD Registry includes all Medicare patients undergoing initial ICD implantation or generator replacement in patients with a primary prevention indication, although 80% of all ICDs implanted for secondary prevention indications are currently being reported.[22] Adverse events are prospectively defined and captured from the perioperative period to hospital discharge. Of 224,233 patients undergoing an initial implantation, the overall complication rate was 3.2% with a major complication rate of 1.2%.[22] Patients with an initial single-chamber ICD had an overall 2.0% complication rate, those with a dual chamber ICD had a 3.0% rate, and those with a CRT-ICD had a 4.3% rate. Patients implanted at hospitals with the highest quartile of annual ICD volume had the lowest total and major complication rates. In-hospital mortality was 0.41%, which included all deaths and not just those that clearly occurred as a direct result of the procedure. Further analysis of the NCDR data demonstrated that the complication rate was lowest if the implanting physician was an electrophysiologist, even while controlling for physician volume.[23]

A retrospective analysis of Medicare data from 2002 to 2005, examined 8,581 patients undergoing ICD implantation.[24] Complication rates decreased from 18.8% in 2002 to 14.2% in 2005, coinciding with an increase of 1,644 implants in 2002 to 2,374 in the first three-quarters of 2005. Most of these complications occurred during the initial hospitalization or within 1 day of discharge. There was a slightly higher rate of complications observed in women compared with men (12.1% vs 10.3% respectively, $P = .03$). Predictors of a higher rate of complications included chronic lung disease, dementia, renal disease, and implantation by a thoracic surgeon. Interestingly, history of heart failure and outpatient implantation were associated with a lower complication rate.

In another retrospective review, complication rates were identified among 31,000 Medicare beneficiaries receiving an ICD or CRT in a 12-month period. A total in-hospital complication rate of 10.8% with ICDs and CRTs was reported.[25] There was a higher rate of a device infection (1.4% vs 0.7%, $P<.0001$) and mechanical complication of the system in those receiving an ICD versus CRT (4.8% vs 3.8%, $P<.001$), although the need for a lead or pocket revision (1.8% vs 1.2%, $P<.001$) and the incidence of pocket hematoma or hemorrhage (2.5% vs 3.4%, $P<.0001$) was greater with a CRT. There was no significant difference in in-hospital mortality (0.9% vs 1.1%) between ICD and CRT implants.

Investigators from 18 centers in Ontario, Canada, reported 45-day outcomes of 3,340 patients undergoing initial ICD implants.[26] Of these, 7.4% experienced any complication, with 4.1% having a major complication. Multivariate predictors of major complications included female sex, use of class I or class III antiarrhythmic agents, left ventricular end-systolic dimension equal to or greater than 45 mm, and use of CRT or dual-chamber ICD versus single-chamber ICD. Those patients who had a major complication had a significantly higher 45-day mortality (hazard ratio 3.70, 95% CI 1.64–8.33) compared with those with no complication, and those with a direct implant-related complication had the highest 45-day mortality (hazard ratio 24.89, 95% CI 2.11–294.26).

Finally, three German studies reported periprocedural complications occurring in 10% to 17% of patients, 3% to 5% of whom needed an operative revision.[27–29]

COMPLICATIONS ASSOCIATED WITH ICD GENERATOR REPLACEMENT

Generator changes are typically thought of as easier to perform and associated with lower risk than initial implants, but they present their own unique set of complications. This includes inadvertent damage to previously placed leads, the unanticipated finding of lead dysfunction, and a possibly higher infection rate and overall complication rate.[24,30] Several studies have shown complication rates associated with generator changes ranging between 1.2% and 8.2%.[31–33]

The only prospective data regarding complications associated with cardiovascular implantable electronic device (CIED) generator replacement comes from the REPLACE Registry.[34] This study examined prespecified 6-month complications rates in 1,744 patients undergoing either a pacemaker or ICD generator replacement. Of these, 1031 patients had a planned generator replacement only, while 713 patients had a planned lead addition in combination with a generator replacement. In patients with generator replacement only, the 6-month major and minor complications rates were 4.0% and 7.4%, respectively. Lead malfunction (1.0%) and major hematoma (0.7%) were the most common major complications reported. No deaths related to the procedure were observed. Overall, complications were higher with the more complex devices: CRTs (15.3%), ICDs (12.0%), and pacemakers (8.5%).

Of the 713 patients with an added or revised lead, the periprocedural major event rate was 2.4% and overall 6-month major and minor complication rates were 15.3% and 7.6%, respectively. Eight patient deaths (1.1%) reported were considered directly related to the procedure. Overall, the 6-month major complication rate associated with a transvenous left ventricular lead placement or revision was the highest at 18.7%, possibly reflecting the underlying advanced cardiac disease of the patients receiving CRTs.

In a retrospective analysis of 451 Canadian patients undergoing elective generator change for an ICD generator under an advisory, 9.1% had any complication and 5.9% had a major complication requiring reoperation, over a follow-up of 326 plus or minus 203 days.[35] Significantly, 2.2% developed an ICD infection needing device extraction, and there were two postextraction deaths.

TIME COURSE AND TYPES OF COMPLICATIONS
Perioperative Complications

Perioperative complications are generally considered as those occurring during the actual procedure or recognized within the early periprocedural time-period, usually 24 hours. The types of complications occurring in the perioperative time are summarized in **Table 2** . Pneumothorax is reported in 0.5% to 2.0% of cases and may be affected by the venous access technique, occurring most frequently with subclavian vein access (**Fig. 1**).[23,24,27,34,36,37] Men may have a lower risk of pneumothorax than women.[24] Rarely, arterial puncture or perforation of the superior vena cava or large veins by a sheath or guidewire will lead to a right sided hemopneumothorax or hemomediastinum.[26,34] An air embolus can occur when air is sucked through the puncture needle or the introducer sheath's hemostatic valve. An arterial-venous fistula may develop if the artery is inadvertently punctured during venous access. This can be a particularly ominous situation if a subsequent lead extraction is performed.

Lead-related perforation can occur acutely during the procedure, resulting in a pericardial effusion or cardiac tamponade.[24,26,27,36–38] In some

situations, pericardiocentesis and, rarely, open surgical repair may be necessary (**Fig. 2**). The lead may protrude into the lung or cause chest wall discomfort due to mechanical irritation of the lead or due to pacing stimulation. Alternatively, a lead may perforate through the septum into the left ventricle, or the screw of an active fixation atrial lead may enter the right pleural space and cause a right-sided pneumothorax and/or hemothorax.[57]

It is possible that smaller caliber right-ventricular ICD leads are associated with a higher risk of perforation as these leads have a greater force per unit area at their tip compared with larger ICD leads.[58,59] Active fixation leads have a higher perforation risk compared with passive fixation leads.[39,60] In a pacemaker population from the Mayo Clinic, 1.2% of patients developed pericardial effusions and symptoms consistent with pacemaker lead perforation.[39] The use of a lead with an active fixation mechanism increased the perforation risk compared with a passive fixation lead (hazard ratio 2.5, 95% CI 1.4–3.8). Other predictors of perforation included use of a temporary pacemaker lead and steroid use. In contrast, a right ventricular systolic pressure above 35 mm Hg was associated with a lesser perforation risk, possibly explained by associated right ventricular hypertrophy. It is important to recognize that lead perforation may present late after implantation.[40,41] Patients may present with signs of pleuritic chest pain, chest or diaphragmatic pacing stimulation, or cardiac tamponade. However, not all patients will present with a pericardial effusion and some patients may have no symptoms. Perforation may only be noticed due to an alteration in lead performance or appearance of the leads on chest radiograph (**Fig. 3**). Although a "partial" perforation of the lead-tip screw may be present, this situation may not necessitate lead position replacement if lead characteristics are normal and the symptoms resolve with conservative therapy.[61] It is likely that there is a higher rate of perforation than reported, but that patients are asymptomatic. In a study of 100 patients with a CIED, 15% of atrial leads and 6% of ventricular leads had CT scan evidence of lead perforation.[62]

Lead perforation and/or dissection of the coronary sinus and is a well described complication of CRT implantation (video 1, CS dissection-perforation, at www.cardiacEP.theclinics.com). Although of less concern than initially thought, this complication may lead to cardiac tamponade in rare circumstances.[14–17,19,21,27]

Stroke occurs rarely during ICD implantation, due to either unintended arterial puncture or due to left atrial or left ventricular placement of a lead (**Fig. 4**, video 2, lead crossing PFO, at www.cardiacEP.theclinics.com). Another potential cause of

Table 2
Complication rates by type and time of occurrence

Periprocedural	
Resulting from procedural mechanical events	
Pneumothorax[23,24,27,32,34,36,37]	0.5%–2%
Hemothorax[26,34]	0.1%–0.4%
Lead perforation with pericarditis, pericardial effusion, or tamponade[24,26,27,31,36–41]	0.1%–1.5%
RBBB or CHB from lead manipulation[14,18]	<0.1%–0.9%
Coronary sinus dissection or perforation[14–17,19,21,27]	0.1%–2%
IV contrast or other drug reaction[23]	<0.1%–0.1%
Hemomediastinum	Rare
Air embolus	Rare
Arterial stick or lead placement	Rare
Lead crossing PFO or ASD or placed in CS	Rare
Damage to leads during generator change or lead addition[34]	Up to 1%
Clinical events	
Death[14,22,26,27,34]	0.2%–1.1%
Atrial or ventricular arrhythmias[14,26,36]	<0.1%–1.5%
Myocardial infarction[23]	<0.1%
Stroke[23,27]	<0.1%–0.2%
Pulmonary edema[26]	0.6%
Cardiogenic shock[26]	0.2%
Nerve injury[23]	<0.1%
Pulmonary embolus	Rare
Local anesthesia overdose or injection into vessel	Rare
Apnea[34]	Rare
Operator errors	
Loose set screw[27,34]	<0.1%–0.7%
Retained products	Rare
Placing lead in wrong header port[34]	Rare
Lost guidewires in vessels	Rare

Early postprocedural	
Resulting from procedural mechanical events	
Lead dislodgement[27,28,34,42]	1.0%–6.6%
Diaphragm stimulation[14,15,18]	0.4%–2.2%
Delayed perforation of leads[31,40,41]	Rare
Clinical events	
Symptomatic subclavian vein thrombosis[14,27,34]	0.2%–0.7%
AV fistula[23]	<0.1%
Pocket pain[28,36,42]	1%–5%
Hematoma or bleeding[23,24,26–28,34,37]	0.9%–10%
Superficial cellulitis, wound dehiscence, pocket infection, blood stream infection, device endocarditis, or sepsis[23,24,28,34,42–53]	0.3%–7.9%
Thoracic duct injury with chylothorax or lymphatic fistula	Rare
Renal dysfunction from IV contrast	Rare
Pulmonary embolus	Rare

Late postprocedural	
Device malfunction[54]	5.6%–52.5% per 1000 person-y
Lead failure and need for intervention[55]	40% at 8 y
Device migration[14,27,28,36]	0.6%–1.9%
Symptomatic subclavian vein thrombosis[14,27,34]	0.2%–0.7%
Pocket pain[28,36,42]	1%–5%
Tricuspid valve damage[56]	≤25%
Frozen shoulder[27,36]	<0.1%–1.2%
Erosion, pocket infection, blood stream infection, device endocarditis, or sepsis[23,24,28,34,42–53]	0.3%–7.9%
Twiddler syndrome	Rare
SVC syndrome	Rare
AV fistula[23]	<0.1%
Keloid or hypertrophic scar	Unknown

Abbreviations: AV, arteriovenous; ASD, atrial septal defect; CHB, complete heart block; CS, coronary sinus; IV, intravenous; PFO, patent foramen ovale; RBBB, right bundle branch block; SVC, superior vena cava.

stroke is the development of right atrial or ventricular lead thrombus that undergoes embolization across an atrial septal defect or patent foramen ovale. Finally, strokes can occur due to conversion of atrial fibrillation during defibrillation threshold testing in a patient with an unrecognized left atrial thrombus.

Pulmonary emboli can occur due to deep venous thrombosis in the upper extremity or a thrombus that forms on the lead. There is limited data

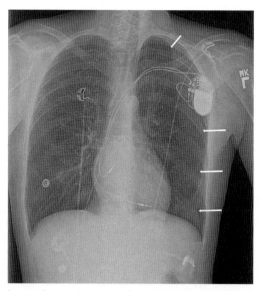

Fig. 1. Chest radiograph of a left-sided pneumothorax.

regarding the frequency of lead-related thrombosis, but clinical experience suggests that the incidence of lead-related pulmonary emboli is low. In one study, 21% of patients with a device had a lead thrombus but none developed symptomatic pulmonary embolism.[42]

Operator error such as retained products, including a sponge, wire, or sheath, can occur (**Fig. 5**). Device–lead interface problems include placing the lead in the wrong port on the header or failure to secure the set-screw correctly, leading to noise on the lead and inappropriate sensing.[27]

Rhythms disturbances as a direct consequence of the procedure include complete heart block during lead placement, particularly in patients with a preexisting left bundle brunch block,[14,18] and ventricular arrhythmias due to mechanical irritation from lead manipulation, patient clinical instability, or lead dislodgement.[26,36]

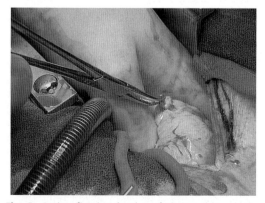

Fig. 2. Active fixation lead perforating through the right ventricle with lead-tip secured with surgical clamp. (*Courtesy of* Lyle Larson, PA-C, PhD.)

Major medical complications can occur in the periprocedural period. Even a "simple" procedure in a patient with significant cardiac disease and comorbidities can result in adverse clinical events that, although not directly caused by the procedure, are precipitated by its occurrence. This includes apnea, hypotension, cardiac arrest, acute coronary ischemia, pulmonary edema, and worsened heart failure.[22,26,27,34,36]

Early Postoperative Complications

Hematoma is a frequent complication of device placement and generator change, especially in the setting of more potent antiplatelet agents.[23,24,26–28,34,37] There is a trend toward implantation of patients while on therapeutic warfarin dosing, as the incidence of hematoma may be lower than on unfractionated heparin for patients who must maintain anticoagulation.[63,64] Generally, even a tense hematoma can be managed conservatively with pressure dressings and pain control. Reentering a pocket increases the risk of infection[43,44,65] and should only be considered if wound dehiscence, skin necrosis, or continued expansion occurs.

Patients may develop pocket pain, which is often due to migration of the generator into the axilla or breast (**Fig. 6**), compression of adjacent structures, or abutting of the generator against the clavicle or humeral head. Moving the device may be necessary.[28,36,42] There should be a high degree of suspicion for infection if a patient complains of persistent pain well past the time when surgical-related pain should have resolved and an obvious source of local pressure on adjacent structures is not obvious.

Diaphragmatic stimulation is possible with any lead, either with capturing a phrenic nerve or with direct diaphragm stimulation. This situation often requires lead repositioning to manage. Because the left phrenic nerve overlies the left ventricle, there is a higher rate of diaphragm stimulation with CRT.[14,21] It is also possible with unipolar pacing to stimulate the pectoralis muscle.

Heart failure decompensation may not occur acutely during the procedure, but may occur up to a few weeks afterward[2] and is more common in CRT implantations due to the more advanced heart failure in these patients.[14,17,21]

Late Follow-up

Complications as a direct consequence of the surgical procedure, as well as medical complications precipitated by the procedure, may be observed weeks to years later.

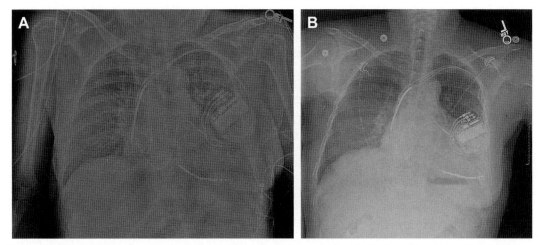

Fig. 3. (*A*) Chest radiograph of a biventricular ICD taken the day after implant. (*B*) Chest radiograph 1 week later. The right ventricular ICD lead has perforated and moved significantly leftward.

Venous occlusion occurs chronically in 18% to 50% of patients[66] and can be identified by unilateral arm edema or pain, chest wall collateral vessels, or may be asymptomatic. The first recognition of venous occlusion may be when venous access is attempted with a new lead implantation. Rarely, venous occlusion happens at the level of the superior vena cava. This usually happens in patients with multiple abandoned leads or infection with vegetation. It is also seen with more frequency in patients with a prior Mustard or Senning repair for transposition of the great arteries.[67]

Clinically manifest tricuspid regurgitation or stenosis may occur due to lead perforation of a valve leaflet, restricted closing of the valve orifice by the lead, lead entanglement in the tricuspid valve apparatus, or fibrous adhesion of the lead to the valve.[68] In a study of 248 patients with

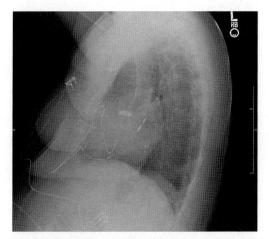

Fig. 4. Lateral chest radiograph of an atrial lead coursing posterior into the left atrium.

a CIED, 74 of whom had an ICD, 24.2% had worsening of tricuspid regurgitation (TR).[56] Five percent of these had mild TR at baseline but developed moderately severe or severe TR within 1 year of implantation. Worsening TR occurred more frequently in those receiving an ICD versus a pacemaker (32.4% vs 20.7%, *P*<.05).

Lead-Related Complications

One of the most common ICD-related complications is lead dislodgement or lead failure. Lead dislodgement may occur anytime from immediately after implant to several months postimplant. Lead dislodgement is reported to occur in as many as 6.6% of newly implanted ICD leads. Not surprisingly, the risk increases with more leads implanted.[26–28,34,42] Lead dislodgement can be macro-dislodgement, such as an atrial lead falling into the ventricle, or a micro-dislodgement only noted because of abnormal sensing or capture threshold. Coronary sinus left ventricular lead dislodgement occurs more frequently, reported up to 7.9%.[14,15,17–19,21,34] Management of a lead dislodgement most often will require a repositioning of the lead. Although some implanters try to reduce the chances of lead dislodgement by having the patient use a sling to keep the arm immobilized, this may increase the chance of a frozen shoulder developing.[27,36]

The rate of lead failure, due to fracture, insulation breach, pacing exit block, poor sensing, or other causes, increases with time and may be as high as 40% at 8 years.[55,69] Improvements in lead design are directed at improved lead longevity, as well as improved stability, handling characteristics, and electrical properties. Unfortunately, not all

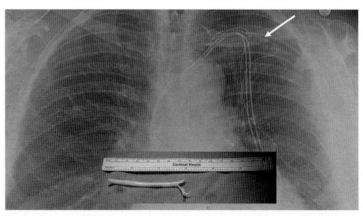

Fig. 5. Chest radiograph of a portion of a retained tear-away sheath. The patient later developed a device infection and the sheath was removed (inset).

leads prove reliable, as has been seen with several of the more recently developed ICD leads.[70,71]

The management of a lead with a high failure rate is difficult as reoperation is not without its own set of risks. In a multicenter Canadian study of 469 patients with Sprint Fidelis (Medtronic, Minneapolis, MN, USA) leads undergoing revision, 14.5% of patients experienced a complication, 7.25% of which were major.[72] Over 6% had a complication that necessitated another surgery and 1.9% developed infection needing removal.

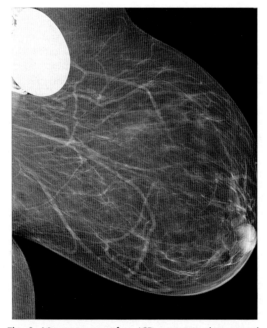

Fig. 6. Mammogram of an ICD generator inappropriately implanted superficially into breast tissue (rather than placed on pectoral muscle), which caused pain.

Infectious Complications

ICD infections may be classified as localized pocket infections, erosion, or lead-related endocarditis (**Fig. 7**, video 3, lead vegetation, at www.cardiacEP.theclinics.com). Depending on whether both pacemakers and ICDs are included, the length of follow-up, the location of the pulse generator, transvenous versus epicardial lead positions, and concomitant cardiac surgery, the CIED infection rate ranges between 0.03% and 7.9%.[23,24,28,34,42–53]

Although the number of initial CIED implantations has risen, it is exceeded by the rate of rise of CIED infections as a percentage of new CIED implantations.[73,74] Voigt and colleagues[74] estimated an increase in CIED infections from 8273 to 12,979 between 2004 and 2006, with the rate of CIED infections compared with the rate of new implants rising from 4.1% to 5.8%.

Several studies have demonstrated that a generator change is associated with a 1.8-fold to 3.7-fold higher risk of infection compared with initial

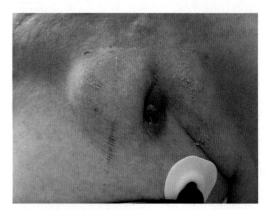

Fig. 7. ICD pocket infection.

implantation.[30,44,47,49,75] In the REPLACE registry, however, the overall infection rates were low— 1.4% for the 1,031 patients who had a generator replacement without a new lead added and 1.1% for the 713 patients with a lead added or revised.[34] Ten patients in the study required complete extraction of the CIED system. The lower identified infection rates in this study may reflect follow-up limited to 6 months.

Most infections usually present within 1 year of the last procedure and often within the first 90 days, but a significant proportion can occur after 1 year.[43–45,48] Analysis of the SCD-HeFT study demonstrated that at 30 days, 23% of infections had been identified, 55% by between 1 and 12 months, and 23% by 12 months.[6]

Several risk factors for infection have been identified. Hemodialysis and diabetes have been the most consistent risk factors, though coronary artery disease, pulmonary disease, use of oral anticoagulation or steroids, presence of a central venous catheter, fever within 24 hours of implant, and use of a temporary pacemaker wire may also affect risk.[43,44,46,49,76–78] Older age may be a risk factor for infection,[75] but younger patients, such as those with congenital heart disease, will undergo multiple generator replacements and lead revisions over their lifetime; the infectious risk may turn out to be higher risk in these individuals.

A few reports suggest a greater infectious risk with more leads,[45,77] but it is not known if the practice of extracting abandoned leads reduces the chances of future infection. A longer procedural time and need for early reintervention, such as that caused by a hematoma or lead dislodgement, also increases infection risk.[43,44,65] It is likely that pectoral generators have a lower infection rate than abdominal devices.[52,79]

Finally, procedure-related factors can increase infectious risk. Lack of periprocedural antibiotics within 2 hours of skin incision increases the chances of device infection.[44,65,75,76,80] Preprocedure skin cleansing with chlorhexidine has been associated with a lower rate of device infection.[34,52] Irrigation of the pocket is often completed to reduce infection, though it is not clear whether antibiotics are needed in the irrigation solution versus saline only.[81,82]

Approximately, 60% to 80% of CIED infections are due to Staphylococcus aureus or coagulase negative Staphylococci.[42,43,48,49,75,76] Around 50% of patients with a CIED who develop S aureus bacteremia will develop a secondary seeding of the CIED.[46]

One large study of CIED infections showed that non-Staphylococcal species, including gram negative bacteria or fungi, present later than those

with Staphylococcus, on average, 2 years from the last device manipulation.[83] The clinical course appears less virulent with a lower rate of lead endocarditis.

Management of CIED infections has been summarized in a recent American Heart Association scientific statement.[76] The entire device, including the leads, whether active or abandoned, should be extracted. This should be performed by experienced operators using specialized equipment, if needed.

FINANCIAL ASPECTS OF ICD COMPLICATIONS

The financial implications of ICD complications can be significant. In 31,000 Medicare beneficiaries receiving an ICD or CRT, after adjusting for baseline covariates, an ICD complication increased hospital costs $7251 per patient and hospital length of stay by 3.4 days.[25] The additional cost and length of stay varied by type of complication, including pericardial effusion or tamponade ($8249, 1.9 days), hematoma or hemorrhage ($6995, 3.1 days), mechanical complication with lead or pocket revision ($5436, 1.3 days), and pneumothorax ($5301, 2.9 days).

Using an administrative claims database of 26,877 hospitalizations,[84] the presence of any complication led to an increased total cost of hospitalization of $5643 to $13,547 with an increased length of stay of 5 to 9 days.[84] A 1996 study from Barnes Hospital in St Louis, Missouri examined hospital costs related to CIED complications, almost all of which were pacemakers.[85] On average, a pacemaker complication led to an additional 2.5 days in the hospital and increase of $10,583 plus or minus $12,222 in hospital costs.

The costs associated specifically with CIED-related infections are also significant. The average hospital length of stay can range from 8 to 20 days and[10,37,38] total costs range from $24,000 to $130,000.[25,45,74,85,86]

SUMMARY

Device-based therapy is life-saving in many patients with symptomatic bradycardia or tachycardia and results of clinical trials support the use of ICD and CRT therapy in the management of heart failure. These benefits notwithstanding, the impact of device-related complications is significant. Whereas individually, the majority of complications occur only rarely, the chance of any complication occurring can be substantial. Complications lead to increased risk of significant morbidity and mortality, length of hospitalization, and health care costs. Research directed at decreasing complications is critical. Increased battery longevity will reduce the number of times a pocket will be opened. Efforts focused on reducing lead-related complications and CIED-associated infections are all important. Knowing that complications increase with devices that are more complex should prompt careful consideration of the risks versus benefits. For patients who need devices that are more complex, particularly CRT, considerations should include optimizing the patient's medical issues, particularly heart failure status, before implantation and avoiding implantation in patients with such advanced disease that the benefit is unlikely to outweigh the risk.

VIDEOS

Videos related to this article can be found online at doi:10.1016/j.ccep.2011.05.005.

REFERENCES

1. Moss AJ, Hall WJ, Cannom DS, et al. Improved survival with an implanted defibrillator in patients with coronary disease at high risk for ventricular arrhythmia. Multicenter Automatic Defibrillator Implantation Trial Investigators. N Engl J Med 1996;335(26):1933–40.

2. Moss AJ, Zareba W, Hall WJ, et al. Prophylactic implantation of a defibrillator in patients with myocardial infarction and reduced ejection fraction. N Engl J Med 2002;346(12):877–83.

3. Bansch D, Antz M, Boczor S, et al. Primary prevention of sudden cardiac death in idiopathic dilated cardiomyopathy: the Cardiomyopathy Trial (CAT). Circulation 2002;105(12):1453–8.

4. Kadish A, Dyer A, Daubert JP, et al. Prophylactic defibrillator implantation in patients with nonischemic dilated cardiomyopathy. N Engl J Med 2004; 350(21):2151–8.

5. Hohnloser SH, Kuck KH, Dorian P, et al. Prophylactic use of an implantable cardioverter-defibrillator after acute myocardial infarction. N Engl J Med 2004; 351(24):2481–8.

6. Ravindran BK, Poole JE, Johnson GW, et al. Timing of device-specific ICD complications: analysis of the Sudden Cardiac Death in Heart Failure Trial (SCD-HeFT). [abstract]. Heart Rhythm 2010;7(5 Suppl 1):S9.

7. Steinbeck G, Andresen D, Seidl K, et al. Defibrillator implantation early after myocardial infarction. N Engl J Med 2009;361(15):1427–36.

8. Kron J, Herre J, Renfroe EG, et al. Lead- and device-related complications in the antiarrhythmics versus implantable defibrillators trial. Am Heart J 2001; 141(1):92–8.

9. Connolly SJ, Gent M, Roberts RS, et al. Canadian implantable defibrillator study (CIDS): a randomized trial of the implantable cardioverter defibrillator against amiodarone. Circulation 2000;101(11):1297–302.

10. Kuck KH, Cappato R, Siebels J, et al. Randomized comparison of antiarrhythmic drug therapy with implantable defibrillators in patients resuscitated from cardiac arrest: the Cardiac Arrest Study Hamburg (CASH). Circulation 2000;102(7):748–54.

11. Abraham WT, Fisher WG, Smith AL, et al. Cardiac resynchronization in chronic heart failure. N Engl J Med 2002;346(24):1845–53.

12. Cazeau S, Leclercq C, Lavergne T, et al. Effects of multisite biventricular pacing in patients with heart failure and intraventricular conduction delay. N Engl J Med 2001;344(12):873–80.

13. Knight BP, Desai A, Coman J, et al. Long-term retention of cardiac resynchronization therapy. J Am Coll Cardiol 2004;44(1):72–7.

14. Leon AR, Abraham WT, Curtis AB, et al. Safety of transvenous cardiac resynchronization system implantation in patients with chronic heart failure: combined results of over 2,000 patients from a multicenter study program. J Am Coll Cardiol 2005;46(12):2348–56.

15. Abraham WT, Young JB, Leon AR, et al. Effects of cardiac resynchronization on disease progression in patients with left ventricular systolic dysfunction, an indication for an implantable cardioverter-defibrillator, and mildly symptomatic chronic heart failure. Circulation 2004;110(18):2864–8.

16. Bristow MR, Saxon LA, Boehmer J, et al. Cardiac-resynchronization therapy with or without an implantable defibrillator in advanced chronic heart failure. N Engl J Med 2004;350(21):2140–50.

17. Cleland JG, Daubert JC, Erdmann E, et al. The effect of cardiac resynchronization on morbidity and mortality in heart failure. N Engl J Med 2005; 352(15):1539–49.

18. Linde C, Abraham WT, Gold MR, et al. Randomized trial of cardiac resynchronization in mildly symptomatic heart failure patients and in asymptomatic patients with left ventricular dysfunction and previous heart failure symptoms. J Am Coll Cardiol 2008;52(23):1834–43.

19. Moss AJ, Hall WJ, Cannom DS, et al. Cardiac-resynchronization therapy for the prevention of heart-failure events. N Engl J Med 2009;361(14):1329–38.

20. Bardy GH, Lee KL, Mark DB, et al. Amiodarone or an implantable cardioverter-defibrillator for congestive heart failure. N Engl J Med 2005;352(3):225–37.

21. Gras D, Bocker D, Lunati M, et al. Implantation of cardiac resynchronization therapy systems in the CARE-HF trial: procedural success rate and safety. Europace 2007;9(7):516–22.

22. Freeman JV, Wang Y, Curtis JP, et al. The relation between hospital procedure volume and complications of cardioverter-defibrillator implantation from the implantable cardioverter-defibrillator registry. J Am Coll Cardiol 2010;56(14):1133–9.

23. Curtis JP, Luebbert JJ, Wang Y, et al. Association of physician certification and outcomes among patients receiving an implantable cardioverter-defibrillator. JAMA 2009;301(16):1661–70.

24. Al-Khatib SM, Greiner MA, Peterson ED, et al. Patient and implanting physician factors associated with mortality and complications after implantable cardioverter-defibrillator implantation, 2002–2005. Circ Arrhythm Electrophysiol 2008;1(4):240–9.

25. Reynolds MR, Cohen DJ, Kugelmass AD, et al. The frequency and incremental cost of major complications among Medicare beneficiaries receiving implantable cardioverter-defibrillators. J Am Coll Cardiol 2006;47(12):2493–7.

26. Lee DS, Krahn AD, Healey JS, et al. Evaluation of early complications related to De Novo cardioverter defibrillator implantation insights from the Ontario ICD database. J Am Coll Cardiol 2010;55(8):774–82.

27. Alter P, Waldhans S, Plachta E, et al. Complications of implantable cardioverter defibrillator therapy in 440 consecutive patients. Pacing Clin Electrophysiol 2005;28(9):926–32.

28. Gradaus R, Block M, Brachmann J, et al. Mortality, morbidity, and complications in 3344 patients with implantable cardioverter defibrillators: results from the German ICD Registry EURID. Pacing Clin Electrophysiol 2003;26(7 Pt 1):1511–8.

29. Kleemann T, Becker T, Strauss M, et al. Perioperative complications and hospital outcome in 1428 patients undergoing first implantation of an implantable cardioverter defibrillator: A single center experience from 1992 to 2009. [abstract]. Heart Rhythm 2010; 7:S9.

30. Borleffs CJ, Thijssen J, de Bie MK, et al. Recurrent implantable cardioverter-defibrillator replacement is associated with an increasing risk of pocket-related complications. Pacing Clin Electrophysiol 2010;33(8):1013–9.

31. Costea A, Rardon DP, Padanilam BJ, et al. Complications associated with generator replacement in response to device advisories. J Cardiovasc Electrophysiol 2008;19(3):266–9.

32. Kapa S, Hyberger L, Rea RF, et al. Complication risk with pulse generator change: implications when reacting to a device advisory or recall. Pacing Clin Electrophysiol 2007;30(6):730–3.

33. Moore JW 3rd, Barrington W, Bazaz R, et al. Complications of replacing implantable devices in response to advisories: a single center experience. Int J Cardiol 2009;134(1):42–6.

34. Poole JE, Gleva MJ, Mela T, et al. Complication rates associated with pacemaker or implantable cardioverter-defibrillator generator replacements and upgrade procedures. results from the REPLACE registry. Circulation 2010;122(16):1553–61.

35. Gould PA, Gula LJ, Champagne J, et al. Outcome of advisory implantable cardioverter-defibrillator replacement: one-year follow-up. Heart Rhythm 2008;5(12):1675–81.

36. Rosenqvist M, Beyer T, Block M, et al. Adverse events with transvenous implantable cardioverter-defibrillators: a prospective multicenter study. European 7219 Jewel ICD investigators. Circulation 1998;98(7):663–70.

37. Takahashi T, Bhandari AK, Watanuki M, et al. High incidence of device-related and lead-related complications in the dual-chamber implantable cardioverter defibrillator compared with the single-chamber version. Circ J 2002;66(8):746–50.

38. Molina JE. Perforation of the right ventricle by transvenous defibrillator leads: prevention and treatment. Pacing Clin Electrophysiol 1996;19(3):288–92.

39. Mahapatra S, Bybee KA, Bunch TJ, et al. Incidence and predictors of cardiac perforation after permanent pacemaker placement. Heart Rhythm 2005; 2(9):907–11.

40. Ellenbogen KA, Wood MA, Shepard RK. Delayed complications following pacemaker implantation. Pacing Clin Electrophysiol 2002;25(8):1155–8.

41. Khan MN, Joseph G, Khaykin Y, et al. Delayed lead perforation: a disturbing trend. Pacing Clin Electrophysiol 2005;28(3):251–3.

42. Pfeiffer D, Jung W, Fehske W, et al. Complications of pacemaker-defibrillator devices: diagnosis and management. Am Heart J 1994;127(4 Pt 2): 1073–80.

43. Romeyer-Bouchard C, Da Costa A, Dauphinot V, et al. Prevalence and risk factors related to infections of cardiac resynchronization therapy devices dagger. Eur Heart J 2010;31(2):203–10.

44. Klug D, Balde M, Pavin D, et al. Risk factors related to infections of implanted pacemakers and cardioverter-defibrillators: results of a large prospective study. Circulation 2007;116(12):1349–55.

45. Nery PB, Fernandes R, Nair GM, et al. Device-related infection among patients with pacemakers and implantable defibrillators: incidence, risk factors, and consequences. J Cardiovasc Electrophysiol 2010;21(7):786–90.

46. Uslan DZ, Sohail MR, St Sauver JL, et al. Permanent pacemaker and implantable cardioverter defibrillator infection: a population-based study. Arch Intern Med 2007;167(7):669–75.

47. Trappe HJ, Pfitzner P, Klein H, et al. Infections after cardioverter-defibrillator implantation: observations in 335 patients over 10 years. Br Heart J 1995; 73(1):20–4.

48. Samuels LE, Samuels FL, Kaufman MS, et al. Management of infected implantable cardiac defibrillators. Ann Thorac Surg 1997;64(6):1702–6.

49. Lekkerkerker JC, van Nieuwkoop C, Trines SA, et al. Risk factors and time delay associated with cardiac device infections: Leiden device registry. Heart 2009;95(9):715–20.

50. Shahian DM, Williamson WA, Martin D, et al. Infection of implantable cardioverter defibrillator systems: a preventable complication? Pacing Clin Electrophysiol 1993;16(10):1956–60.

51. Kelly PA, Cannom DS, Garan H, et al. The automatic implantable cardioverter-defibrillator: efficacy, complications and survival in patients with malignant ventricular arrhythmias. J Am Coll Cardiol 1988; 11(6):1278–86.

52. Uslan DZ, Gleva MJ, Mela T, et al. Infections following cardiovascular implantable electronic device replacement: results from the REPLACE registry (abstract). Heart Rhythm 2010;7(5 Suppl 1):S252.

53. Peterson PN, Daugherty SL, Wang Y, et al. Gender differences in procedure-related adverse events in patients receiving implantable cardioverter-defibrillator therapy. Circulation 2009;119(8):1078–84.

54. Maisel WH. Pacemaker and ICD generator reliability: meta-analysis of device registries. JAMA 2006; 295(16):1929–34.

55. Kleemann T, Becker T, Doenges K, et al. Annual rate of transvenous defibrillation lead defects in implantable cardioverter-defibrillators over a period of >10 years. Circulation 2007;115(19):2474–80.

56. Kim JB, Spevack DM, Tunick PA, et al. The effect of transvenous pacemaker and implantable cardioverter defibrillator lead placement on tricuspid valve function: an observational study. J Am Soc Echocardiogr 2008;21(3):284–7.

57. Rosman J, Shapiro MD, Hanon S. Pneumomediastinum and right sided pneumothorax following dual chamber-ICD implantation. J Interv Card Electrophysiol 2006;17(2):157–8.

58. Ellis CR, Rottman JN. Increased rate of subacute lead complications with small-caliber implantable cardioverter-defibrillator leads. Heart Rhythm 2009; 6(5):619–24.

59. Danik SB, Mansour M, Singh J, et al. Increased incidence of subacute lead perforation noted with one implantable cardioverter-defibrillator. Heart Rhythm 2007;4(4):439–42.

60. Sterlinski M, Przybylski A, Maciag A, et al. Subacute cardiac perforations associated with active fixation leads. Europace 2009;11(2):206–12.

61. Levy Y, Shovman O, Granit C, et al. Pericarditis following permanent pacemaker insertion. Isr Med Assoc J 2004;6(10):599–602.

62. Hirschl DA, Jain VR, Spindola-Franco H, et al. Prevalence and characterization of asymptomatic pacemaker and ICD lead perforation on CT. Pacing Clin Electrophysiol 2007;30(1):28–32.

63. Ahmed I, Gertner E, Nelson WB, et al. Continuing warfarin therapy is superior to interrupting warfarin with or without bridging anticoagulation therapy in patients undergoing pacemaker and defibrillator implantation. Heart Rhythm 2010;7(6):745–9.

64. Tolosana JM, Berne P, Mont L, et al. Preparation for pacemaker or implantable cardiac defibrillator implants in patients with high risk of thromboembolic events: oral anticoagulation or bridging with intravenous heparin? A prospective randomized trial. Eur Heart J 2009;30(15):1880–4.

65. de Oliveira JC, Martinelli M, Nishioka SA, et al. Efficacy of antibiotic prophylaxis before the implantation of pacemakers and cardioverter-defibrillators: results of a large, prospective, randomized, double-blinded, placebo-controlled trial. Circ Arrhythm Electrophysiol 2009;2(1):29–34.

66. Rozmus G, Daubert JP, Huang DT, et al. Venous thrombosis and stenosis after implantation of pacemakers and defibrillators. J Interv Card Electrophysiol 2005;13(1):9–19.

67. Emmel M, Sreeram N, Brockmeier K, et al. Superior vena cava stenting and transvenous pacemaker implantation (stent and pace) after the Mustard operation. Clin Res Cardiol 2007;96(1):17–22.

68. Lin G, Nishimura RA, Connolly HM, et al. Severe symptomatic tricuspid valve regurgitation due to permanent pacemaker or implantable cardioverter-defibrillator leads. J Am Coll Cardiol 2005;45(10): 1672–5.

69. Borleffs CJW, van Erven L, van Bommel RJ, et al. Risk of failure of transvenous implantable cardioverter-defibrillator leads. Circ Arrhythm Electrophysiol 2009;2(4):411–6.

70. Ellenbogen KA, Wood MA, Shepard RK, et al. Detection and management of an implantable cardioverter defibrillator lead failure: incidence and clinical implications. J Am Coll Cardiol 2003;41(1):73–80.

71. Hauser RG, Hayes DL. Increasing hazard of Sprint Fidelis implantable cardioverter-defibrillator lead failure. Heart Rhythm 2009;6(5):605–10.

72. Parkash R, Crystal E, Bashir J, et al. Complications associated with revision of Sprint Fidelis leads: report from the Canadian Heart Rhythm Society Device Advisory Committee. Circulation 2010;121(22):2384–7.

73. Cabell CH, Heidenreich PA, Chu VH, et al. Increasing rates of cardiac device infections among Medicare beneficiaries: 1990–1999. Am Heart J 2004;147(4):582–6.

74. Voigt A, Shalaby A, Saba S. Continued rise in rates of cardiovascular implantable electronic device infections in the United States: temporal trends and causative insights. Pacing Clin Electrophysiol 2010;33(4):414–9.

75. Cengiz M, Okutucu S, Ascioglu S, et al. Permanent pacemaker and implantable cardioverter defibrillator infections: seven years of diagnostic and therapeutic experience of a single center. Clin Cardiol 2010;33(7):406–11.

76. Baddour LM, Epstein AE, Erickson CC, et al. Update on cardiovascular implantable electronic device infections and their management: a scientific

statement from the American Heart Association. Circulation 2010;121(3):458–77.

77. Sohail MR, Uslan DZ, Khan AH, et al. Risk factor analysis of permanent pacemaker infection. Clin Infect Dis 2007;45(2):166–73.

78. Bloom H, Heeke B, Leon A, et al. Renal insufficiency and the risk of infection from pacemaker or defibrillator surgery. Pacing Clin Electrophysiol 2006;29(2): 142–5.

79. Mela T, McGovern BA, Garan H, et al. Long-term infection rates associated with the pectoral versus abdominal approach to cardioverter- defibrillator implants. Am J Cardiol 2001;88(7):750–3.

80. Da Costa A, Kirkorian G, Cucherat M, et al. Antibiotic prophylaxis for permanent pacemaker implantation: a meta-analysis. Circulation 1998;97(18): 1796–801.

81. Belott PH, Reynolds DW. Permanent pacemaker and implantable cardioverter-defibrillator implantation. In: Ellenbogen KA, Kay GN, Lau CP, et al, editors. Clinical cardiac pacing, defibrillation, and resynchronization therapy. 3rd edition. Philadelphia: Saunders Elsevier; 2007. p. 561–651.

82. Lakkireddy D, Valasareddi S, Ryschon K, et al. The impact of povidone-iodine pocket irrigation use on pacemaker and defibrillator infections. Pacing Clin Electrophysiol 2005;28(8):789–94.

83. Viola GM, Awan LL, Darouiche RO. Nonstaphylococcal infections of cardiac implantable electronic devices. Circulation 2010;121(19):2085–91.

84. Swindle JP, Rich MW, McCann P, et al. Implantable cardiac device procedures in older patients: use and in-hospital outcomes. Arch Intern Med 2010; 170(7):631–7.

85. Ferguson TB Jr, Ferguson CL, Crites K, et al. The additional hospital costs generated in the management of complications of pacemaker and defibrillator implantations. J Thorac Cardiovasc Surg 1996;111(4):742–51 [discussion 51–2].

86. Kurtz SM, Lau E, Ochoa JA, et al. Fifteen-year trends in the infection burden for pacemakers and ICDs in the United States. Heart Rhythm 2010;7(5 Suppl 1):S57.

Total Subcutaneous Defibrillators: The Current Status and Future Prospect of a New Technology

Marwan Refaat, MD, Samir Saba, MD, FHRS*

KEYWORDS

- Defibrillators • Subcutaneous
- Implantable cardioverter-defibrillator
- Treatment outcome

Sudden cardiac death (SCD) is defined as an unexpected death from a cardiac cause generally within 1 hour of onset of symptoms. The event is referred to as sudden cardiac arrest (SCA) if an intervention such as defibrillation restores circulation. SCD remains a major public health concern, affecting annually more than 3 million people worldwide and accounting for up to 450,000 deaths in the United States, which represents 15% of all deaths.[1] About half of all SCDs occur out of the hospital setting, and, of those, about 40% are unwitnessed. Most victims of SCD have coronary artery disease (80%), whereas the rest of them have other forms of acquired or inherited cardiomyopathies (15%) or intrinsic cardiac conduction system abnormalities.[2] Clinical factors used to predict sudden death include a prior history of aborted sudden death, left ventricular dysfunction, and the diagnosis of inherited syndromes associated with arrhythmias such as hypertrophic cardiomyopathy, arrhythmogenic right ventricular cardiomyopathy, long QT syndrome, the Brugada syndrome, and others.[3]

Implantable cardioverter-defibrillators (ICDs) constitute an effective therapy for protection against death in survivors of SCA and in those at risk for SCD based on poor left ventricular function.[4–10] The use of conventional ICDs is, however, associated with complications at the time of device and transvenous lead insertions as well as during follow-up. These complications, which include device and lead failures, vascular occlusions, inappropriate shocks, and others, contribute to increased patient morbidity, worsened quality of life, and increased cost to the health care system.[11,12] In this article, the authors discuss the totally subcutaneous ICD (SC-ICD) system that was designed to provide an alternative to transvenous electrodes in patients who do not require cardiac pacing. The authors also discuss the promises and shortcomings of this new device technology compared with the conventional transvenous implantable defibrillator system and review the experience up-to-date with the SC-ICD.

RATIONALE AND ADVANTAGES OF THE SC-ICD

Implanting devices such as transvenous ICD systems require a set of skills that only trained cardiac electrophysiologists and some cardiothoracic surgeons possess. Few years ago, there was concern regarding the lack of availability of experienced implanters of conventional intravenous

Disclosures: Dr Saba received research support from Medtronic, Boston Scientific, and St Jude Medical and is a consultant for St Jude Medical and Spectranetics Inc.
Cardiovascular Electrophysiology Section, University of Pittsburgh, Pittsburgh, PA, USA
* Corresponding author. Cardiac Electrophysiology, Cardiovascular Electrophysiology Section, University of Pittsburgh Medical Center, 200 Lothrop Street, PUH B535, Pittsburgh, PA 15213.
E-mail address: sabas@upmc.edu

Card Electrophysiol Clin 3 (2011) 403–408
doi:10.1016/j.ccep.2011.05.006
1877-9182/11/$ – see front matter © 2011 Published by Elsevier Inc.

ICD systems in the face of exponentially expanding indications. Therefore, there was a perceived need for simplified SC-ICD systems that could deliver lifesaving shocks and could be implanted by less-experienced implanters, including interventional and even general cardiologists. This perception was a major initial impetus in the development of the SC-ICD.

The use of conventional ICDs is associated with complications during transvenous lead insertion, such as pneumothorax, hemothorax, and cardiac tamponade. Postoperatively, complications along the lines of ICD system infections, lead failures, or recalls also take place[13] and are even more pronounced after device system changeouts or upgrades for which infections and vascular occlusions are more common than with original fresh implantations, leading to the relocation of the ICD system to the contralateral prepectoral area, to lead tunneling, or to the higher risk procedures of chronic lead extractions.[14,15]

Because achieving and maintaining venous access remains a challenge with conventional ICD implantations, the SC-ICD presents an alternative technique that can help avoid most of the aforementioned complications. SC-ICD also offers a needed solution to the problem of limited or no venous access to the heart in patients who would otherwise be considered for the placement of epicardial shocking pads via thoracotomy.

The SC-ICD presents other advantages that deserve mentioning. First, the device can be implanted without the need for fluoroscopic guidance, thus limiting radiation exposure to patients and operators. Second, in the event of device system infection, explantation of the SC-ICD and associated lead does not involve the cardiac or vascular compartments and, therefore, is technically easier and confers lower risk of mortality and major complications to the patient. Last, reports suggest a lower risk of myocardial injury from shock delivery with the SC-ICD compared with the conventional ICD.[16] Although this finding remains unconfirmed in other studies, the authors mention it in this article for completion.

SHORTCOMINGS OF THE SC-ICD

Despite its many established and potential advantages, the SC-ICD presents some considerable disadvantages that have dampened the excitement for it. By virtue of the absence of a lead or electrode that is in direct contact with the myocardium on either the endocardial or epicardial surface, the SC-ICD cannot provide backup pacing in the event of bradycardia developing spontaneously or in the immediate postshock phase. Also, the lack of pacing capability in the SC-ICD commits the patient to receiving an energy discharge in response to sustained arrhythmias without the benefit of antitachycardia pacing, which may save the patient the physical and emotional pains of receiving a shock as well as preserve device battery life.

From the device sensing perspective, the SC-ICD may lack specificity in identifying arrhythmias and ascertaining their chamber of origin. Compared with dual-chamber conventional devices, SC-ICDs do not sample atrial events and are, therefore, less likely to correctly discriminate between ventricular and supraventricular arrhythmias. Also, the rate of false oversensing of events is likely higher with subcutaneous as opposed to intracardiac electrodes. Although this oversensing has been suggested by small retrospective clinical trials,[17] given the currently limited clinical experience with the SC-ICD, these disadvantages remain speculative and ought to be examined prospectively in larger groups of patients.

More confirmed is the fact that, compared with the conventional ICD, SC-ICDs have higher defibrillation thresholds (DFTs) for termination of ventricular fibrillation. In one study,[18] the energy requirement was 36.6 J with the SC-ICD compared with 11.1 J with conventional transvenous systems. Also, although completely subcutaneous, the SC-ICD implantation technique involves multiple incisions and lead tunnelings. It, therefore, remains fairly complex and may be associated with significant complications such as system infection or erosion and lead failure, dislodgement, or deformation even in the hands of experienced implanters. In one report,[17] the survival of the SC-ICD system was shorter than that of conventional intravenous systems. A retrospective review of all subjects undergoing ICD placement at the Children's Hospital in Boston from January 2000 to February 2009 examined 78 patients in the transvenous ICD group who were matched by the type of cardiac disease and implant date to 39 patients in the nontransvenous group in a 2:1 ratio. The indications for a nontransvenous system included small patient size (n = 21), systemic venous access problems (n = 9), intracardiac shunt (n = 4), implant at the time of cardiovascular surgery with thoracotomy (n = 4), and tricuspid valve abnormality (n = 1). Survival of ICD systems using nontransvenous defibrillation coils was significantly shorter than that with transvenous ICD systems, with a system survival at 12, 24, and 36 months of 73%, 55%, and 49%, respectively, in the nontransvenous group compared with 91%, 83%, and 76%, respectively, in the transvenous group (P = .003).

A multivariable Cox proportional hazards model revealed that the nontransvenous approach was an independent predictor of system failure (hazard ratio, 2.9; $P = .04$). The rate of total unanticipated interventions was also higher in the nontransvenous group than in the transvenous group (18 vs 6 per 1000 person-months).

The perceived need for more ICD system implanters, which surfaced at the time of expanding indications of defibrillators mainly for the primary prevention of SCD and which constituted one of the rationales for developing a simpler totally subcutaneous defibrillator, may have been overestimated. Except in designated underserved areas, the current need for device implantations seems to be adequately met by the numbers of intravascular implanters.

EXPERIENCE WITH THE SC-ICD
Pediatric Data

The use of transvenous ICD leads in small children is problematic, given the size discrepancy between the venous access and the available lead systems. The addition of subcutaneous array leads has been proved to be reliable in increasing the safety margin of effective defibrillation.[19] To avoid the placement of epicardial defibrillation pads and their possible complications, such as constrictive pericarditis and crinkling of the patch electrode, Cannon and colleagues[20] proposed the use of an SC-ICD coil directly into the pericardial sac through a full thoracotomy. Many effective and less-invasive nonvascular ICD implantation techniques in children have also been reported.[21,22] Bové and colleagues[22] proposed a method of implanting a cardioverter-defibrillator without the need for thoracotomy based on the subxiphoid insertion of an epicardial bipolar ventricular pacing and sensing lead, an active can placed in the abdomen, and a subcutaneous array tunneled along the left thoracic wall as a shocking electrode. This technique offers the advantage of an effective and minimally invasive ICD with wide applicability for children, independent of their size and cardiac status. Although few patients were examined in this study, its results revealed maintenance of acceptably low DFTs in short follow-up.

Best Subcutaneous Shocking Vector and DFTs

Exploration of novel and efficient electrode configurations is important in the development of the SC-ICDs and their implantation procedures. Image-based finite element models (FEMs) of an adult man were used to predict the myocardial electric field generated during defibrillation shocks (pseudo-DFT) in various subcutaneous electrode positions to determine factors affecting optimal lead positions for SC-ICD.[23] Generator location, lead location, length, geometry, orientation, as well as spatial relation of electrodes to ventricular mass were systematically varied. A total of 122 single-electrode/array configurations and 28 dual-electrode configurations were simulated. Favorable alignment of lead-generator vector with ventricular myocardium and increased lead length were the most important favorable factors correlated with lower pseudo-DFTs, accounting for 70% of the predicted variation ($R^2 = 0.70$, each factor $P<.05$). This FEM modeling suggested that the choice of configurations that maximize shock vector alignment with the center of myocardial mass and the use of longer leads result in lower DFTs.

The device configuration and energy requirements were investigated in 2 short-term clinical trials, in which 4 system designs underwent short-term testing in 78 patients.[18] The best-performing design was then tested in 49 additional patients to determine the SC-ICD DFT compared with the standard transvenous ICD. After a pilot study to evaluate the long-term use of the SC-ICD system in 6 patients, a final single-group clinical trial was performed in 55 patients. After initial testing, the optimal configuration for the SC-ICD system included a parasternal electrode and a left lateral thoracic pulse generator (**Fig. 1**). Device insertion was guided by anatomic landmarks only, with no need for fluoroscopy. This configuration was as effective as the conventional transvenous ICD in terminating episodes of induced ventricular fibrillation. In 2 consecutive tests, induced episodes of ventricular fibrillation were effectively converted using 65-J shocks in 58 of 59 (98%) patients.[18]

The Dedicated Totally Subcutaneous Defibrillator

The only dedicated SC-ICD currently manufactured and used in clinical trials is made by Cameron Health Inc (San Clemente, CA, USA; **Fig. 2**). This SC-ICD system consists of 2 implantable elements, a pulse generator (SQ-RX) and a subcutaneous lead (Q-TRAK). A single-use tunneling tool (Q-GUIDE) is used for positioning the subcutaneous lead. The subcutaneous lead has 2 sensing electrodes, A and B, and one 8-cm defibrillation coil between these electrodes. The pulse generator is also a sensing electrode (electrode C). There are, therefore, 3 possible sensing vectors: A–B, A–C, and B–C. This SC-ICD uses the subcutaneous electrocardiogram (ECG) to monitor heart rhythm and detect ventricular arrhythmias. The algorithm chooses the best of the 3 sensing vectors, taking

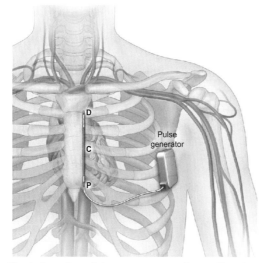

Fig. 1. Location of the components of a totally subcutaneous ICD in situ. The distal and proximal sensing electrodes (D and P, respectively) of the device system are shown, with the left lateral pulse generator and an 8-cm parasternal coil electrode (C). (*Adapted from* Bardy GH, Smith WM, Hood MA, et al. An entirely subcutaneous implantable cardioverter-defibrillator. N Eng J Med 2010;363:36–44; with permission.)

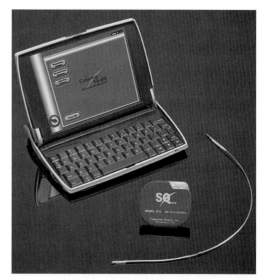

Fig. 2. Components of the totally subcutaneous defibrillator made by Cameron Health Inc. (San Clemente, CA, USA) are shown, including the implantable device, the subcutaneous lead, and the programmer. (*Courtesy of* Cameron Health Inc, San Clemente, CA, USA; with permission.)

into consideration the subcutaneous waveforms, including the QRS to T-wave amplitude. Preoperatively, a 3-lead surface ECG is recorded as a surrogate for the subcutaneous ECG. The 3-surface ECG electrodes are placed in the expected positions of the subcutaneous electrodes to confirm that the ECG signals are suitable for the SC-ICD. The implantation of this device consists in making a 6-cm incision above the left fifth intercostal space in the midaxillary line. A subcutaneous pocket, sufficient to accommodate the generator, is then made below the incision. A 2-cm horizontal incision is also made immediately to the left of the xiphoid/sternum with dissection down to the muscle. The Q-GUIDE tunneling tool is pushed subcutaneously from the xiphoid incision to the pocket and attached to the suture hole in the tip of the lead by a loop of silk suture. The tip of the lead is then pulled subcutaneously by the Q-GUIDE from the generator pocket through the lower sternal wound until the proximal electrode (B) lies within the xiphoid wound. The lead is secured to the underlying muscle within the xiphoid wound just proximal to electrode B. The distal remainder of the lead is then placed on the surface of the left chest 1 to 2 cm lateral of the midline. A 2-cm vertical incision is made where the distal tip is located. The Q-GUIDE is pushed subcutaneously, and the tip of the lead is pulled into the upper sternal wound. The lead tip is secured to the underlying muscle.

The generator is connected to the proximal end of the lead and secured within the subcutaneous pocket. The deep layers of all 3 incisions are then closed.

Long-Term Experience with the Subcutaneous Defibrillator

As mentioned earlier, the SC-ICD had a high rate of termination of ventricular fibrillation episodes induced at the time of device implantation and, therefore, seems to be safe and effective for detecting and converting ventricular fibrillation. A total of 55 patients implanted with the SC-ICD were followed up for a mean of 10 ± 1 months, during which the device successfully detected and converted 12 of 12 episodes of spontaneous sustained ventricular tachyarrhythmias. Complications from the procedure included infections involving the device implantation pocket in 2 patients and 4 lead dislodgements requiring system revisions.[18]

THE SC-ICD: A MAJOR STEP FORWARD OR A NICHE THERAPY

The SC-ICD constitutes a novel ICD technology that offers an alternative to operators and to the patients they care for. It is the opinion of the authors that the SC-ICD niche will clearly be established for those patients with limited or no venous access who also do not require pacing.

Given the limited clinical experience and short follow-up with the currently available SC-ICD system, it is not yet clear whether the SC-ICD will become a viable alternative for most patients who need protection with an ICD. Many questions still need to be answered. How specific is the sensing in this defibrillator system? How important is ventricular pacing in the early postshock period? How durable is the SC-ICD over long follow-up periods in a large number of patients? Based on the answer to these questions and the future performance of the SC-ICD in clinical trials, this technology may grow exponentially to become the mainstream device system for patients at risk of SCD or may remain limited in its scope and reserved to those patients with no vascular access, just as an alternative to cardiac surgery. Further development and testing are needed, ultimately, including randomized, multicenter, noninferiority clinical trials comparing SC-ICDs with transvenous ICDs.

The future of the SC-ICD will also be determined by the rate of development and success of competing technologies such as the intravascular lead extraction tools. Although the SC-ICD could potentially reduce or eliminate problems such as failure to achieve vascular access, intravascular injury, and lead failure requiring difficult procedures for extraction and replacement, improvement in conventional ICD implantation and explantation tools and techniques may strip the SC-ICD from most of these potential advantages.

From the physicians' and operators' perspective, these competing technologies are exciting because they will surely bring better tools and alternatives for an improved patient care delivery.

REFERENCES

1. Zheng ZJ, Croft JB, Giles WH, et al. Sudden death in the United States, 1989 to 1998. Circulation 2001; 104:2158–63.

2. Zipes DP, Wellens HJ. Sudden cardiac death. Circulation 1998;98:2334–51.

3. Frangiskakis JM, London B. Targeting device therapy: genomics of sudden death. Heart Fail Clin 2010;6(1):93–100.

4. The Antiarrhythmic Versus Implantable Defibrillator (AVID) Investigators. A comparison of antiarrhythmic-drug therapy with implantable defibrillators in patients resuscitated from near-fatal ventricular arrhythmias. N Engl J Med 1997;337:1576–83.

5. Connolly SJ, Gent M, Roberts RS, et al. Canadian Implantable Defibrillator Study (CIDS). A randomized trial of the implantable cardioverter defibrillator against amiodarone. Circulation 2000;101:1297–302.

6. Kuck K-H, Cappato R, Siebels J, et al. Randomized comparison of antiarrhythmic drug therapy with implantable defibrillators in patients resuscitated from cardiac arrest: the Cardiac Arrest Study Hamburg (CASH). Circulation 2000;102:748–54.

7. Moss AJ, Hall WJ, Cannom DS, et al. Improved survival with an implanted defibrillator in patients with coronary disease at high risk for ventricular arrhythmia. N Engl J Med 1996;335:1933–40.

8. Buxton AE, Lee DL, Fisher JD, et al. A randomized study of the prevention of sudden death in patients with coronary artery disease. N Engl J Med 1999; 341:1882–90.

9. Moss AJ, Zareba W, Hall WJ, et al, Multicenter Automatic Defibrillator Implantation Trial II Investigators. Prophylactic implantation on a defibrillator in patients with myocardial infarction and reduced ejection fraction. N Engl J Med 2002;346:877–83.

10. Bardy GH, Lee KL, Mark DB, et al. Amiodarone or an implantable cardioverter-defibrillator for congestive heart failure. N Engl J Med 2005;352:225–37.

11. Korte T, Jung W, Spehl S, et al. Incidence of ICD lead related complications during long-term follow-up: comparison of epicardial and endocardial electrode systems. PACE 1995;18:2053–61.

12. Lickfett L, Bitzen A, Arepally A, et al. Incidence of venous obstruction following insertion of an implantable cardioverter defibrillator: a study of systematic contrast venography on patients presenting for their first elective ICD generator replacement. Europace 2004;6:25–31.

13. Maisel WH. Implantable cardioverter-defibrillator lead complication: when is an outbreak out of bounds? Heart Rhythm 2008;5(12):1673–4.

14. Byrd CL, Wilkoff B, Love CJ, et al. Intravascular extraction of problematic or infected permanent pacemaker leads: 1994–1996, U.S. Extraction Database, MED institute. PACE 1999;22:1348–57.

15. Wazni O, Epstein LM, Carrillo RG, et al. Lead extraction in the contemporary setting: the LExICon study: an observational retrospective study of consecutive laser lead extractions. J Am Coll Cardiol 2010;55(6): 579–86.

16. Killingsworth CR, Litovsky SH, Melnick SB, et al. Shocks delivered via a subcutaneous defibrillation system cause less acute injury than transvenous leads in swine. Heart Rhythm 2010;7(5):S186.

17. Radbill AE, Triedman JK, Berul CI, et al. System survival of nontransvenous implantable cardioverter-defibrillators compared to transvenous implantable cardioverter-defibrillators in pediatric and congenital heart disease patients. Heart Rhythm 2010;7(2): 193–8.

18. Bardy GH, Smith WM, Hood MA, et al. An entirely subcutaneous implantable cardioverter-defibrillator. N Engl J Med 2010;363:36–44.

19. Osswald BR, De Simone R, Most S, et al. High defibrillation threshold in patients with implantable

defibrillator: how effective is the subcutaneous finger lead? Eur J Cardiothorac Surg 2009;35:489–92.

20. Cannon BC, Friedman RA, Fenrich AL, et al. Innovative techniques for placement of implantable cardioverter defibrillator leads in patients with limited venous access to the heart. PACE 2006;29:181–7.

21. Gradaus R, Hammel D, Kotthoff D, et al. Non-thoracotomy implantable cardioverter defibrillator placement in children: use of subcutaneous array leads and abdominally placed implantable cardioverter

defibrillators in children. J Cardiovasc Electrophysiol 2001;12:256–360.

22. Bové T, François K, De Caluwe W, et al. Effective cardioverter defibrillator implantation in children without thoracotomy: a valid alternative. Ann Thorac Surg 2010;89:1307–9.

23. Jolley M, Stinstra J, Tate J, et al. Finite element modeling of subcutaneous implantable defibrillator electrodes in an adult torso. Heart Rhythm 2010; 7(5):692–8.

Lead Fracture: Incidence, Diagnosis and Preventing Inappropriate ICD Therapy

Jayanthi N. Koneru, MBBS[a], Karoly Kaszala, MD, PhD[a,b],
Jose F. Huizar, MD[a,b], Kenneth A. Ellenbogen, MD, FAHA, FHRS[a,*]

KEYWORDS

• ICD • Lead fracture • Lead integrity algorithm

In the last decade, multiple prospective multicenter studies have shown a survival benefit with implantable cardiac defibrillators (ICD) therapy in patients with impaired left ventricular function as well as in patients with a high risk of ventricular arrhythmias such as Brugada syndrome, severe hypertrophic cardiomyopathy, long QT syndrome, and arrhythmogenic right ventricular dysplasia.[1–4] This has resulted in an increase in the number of ICD implantations for primary prevention of sudden cardiac death. Accurate and effective ICD function is predicated on sensing intracardiac electrical activity and subsequent appropriate interpretation by device algorithms. Ventricular sensing is the process by which pacemakers and ICDs identify electrical signals representing ventricular depolarization as local intracardiac electrograms (EGMs). Sensing of signals that do not represent local depolarizations is referred to as "oversensing". Ventricular oversensing may be caused by signals from either an ICD lead fracture or connection issues or physiologic signals (eg, T-waves, myopotentials) or electromagnetic interference.[5,6] Oversensing is responsible for approximately one-third of inappropriate shocks during long-term follow-up of ICD patients.[2] Inappropriate shocks not only cause significant psychological and physical distress

but may also cause at least transient myocardial dysfunction in patients who often already have decreased left ventricular function.[7] Integrity of the sensing circuit is of paramount importance for appropriate arrhythmia detection by the ICD. The weakest link in this circuit is the ICD lead and the most common manifestation of lead failure is lead fracture. This article discusses the incidence and causative factors of lead fracture and diagnostic strategies and therapeutic options for this important clinical problem.

ENGINEERING ASPECTS OF LEAD FAILURE

Early transvenous ICD leads were based on coaxial design wherein each of the conductors is coiled around the central cathodal coil conductor and separated by insulation. Examples of such leads include Medtronic 6936, St. Jude Medical Ventritex TVL RV 01, and the Guidant ENDOTAK 0073/75 (**Fig. 1**). Given that coaxial leads were more prone to lead fracture, manufacturers have developed a multilumen design. Similar to the coaxial design, a central coil conductor is used as the cathode allowing for stylet insertion and provides the extendable-retractable active fixation mechanism. Another design innovation is the use

[a] Cardiac Electrophysiology, Division of Cardiology, Medical College of Virginia/Virginia Commonwealth University, Gateway Building, 3rd Floor, PO Box 980053, Richmond, VA 23298–0053, USA
[b] Cardiac Electrophysiology, Division of Cardiology, McGuire VA Medical Center, Medical College of Virginia, Gateway Building, 3rd Floor, PO Box 980053, Richmond, VA 23298–0053, USA
* Corresponding author.
E-mail address: kellenbogen@mcvh-vcu.edu

Card Electrophysiol Clin 3 (2011) 409–420
doi:10.1016/j.ccep.2011.05.007
1877-9182/11/$ – see front matter © 2011 Published by Elsevier Inc.

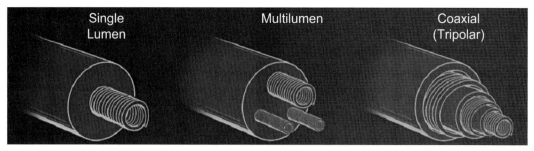

Fig. 1. Different lead designs.

of compression lumens that may protect against fracture by absorbing crush stress. The technique of "resistance spot welding" has been implicated as one of the failure mechanisms for the Medtronic Sprint Fidelis lead. However, this assertion is not substantiated by the manufacturer's returned product analysis (RPA). It has been argued that smaller lead diameter is more likely to cause early lead failure than larger leads.[8] The initial design of the conductor-to-terminal ring interface of the EN-DOTAK DSP Model 0125 lead (Guidant/CPI) had a flexion point that resulted in damage to the conductor and insulation. This lead was placed on advisory in 1999 due to a problem with the long IS-1 terminal pin connector. In a series of patients, this design characteristic resulted in a 3.5% incidence of lead fracture over a 31-month follow-up period. The high fracture rate necessitated a design modification that allowed the connection point to be contained inside the header, thus protecting a vulnerable flexion point.[9]

A unique failure mode was identified in a coaxial lead, the Medtronic Transvene (model 6936). According to the manufacturer, approximately 23,700 were implanted and some of them are still in active clinical use. Dorwarth and colleagues[10] reported a 62% lead survival at 8 years with no relationship between lead survival and patient factors or implant technique. A registry study conducted by the US Food and Drug Administration to evaluate the causes of long-term failure of the 6936 lead reported that 76% of lead failures were heralded by oversensing, and two-thirds of these resulted in inappropriate shocks. It was also noted that, in most cases of oversensing, leads had insulation defects or fractures of a pace-sense conductor. High-voltage coil fracture was not as common in the registry data as it was in the manufacturer's RPA. The same study reported that the middle layer of Polyurethane 80A was more likely to fail than the outer layer.[11] Metal ion oxidation (MIO) is the purported mechanism of failure of the middle layer. A distinctive clinical presentation of this lead was oversensing

after an ICD shock that resulted in additional inappropriate shocks.

The magnitude of clinical problem caused by the Medtronic Transvene lead is small compared with the problem of lead failure of the Medtronic Sprint Fidelis lead. The vast majority of these leads were model 6949, which is a dual coil, active-fixation lead. The manufacturer's RPA reveals that conductor fracture is the predominant (90%) cause of failure with fractures of the proximal RV coil or DF-1 connector segment. The two sites of conductor fractures have been localized to the distal portion of the lead (conductor cable) near the anode and at the proximal portion of the lead (conductor coil) near the anchoring sleeve. The "stiffness transition and seal zone" is the area where the relatively flexible lead body transitions to the rigid sleeve head. This might be a weak-link in the lead design and may have contributed to the fracture mechanism.[12] Of the proximal coil fractures, 60% have occurred adjacent to the anchoring sleeve and 30% have occurred within the sleeve and the yoke (**Fig. 2**).

INCIDENCE OF LEAD FRACTURE AND SCOPE OF THE PROBLEM

With increasing number of ICDs being implanted in patients with longer life expectancy, even more leads will be at risk of failure in the future. Kleemann and colleagues[13] analyzed the long-term reliability of implantable cardioverter-defibrillator leads and assessed the annual rate of transvenous defibrillation lead defects. They found that, in 990 patients who underwent first implantation of an ICD between 1992 and May 2005 with a median follow-up time of 934 days, 148 (15%) defibrillation leads failed. They estimated lead survival rates at 5 and 8 years after implantation to be 85% and 60%, respectively, and the annual failure rate for transvenous ICD leads increased progressively with time after implantation and reached 20% in 10-year-old leads. The major causes of lead failure were insulation defects (56%), lead fractures (12%), loss

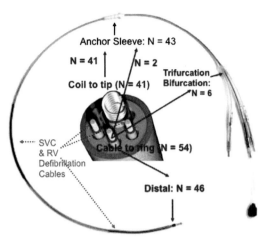

Fig. 2. Implantable cardioverter-defibrillator lead. (*Reproduced from* Swerdlow CD, Gunderson BD, Ousdigian KT, et al. Downloadable algorithm to reduce inappropriate shocks caused by fractures of implantable cardioverter-defibrillator leads. Circulation 2008;118(21):2122–9; with permission.)

of ventricular capture (11%), abnormal lead impedance (10%), and sensing failure (10%). Although ICD lead failure is not a new problem, it has become a subject of intense focus after Medtronic voluntarily discontinued the sale of Sprint Fidelis leads in October 2007 because of an increased rate of lead fractures. As of January 2009, approximately 229,000 Sprint Fidelis leads remain implanted worldwide.[14] The Medtronic Sprint Fidelis leads (models 6930, 6931, 6948, 6949) are 6.6-F bipolar high-voltage ICD leads, first introduced in September 2004. A retrospective analysis of a large patient dataset demonstrated that the hazard of fracture increased exponentially over time, by a power of 2.13 and the 3-year Fidelis survival rate was 90.8%, lower than that for most other ICD leads. These investigators have estimated the annual risk of failure is 3.6% and postulated that it may continue to increase over time.[15]

DIAGNOSIS OF LEAD FRACTURE AND DIFFERENTIAL DIAGNOSIS OF NOISE IN ICDs

To reduce untoward clinical consequences such as inappropriate shocks or failure to deliver bradycardia pacing, early detection of lead defects is of paramount importance. One of the characteristic features of lead fracture is detection of "noise" on the electrograms, secondary to oversensing. However, not all electrograms with noise signify lead fracture. In order to aid the clinician in diagnosing the cause of noise, the authors present a differential diagnosis and clues to identify various causes of noise (**Box 1**).

> **Box 1**
> **Differential diagnosis of noise on electrograms in a cardiovascular implantable electronic device**
>
> *Electromagnetic interference (EMI)* **Fig. 3**
> - Noise on all channels
> - History of encounter with a source of EMI
>
> *Lead or connector problem (header-adapter or setscrew)*
> - It occurs during a small fraction of the cardiac cycle (<10%)
> - It often saturates the amplifier
> - Pacing lead impedance is abnormal and intermittent
> - Chest radiograph may reveal a loose setscrew or inadequate pin position
>
> *Lead fracture or insulation breach*
> - Abnormally high or low impedance
> - May have evidence of fracture on chest radiograph
> - Pocket manipulation may produce noise
> - Intermittent with variable amplitude often saturating the amplifier
>
> *Skeletal muscle oversensing* **Figs. 4–6**
> - Provocative isometric upper extremity exercise and straining reproduces noise
> - Removal of can from sensing circuit results in absence of noise
>
> *Diaphragmatic oversensing*
> - Noise typically seen on the ventricular electrogram and rarely on the shock electrograms
> - More common with integrated bipolar lead
> - Deep breathing, Valsalva and coughing reproduces noise
> - Typically less than 50% of cycle length

NONINVASIVE MANAGEMENT OF LEAD FRACTURE

The objectives of noninvasive management include confirmation of the diagnosis of lead fracture and avoidance of inappropriate therapy. Careful analysis of stored electrograms, arrhythmia logs, and lead parameters often enable clinicians to confirm or refute the diagnosis of lead fracture. Unfortunately, in some instances, inappropriate ICD therapies are the first clue to a lead fracture. Prompt diagnosis of lead failure, prevention of inappropriate shocks, and alerting the patient

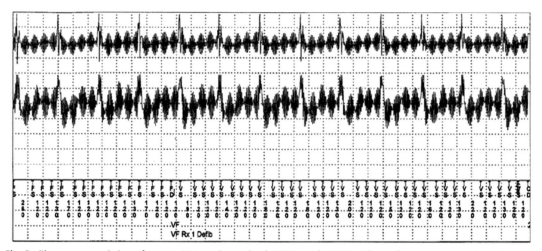

Fig. 3. Electromagnetic interference. Note noise on both EGM1 and EGM2 with resultant erroneous detection and high-voltage therapy of ventricular fibrillation (VF).

and physician to a lead fracture can be achieved by certain downloadable algorithms. In the following paragraphs, the authors detail the workings of the Lead Integrity Algorithm, available as downloadable software for Medtronic devices.

The authors, in collaboration with Medtronic's scientists and engineers, developed unique automated algorithms to detect and identify ICD lead failures before clinical presentation. One of these early algorithms was developed and tested on patients in an ICD database followed for 435 patient-years.[16] The collaborators used three parameters to predict inner insulation failure in coaxial defibrillation leads: the sensing integrity counter (SIC), nonsustained tachycardia (NST) log, and lead impedance trends. Each of these components, if used alone, resulted in a high false-positive rate. Use of a special algorithm that combined abnormal lead diagnostics dramatically

reduced false positive detections. This algorithm had a sensitivity of 82.8% and a specificity of 100% for identification of lead insulation failure. In other words, there were no false-positive detections. It detected lead failures a median 2 days (1 second to 181 days) before clinical presentation. This algorithm has since been refined but the three original parameters to detect lead failure have performed well.[17]

In August 2008, the Lead Integrity Alert (LIA) download was released for download into almost all models of Medtronic ICDs. The LIA was not developed in response to Fidelis, but devised as a means of monitoring lead function. In 2008, Swerdlow and colleagues[12] published performance data on the modified LIA using a simulated retrospective analysis.

The modified LIA was developed and tested on data sets from patients using diagnostics and

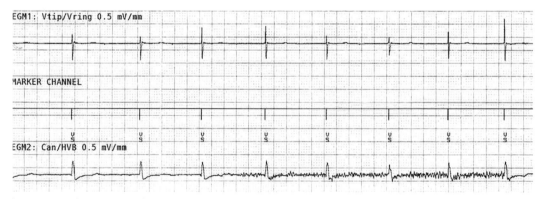

Fig. 4. Pectoral myopotential oversensing: these EGMs were obtained while the patient was performing isometric arm exercises. Note the presence of physiologic oversensing in EGM2, which is derived from a sensing circuit that involves the can. No noise is seen in the rate-sensing Vtip/Vring EGM.

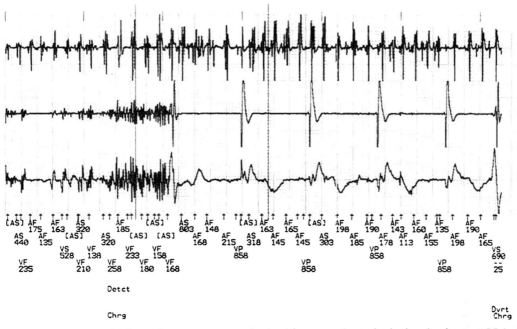

Fig. 5. Pin-port mismatch: these electrograms were obtained from a patient who had an inadvertent DF-1 pin-reversal of the right ventricular and SVC coils in an integrated bipolar lead. Physiologic oversensing occurs secondary to a much larger sensing vector. With the advent of IS-4/DF-4 draft standard for ICD leads, this problem will be minimized.

electrograms from save-to-disk files from leads with fractures verified by analysis of returned, explanted leads as well as electrograms from the CareLink network. It represents a milestone in the development of device enhancements because it was the first ICD monitoring feature that triggered real-time changes in device programming to reduce inappropriate shocks.

How Does the LIA Work?

The LIA was designed to work with existing diagnostics, including pacing impedance and two indicators of nonphysiologic, rapid oversensing. The LIA is triggered by either abnormally high impedance (eg, a dynamic measure based on baseline impedance) or sufficient evidence of nonphysiologic, rapid oversensing. Once the LIA is triggered, it sets the programmed number of intervals to detect (NID) ventricular fibrillation (VF) at 30 of 40 intervals, sounds an audible alert immediately and every 4 hours thereafter, and transmits a wireless, Internet-based alert if enabled (**Fig. 7**). The impedance trigger, designed for chronic leads, uses a threshold based on the average of the most recent weekly maximum and minimum measurements. This threshold is 1000 Ω if the average is less than 700 Ω, 1500 Ω if the average is 700 to 1100 Ω, and 2000 Ω if the average is equal

to or greater than 1100 Ω. The rapid oversensing trigger of the LIA detects nonphysiologic short R-R intervals caused by pace-sense conductor failures via a combination of two criteria based on existing diagnostics: the SIC and NST log. The SIC stores the cumulative number of nonphysiologic short R-R equal to or less than 130 milliseconds. The SIC criterion is satisfied by a count of 30 within 3 days. The NST log stores up to five consecutive sensed events with a cycle-length less than or equal to the ventricular tachycardia detection interval. Most true nonsustained ventricular tachycardias have cycle lengths equal to or greater than 220 milliseconds. The nonsustained tachycardia criterion of the LIA is satisfied by two episodes with an average cycle length of less than or equal to 220 milliseconds in 60 days. The oversensing trigger of the LIA is activated if both the sensing integrity counter and nonsustained tachycardia criteria are fulfilled. This lead-integrity algorithm was tested on data from 15,970 patients with Fidelis leads (including 121 with clinically diagnosed fractures) and 95 other fractured leads confirmed by RPA. The effect of the NID on inappropriate shocks was tested in 92 patients with 927 shocks caused by lead fracture. Increasing the NID reduced inappropriate shocks. The lead-integrity algorithm provided at least a 3-day warning of inappropriate shocks in 76% (95% CI, 66–84) of

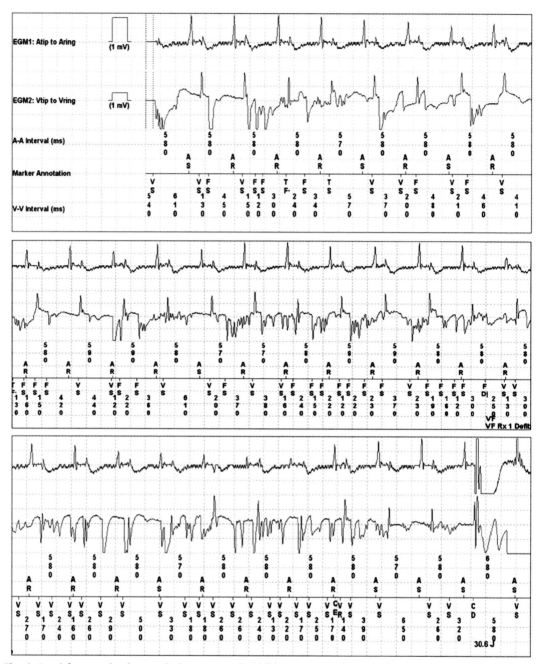

Fig. 6. Lead fracture (*top*), stored electrograms (*middle*), pace-sense (V$_{Tip}$-V$_{Ring}$) electrograms (*bottom*). Atrial (A$_{Tip}$-A$_{Ring}$), and marker channels are shown. VS, TS, and FS are the intervals in sinus, ventricular tachycardia, and VF zones, respectively. FD indicates the detection of VF. Panels are temporally continuous. Pace-sense channel shows intermittent, high-frequency nonphysiologic noise and oversensing. This is characteristic of lead fracture or header-connector problem. Note the very short V-V intervals of 120 milliseconds suggestive of nonphysiologic signals. At the programmed NID 30 of 40, inappropriate detection of VF occurs in the middle panel resulting in an inappropriate shock in the bottom panel.

patients versus 55% (95% CI, 43–64) for optimal impedance monitoring. Its positive predictive value was 72% for lead fractures and 81% for lead fractures or header-connector problems requiring surgical intervention. The false-positive rate was 1 per 372 patient-years of monitoring. This retrospective analysis predicted that a timely response to an alert would be critical because the interval between the LIA alert and the inappropriate shock may be short.[12]

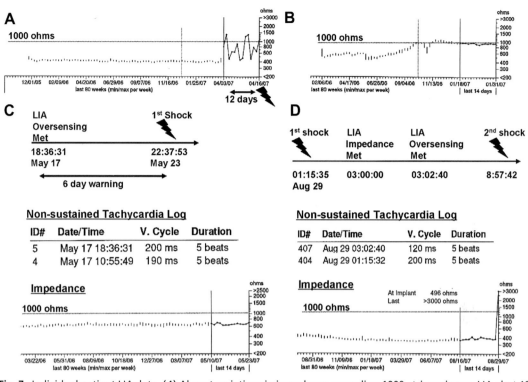

Fig. 7. Individual patient LIA data. (*A*) Abrupt variations in impedance exceeding 1000, triggering an LIA alert 12 days before an inappropriate shock. (*B*) A false-positive LIA impedance trigger gradual with an increase in impedance. (*C*) A true-positive oversensing alert triggered 6 days before an inappropriate shock despite constant impedance. (*D*) The LIA was not triggered before the first inappropriate shock. However, because both impedance and oversensing triggers occurred 1 hour 45 minutes after that shock, the automatic NID increase would have prevented the subsequent shocks 5 hours later. (*Reproduced from* Swerdlow CD, Gunderson BD, Ousdigian KT, et al. Downloadable algorithm to reduce inappropriate shocks caused by fractures of implantable cardioverter-defibrillator leads. Circulation 2008;118(21):2122–9; with permission.)

Effect of Fracture Type on Performance of LIA

In the aforementioned study, of the 95 patients in the RPA group, 41 (43%) had fractures of the coil conductor to the tip electrode and 54 (57%) had fractures of the cable conductor to the ring electrode. **Fig. 2** shows that all coil fractures occurred at the anchor sleeve, whereas 52 of the cable fractures (96%) occurred distally or at the bifurcation or trifurcation. The LIA provided greater warning for cable fractures than coil fractures. However, the incremental benefit of the LIA compared with postadvisory programming was comparable for the two fracture types. For example, 3-day warning increased 22% (from 66% to 88%) for cable fractures and 20% (from 41% to 61%) for coil fractures.

Before the advent of the downloadable RAM-ware for the LIA, the audible alert in Medtronic pulse generators was triggered if abnormal impedance was detected and sounded only once per day (nominally at 8 AM). However, Kallinen and colleagues[18] reported the suboptimal performance of using only the impedance to diagnose lead failure. This result was not surprising given that the least sensitive marker of pace-sense conductor fracture, lead impedance, will miss most Sprint Fidelis lead failures. The authors reported the individual sensitivities of lead impedance, SIC, and NST to detect pace-sense conductor fractures and they were 41%, 79%, and 90%, respectively, in prior bench-testing analyses.

The LIA triggers an audible alert when abnormal impedance *or* noise (based on SIC and NST) is detected on the lead. Unlike the pre-LIA method, the LIA sounds the audible alert immediately and every 4 hours thereafter. In addition, the NID required to detect a tachyarrhythmia is automatically increased to 30 of 40 to reduce the likelihood that lead noise will cause inappropriate shocks. However, the NID for redetection remains at the programmed value. A new LIA version triggers the alert and the NID increase to 30 of 40 when any two of the three criteria (impedance, SIC, NST) are satisfied.[19] Using SIC alone as a marker of noise secondary to lead or connector problems that require surgical intervention will result in a significant number of false-positives. The authors evaluated the cause of frequent SICs in a recent study. To diagnose the cause of oversensing in those patients with frequent SICs, a modified 24-hour digital Holter monitor that recorded ECG, ventricular electrogram, and the ICD Marker Channel (Medtronic) was worn by patients. Recordings were reviewed to determine the causes of oversensing. Patients with confirmed oversensing and adequate data were analyzed. The number of SICs per day and the presence of a NST episode with ventricular mean cycle length equal to or less than 220 milliseconds were retrieved from stored ICD data. Forty-eight patients had a median of 13 SICs per day. Presumed lead-connection issues occurred in only 23% of patients, whereas physiologic oversensing occurred in 77% of patients. A rapid NST was recorded more commonly in patients with lead-connection issues than in those without (9 of 11 vs 1 of 37).[20] Oversensing resulting in frequent, very short intervals typically are caused by either lead-connection issues or physiologic signals. (Fig. 8) Increased SIC counter and the additional finding of rapid NSTs usually indicate a lead-connection issue, even in the absence of impedance abnormalities. This study once again underscores the importance of recognizing that not all oversensing is a lead or lead-connector issue and a meticulous thought process and understanding of sensing function of ICDs is mandatory to avoid unnecessary surgical intervention. The SIC is an oversensing diagnostic intended to facilitate early diagnosis of lead fracture. This study demonstrated that lead or header-connection issues usually present with repetitive, rapid oversensing identified by rapid NSTs, in addition to isolated, rapid oversensing events that increment the SIC. In the absence of rapid NSTs, almost all cases of apparently nonphysiologic short intervals in leads with normal impedance are caused by oversensing combinations of physiologic signals that do not represent true RR intervals.

Clinical Performance of LIA

The new LIA, which incorporates at least two of three (impedance, NST, SIC) parameters, would thus be a more sensitive and specific tool to reduce inappropriate shocks. A prospective single-center study assessed the effectiveness of the LIA algorithm for warning patients of an impending Sprint Fidelis pace-sense conductor fracture and for decreasing the incidence and number of inappropriate shocks.[21] The investigators included all those patients who had Sprint Fidelis leads and Medtronic ICD pulse generators that were implanted and followed at their institution. Patients were evaluated in the clinic every 3 to 4 months or by remote monitoring using the Medtronic CareLink system. When the LIA algorithm was released in August 2008, the RAMware was downloaded to the pulse generator of all patients with Sprint Fidelis leads. Patients and family members were given a demonstration of the audible alerts. The investigators noted that between October 2004 and January 2010 52 (11.3%) of Sprint Fidelis leads failed in the study population. Inappropriate shocks were the first sign of lead failure in 18 (69%) of the 26 patients who did not have the LIA compared with 4 (17%) of 23 patients who had the LIA. Patients who experienced inappropriate shocks without the LIA received an average of 13.2 plus or minus 13.6 inappropriate shocks (range 2–54) versus 3.0 plus or minus 2.0 inappropriate shocks (range 2–6) in patients who had the LIA. The audible alert was effective in only 70% (16 of 23) and 35% (6 of 17) of patients with and without the LIA, respectively, whose alerts were programmed "on". Overall, 8 (32%) of 25 patients whose audible alerts were triggered did not immediately hear or recognize the tone. These findings were in concordance with a recent prospective study that evaluated the efficacy of LIA in ICD leads that RPA testing confirmed fracture.[22] Thus, one can conclude that the LIA appears to be an effective method for detecting most Sprint Fidelis lead fractures and for decreasing the incidence and number of inappropriate shocks.

Compliance with the recommendations from the manufacturer's advisory resulted in fewer inappropriate shocks as reported in a recent single-center experience from Europe. To comply with the advisories, two clinical evaluations were conducted. The effect of the advisories was assessed by the lead failure rate and the occurrence of inappropriate shocks due to lead failure. Three periods were distinguished in the comparison of event rates: lead implantation to advisory 1 (period A), in-between both advisories (period B), and advisory 2 to follow-up (period C). Since 2004, 372 patients received a Medtronic ICD and Sprint Fidelis lead and were followed from first implant (December 2004) to April 2009. The cumulative incidence of lead failure was 3.6% at 21 months and increased to 11.0% at 42 months. After implementation of both advisories, the occurrence of inappropriate shocks due to lead

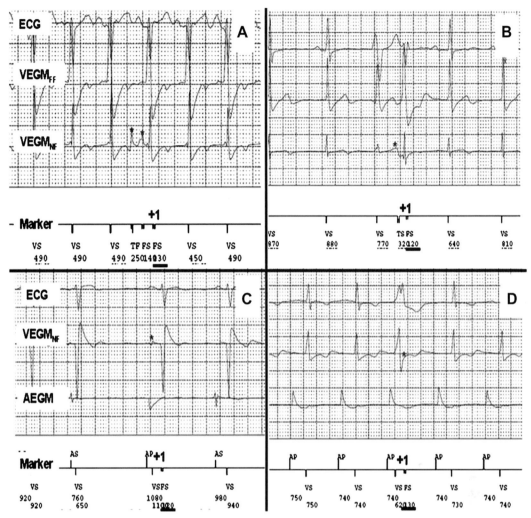

Fig. 8. Telemetry Holter recordings from patients with different types of oversensing. The ECG, atrial electrogram (AEGM), far-field electrogram (VEGMFF), near-field electrogram (VEGMNF), and Marker Channel (Marker) are labeled accordingly. The 120 or 130 milliseconds (*black underline*) would have incremented the SIC by 1 (see + 1). (*A*) Patient with a lead or connection issue. ECG and VEGMFF show normal sinus rhythm. VEGMNF shows the nonphysiologic deflections (*asterisks*) that were oversensed as indicated by the Marker Channel, resulting in short intervals. (*B*) Patient with T wave oversensing followed by correctly sensed premature ventricular complex (PVC). The T wave (*asterisk*) that was oversensed as indicated by the Marker Channel, resulting in a short interval between the T wave and the PVC. (*C*) Patient with P wave oversensing followed by a correctly sensed R wave. Shown is the P wave (*asterisk*) that was oversensed during an atrial pace (AP) as indicated by the Marker Channel, resulting in a short interval between the P wave and the R wave. The cross-chamber blanking after an atrial pace is 30 milliseconds. The atrial pacing pulse is oversensed because the auto-adjusting sensitivity had over 1 second to decay to the programmed sensitivity. (*D*) Patient with double-counting of the PVC. Shown is the PVC (*asterisk*) that was correctly sensed at the leading edge and oversensed at the trailing edge as indicated by the Marker Channel, resulting in a short interval between ventricular sense (VS) and fibrillation sense (FS). An R wave associated with an intraventricular conduction delay or PVC may be sensed at either the leading edge or the trailing edge of the depolarization. (*Reproduced from* Gunderson BD, Swerdlow CD, Wilcox JM, et al. Causes of ventricular oversensing in implantable cardioverter-defibrillators: implications for diagnosis of lead fracture. Heart Rhythm 2010;7(5):626–33; with permission.)

failure decreased from 1.5 per 100 lead-years in period A to 0.8 per 100 lead-years in period C. Thus, the investigators concluded that, despite an increasing risk for Sprint Fidelis lead failure, implementation of the advisories decreased the occurrence of inappropriate shocks due to lead failure.[23]

INVASIVE MANAGEMENT OF LEAD FRACTURE

Once a lead fracture is confirmed, physicians should disable detection of VF to prevent patients from receiving inappropriate shocks. Revision of the ICD system should be undertaken after careful consideration of the risks and benefits of lead extraction. Lead extraction can be done either transvenously or surgically via a median sternotomy. A succinct synopsis of patient selection and safety aspects of transvenous lead extraction specific to the issue of lead fracture follows.

Patient Selection

Every invasive procedure requires a careful balancing of the risks and benefits of the procedure for *that* individual patient. Before extraction, the initial indication for implantation of a cardiac implantable electronic device (CIED) should be reassessed. Patient and device data should be thoroughly analyzed. Pertinent questions include:

- Is the indication for an ICD primary or secondary prevention? If it is a primary prevention device, has the patient ever had appropriate ICD therapy or pacing?
- Is the patient stable enough to go through a high-risk procedure such as lead extraction?
- Is there significant mortality or quality of life benefit with lead extraction and/or subsequent reimplantation?

Decisions should be tailored to the clinical scenario. For example, an infected ICD system in a 20-year-old patient with hypertrophic cardiomyopathy who has had episodes of VF carries a different clinical benefit for lead extraction compared with a failed ICD lead in an 80-year-old patient who has a primary prevention ICD and never received a shock.

There is a significant learning curve associated with performing transvenous pacer-ICD lead extraction. Detailed guidelines regarding who should be performing these procedures, indications for extraction and reimplantation have been developed and are available at the Heart Rhythm Society Web site.[24]

Safety of Transvenous Sprint Fidelis Lead Extraction

Maytin and colleagues[25] recently published a multicenter retrospective analysis of Sprint Fidelis lead extraction data. All the operators in this study were highly experienced (>100 lead extractions per year). A total of 349 leads were extracted in 348 patients—cardio-thoracic surgical assistance was sought twice. There were no deaths related to lead extraction. The fact that this procedure is extremely safe when done by experienced operators does not mean it is extremely safe in every situation and by every electrophysiologist. It behooves all electrophysiologists, when faced with a clinical scenario that entails lead extraction, to analyze if lead extraction is "mandatory, necessary, or discretionary" (the so-called Byrd classification) and to discuss this with their patients before referring for or performing lead extraction.[26]

The results of the LExICon study[27] compared with previous multicenter extraction reports[28,29] suggest that the risks of extraction may be decreasing over time. This is mostly attributable to the advent of new technology—notably the Excimer sheath. It has to be noted that the operators and the centers involved in this study were highly experienced and these results cannot be extrapolated to every electrophysiology laboratory in the country.

Extraction of Abandoned Leads and Reimplantation Versus Insertion of a Pace-Sense Lead

This is a controversial issue in the contemporary electrophysiology community. Spirited, passionate, and well-articulated arguments exist for both strategies.[30,31] Flexibility of thought and belief, predicated on patient preference and safety are of paramount importance. Decisions made with fiduciary diligence are usually acceptable to all parties involved, for there is no incontrovertible answer to every clinical scenario.

SUMMARY

Transvenous ICD leads have made implantation of ICDs a remarkably safe procedure marking a significant engineering achievement that has clinically translated into saving many lives. However, they are also the weakest link in an ICD system and lead fracture is one of the principal reasons for ICD system failure. Inappropriate shocks or asystole in a pacemaker dependent patient, secondary to oversensing are severe consequences of lead fracture. Lead impedance measurements, NST episodes, and SIC aid in its diagnosis. Reprogramming the device once a lead fracture is suspected reduces inappropriate shocks secondary to lead fracture. Although the LIA, which incorporates these elements, prevents inappropriate shocks in most patients with a lead fracture, it does not do so in all cases and is currently only available for Medtronic devices. In the future, improvements in lead design and development of downloadable algorithms by all CIED manufacturers will further improve our ability to tackle this very important clinical problem.

REFERENCES

1. Moss AJ, Zareba W, Hall WJ, et al. Prophylactic implantation of a defibrillator in patients with myocardial infarction and reduced ejection fraction. N Engl J Med 2002;346:877–83.

2. Bardy GH, Lee KL, Mark DB, et al. Amiodarone or an implantable cardioverter-defibrillator for congestive heart failure. N Engl J Med 2005;352:225–37.

3. Bristow MR, Saxon LA, Boehmer J, et al. Cardiac-resynchronization therapy with or without an implantable defibrillator in advanced chronic heart failure. N Engl J Med 2004;350:2140–50.

4. A comparison of antiarrhythmic-drug therapy with implantable defibrillators in patients resuscitated from near-fatal ventricular arrhythmias. The Antiarrhythmics versus Implantable Defibrillators (AVID) Investigators. N Engl J Med 1997;337:1576–83.

5. Rauwolf T, Guenther M, Hass N, et al. Ventricular oversensing in 518 patients with implanted cardiac defibrillators: incidence, complications, and solutions. Europace 2007;9:1041–7.

6. Koneru JN, Dumitru I, Easley AR. Electromagnetic interference from electronic article surveillance system in a patient with a bi-ventricular ICD and a left ventricular assist device. Pacing Clin Electrophysiol 2011;34(2):244–6.

7. Cevik C, Perez-Verdia A, Nugent K. Implantable cardioverter defibrillators and their role in heart failure progression. Europace 2009;11(6):710–5.

8. Borleffs CJ, van Erven L, van Bommel RJ, et al. Risk of failure of transvenous implantable cardioverter-defibrillator leads. Circ Arrhythm Electrophysiol 2009;2(4):411–6.

9. Mera F, DeLurgio DB, Langberg JJ, et al. Transvenous cardioverter defibrillator lead malfunction due to terminal connector damage in pectoral implants. Pacing Clin Electrophysiol 1999;22(12):1797–801.

10. Dorwarth U, Frey B, Dugas M, et al. Transvenous defibrillation leads: high incidence of failure during long-term follow-up. J Cardiovasc Electrophysiol 2003;14(1):38–43.

11. Hauser RG, Cannom D, Hayes DL, et al. Long-term structural failure of coaxial polyurethane implantable cardioverter defibrillator leads. Pacing Clin Electrophysiol 2002;25(6):879–82.

12. Swerdlow CD, Gunderson BD, Ousdigian KT, et al. Downloadable algorithm to reduce inappropriate shocks caused by fractures of implantable cardioverter-defibrillator leads. Circulation 2008;118(21):2122–9.

13. Kleemann T, Becker T, Doenges K, et al. Annual rate of transvenous defibrillation lead defects in implantable cardioverter-defibrillators over a period of >10 years. Circulation 2007;115(19):2474–80.

14. Swerdlow CD, Ellenbogen KA. The changing presentation of implantable cardioverter-defibrillator lead fractures. Heart Rhythm 2009;6(4):478–9.

15. Faulknier BA, Traub DM, Aktas MK, et al. Time-dependent risk of Fidelis lead failure. Am J Cardiol 2010;105(1):95–9.

16. Gunderson BD, Patel AS, Bounds CA, et al. An algorithm to predict implantable cardioverter defibrillator lead failure. J Am Coll Cardiol 2004;44:1898–902.

17. Gunderson BD, Gillberg JM, Wood MA, et al. Development and testing of an algorithm to detect implantable cardioverter-defibrillator lead failure. Heart Rhythm 2006;3:155–62.

18. Kallinen LM, Hauser RG, Lee KW, et al. Failure of impedance monitoring to prevent adverse clinical events caused by fracture of a recalled high-voltage implantable cardioverter-defibrillator lead. Heart Rhythm 2008;5(6):775–9.

19. Patel AS, Gunderson BD, Ousdigian KT, et al. Modification to lead integrity alert improves performance [abstract]. Heart Rhythm 2009;6:S33.

20. Gunderson BD, Swerdlow CD, Wilcox JM, et al. Causes of ventricular oversensing in implantable cardioverter-defibrillators: implications for diagnosis of lead fracture. Heart Rhythm 2010;7(5):626–33.

21. Kallinen LM, Hauser RG, Tang C, et al. Lead integrity alert algorithm decreases inappropriate shocks in patients who have Sprint Fidelis pace-sense conductor fractures. Heart Rhythm 2010;7(8):1048–55.

22. Swerdlow CD, Gunderson BD, Ousdigian KT, et al. Downloadable software algorithm reduces inappropriate shocks caused by implantable cardioverter-defibrillator lead fractures: a prospective study. Circulation 2010;122(15):1449–55.

23. VAN Rees JB, Borleffs CJ, Bax JJ, et al. Implementation of lead safety recommendations. Pacing Clin Electrophysiol 2010;33(4):431–6.

24. Wilkoff BL, Love CJ, Byrd CL, et al, Heart Rhythm Society; American Heart Association. Transvenous lead extraction: Heart Rhythm Society expert consensus on facilities, training, indications, and patient management. Heart Rhythm 2009;6(7):1085–104.

25. Maytin M, Love CJ, Fischer A, et al. Multicenter experience with extraction of the Sprint Fidelis

implantable cardioverter-defibrillator lead. J Am Coll Cardiol 2010;56(8):646–50.

26. Love CJ. Current concepts in extraction of transvenous pacing and ICD leads. Cardiol Clin 2000; 18(1):193–217.

27. Wazni O, Epstein LM, Carrillo RG, et al. Lead extraction in the contemporary setting: the LExICon study: an observational retrospective study of consecutive laser lead extractions. J Am Coll Cardiol 2010;55: 579–86.

28. Kay GN, Brinker JA, Kawanishi DT, et al. Risks of spontaneous injury and extraction of an active fixation pacemaker lead: report of the Accufix Multicenter Clinical Study and Worldwide Registry. Circulation 1999;100:2344–52.

29. Byrd CL, Wilkoff BL, Love CJ, et al. Clinical study of the laser sheath for lead extraction: the total experience in the United States. Pacing Clin Electrophysiol 2002;25:804–8.

30. Henrikson CA, Maytin M, Epstein LM. Think before you pull—not every lead has to come out. Circ Arrhythm Electrophysiol 2010;3(4):409–12.

31. Maytin M, Epstein LM, Henrikson CA. Lead extraction is preferred for lead revisions and system upgrades: when less is more. Circ Arrhythm Electrophysiol 2010;3:413–24.

Cost-effectiveness of Implantable Cardioverter-Defibrillators and Cardiac Resynchronization Therapy

James V. Freeman, MD, MPH, MS[a], Aditya Ullal, BA[b,c],
Mintu P. Turakhia, MD, MAS[a,b,*]

KEYWORDS
- Sudden cardiac death
- Implantable cardioverter-defibrillator • ICD
- Cardiac resynchronization therapy • CRT
- Cost-effectiveness

Since the introduction of implantable cardioverter-defibrillators (ICDs) almost 30 years ago, there has been ongoing debate about the value of ICDs to public health. Randomized trials in the last 15 years have consistently shown the benefit of ICDs for primary prevention of sudden cardiac death (SCD) in patients with heart failure and reduced ejection fraction.[1–7] Similarly, such studies have also revealed benefits of ICDs for secondary prevention in patients with a history of prior ventricular arrhythmias or aborted SCD.[8–10] More recently, clinical trials have shown that cardiac resynchronization therapy with defibrillator function (CRT-D) and cardiac resynchronization therapy without defibrillator function (CRT-P) improves quality of life, heart failure hospitalizations, and/or survival in patients with heart failure (New York Heart Association [NYHA] functional class III and IV, left ventricular

Funding Support: Dr Freeman is supported by an American Heart Association Pharmaceutical Round Table Outcomes Research Development Postdoctoral Fellowship (0875162N). Dr Turakhia is supported by a Veterans Health Services Research & Development Career Development Award (CDA09027-1) and an American Heart Association National Scientist Development Grant (09SDG2250647).
Disclosures: Dr Turakhia serves as a coinvestigator on a research grant from Medtronic, Inc (major), and has received speaking fees (minor) from Medtronic, Inc Dr Turakhia has served as a consultant (minor) to St Jude Medical. The content and opinions expressed are solely the responsibility of the authors and do not necessarily represent the views or policies of the Department of Veterans Affairs.
a Division of Cardiovascular Medicine, Department of Medicine, Stanford University School of Medicine, 300 Pasteur Drive, Falk Building, CVRC 5406, Stanford, CA 94305-5406, USA
b VA Palo Alto Veterans Affairs Health Care System, 3801 Miranda Avenue - 111C, Palo Alto, CA 94304, USA
c University of California at Berkeley, Berkeley, CA 94720, USA
* Corresponding author. VA Palo Alto Veterans Affairs Health Care System, 3801 Miranda Avenue - 111C, Palo Alto, CA 94304.
E-mail address: mintu@stanford.edu

Card Electrophysiol Clin 3 (2011) 421–440
doi:10.1016/j.ccep.2011.05.008

ejection fraction <0.35), and prolonged QRS complex (>120 milliseconds) on optimal medical therapy.[7,11–14] Accordingly, American and international society clinical guidelines have supported the use of ICDs and CRT-P and CRT-D for these patient populations.[15,16]

In response to trial data and guidelines, ICD implantations increased 24% between 1998 and 2002 and continue to increase.[17] After publication of the Sudden Cardiac Death in Heart Failure Trial (SCD-HeFT), the number of eligible Medicare beneficiaries as much as threefold, to almost 500,000.[18] Because of the rising epidemic of coronary heart disease, most notably in India and China, the eligible population worldwide is expected to increase dramatically in coming years. Although the development of new therapeutic modalities such as ICDs drives medical progress, these new therapies also result in significant increases in health care costs.

In the past, the approval and adoption of new medical technologies has required only the demonstration of clinical safety and efficacy. More recently, several health care systems, including those in Australia and the United Kingdom, have begun to use cost-effectiveness analysis as part of their medical technology assessment and coverage determination. However, demonstration of cost-effectiveness is currently not a criterion for local or national coverage determination by Medicare, the largest US health care system payer.[19,20] Nonetheless, it is clear that formal evaluation of cost-effectiveness is an increasingly important field of health care research and evaluation.

COST-EFFECTIVENESS ANALYSIS

Cost-effectiveness analysis is used to determine the clinical benefit of interventions relative to their costs. The value of a new technology like an ICD can be gauged by comparing it with an existing therapy, usually the current standard of care, and calculating the incremental cost-effectiveness ratio (ICER). The ICER is the total net cost of the new therapy compared with the alternative therapy, divided by the total net effectiveness of the new therapy compared with the alternative (**Fig. 1**).[21] Simply stated, the ICER of a therapy is the cost difference per unit of effectiveness gained.

Costs

By definition, the cost valuation of a therapy includes all costs of providing that therapy as well as any downstream costs related to that therapy. The costs associated with a new technology are borne by different parties but analyses are generally conducted from the perspective of society as a whole, taking into account all medical costs irrespective of who bears them (hospital, patient, or a third-party payer). The societal perspective requires that the analysis measures all costs related to any changes in health effects or resource use caused by an intervention. In the case of ICD and CRT devices, this cost includes the cost of the device and its initial implantation, as well as the costs of all related follow-up care, such as device interrogations and generator replacements, and cost of complications. These costs may be offset by cost savings associated with improvement in a patient's health state. Costs not directly associated with medical care, such as lost work productivity, are termed indirect costs and are usually omitted from cost-effectiveness studies. Future costs are usually discounted at a rate of between 2% and 5% per year to calculate the present value of future costs.

Effectiveness

Effectiveness is conventionally measured by the extent to which survival or quality of life is improved. Effectiveness is generally measured as survival in years and quality-adjusted survival measured in quality-adjusted life years (QALYs).[22] QALYs are calculated by multiplying the life expectancy of the patient (in years) by a metric of quality of life. Quality of life is generally measured using scaled units of utility, in which various health states or conditions are assigned a value between 0.00 (death) and 1.00 (ideal health). For example, if a patient spends 2 years in a health condition associated with a utility of 0.6, she has gained $2 \times 0.6 = 1.2$ QALYs. The utility used to calculate QALYs can be obtained using formal elicitation techniques (eg, the standard-gamble) or quality-of-life questionnaires (eg, Minnesota Living with Heart Failure questionnaire).[19,23] As with costs, future clinical effects are often discounted between 1% and 5% per year relative to current health effects to estimate the present value of future effects.

Incremental cost-effectiveness ratio =

$$\frac{(Cost\ for\ therapy\ A) - (Cost\ for\ therapy\ B)}{(Effectiveness\ for\ therapy\ A) - (Effectiveness\ for\ therapy\ B)}$$

Fig. 1. The ICER of a therapy is the cost difference per unit of effectiveness gained.

Additional Cost-effectiveness Concepts

Several additional concepts emerge from the incremental cost-effectiveness equation.[19] First, the choice of comparators is important when assessing a new technology. Cost-effectiveness is a relative measure rather than an absolute measure and can only be determined when compared to a clinically relevant alternative. Second, the ICER is based on assessing the complete costs and benefits of each treatment. A long-term perspective is essential to obtain a complete understanding of costs and benefits, rather than simply initial costs and short-term outcomes. Although it would be ideal to measure costs and effects for the lifetime of the patient, it is most important that the follow-up in the analysis be sufficiently long to capture all of the relevant costs and benefits. Third, the ICER is usually expressed as dollars per life year (LY) or QALY gained, which then should be compared with a benchmark to interpret the result. Several countries, including the United Kingdom and the Netherlands, have defined monetary thresholds for their health care systems beyond which a new technology is not considered cost-effective. Although there is no defined threshold in the United States, most analysts consider less than or equal to $50,000/QALY to be acceptable, which was originally based on the cost of providing renal hemodialysis for 1 year. ICERs over $100,000/QALY are often not considered cost-effective. Cost-effectiveness thresholds vary markedly for different countries depending on the resources available for health care expenditure.[19,24]

Methods to Ascertain Effectiveness and Costs

Estimation of clinical benefit and costs is a critical step in the evaluation of cost-effectiveness, and changes in these estimations can have a dramatic effect on any such analysis. The cost and effectiveness data used to calculate the ICER may be collected alongside the clinical data while conducting a randomized clinical trial (RCT). As with the clinical data obtained from an RCT, the cost data may provide an objective measure of the expenses associated with the intervention that requires no simulation or major assumptions.

The second approach for evaluating the cost-effectiveness of a therapy involves developing a model of the natural history of the disease and the impact of the interventions being studied. Decision models, such as Markov models, can estimate cost and utility by modeling health states related to the interventions being compared.[25,26] A major advantage of this approach is that it can incorporate average costs and outcomes from several published RCTs or meta-analyses of

RCTs. Moreover, sensitivity analyses can be performed by varying the model input variables, either individually or simultaneously as a group, and thereby evaluating the robustness of results across a broad range of cost, utility, and other model assumptions.[19]

Limitations of Trial-based and Model-based Cost-effectiveness Analysis

Trial-based cost-effectiveness analysis has several important limitations. The costs incurred in an RCT are dependent on the characteristics of the patients recruited to the study as well as the clinical centers where the trial is being conducted. The effectiveness of therapies for patients treated in clinical practice may be worse than for patients treated in randomized trials, which generally enroll healthier patients, achieve high levels of patient adherence, and use more careful monitoring and systematic follow-up, particularly among elderly patients. More importantly, RCTs tend to have short durations of follow-up that are generally 1 to 5 years, limiting long-term evaluation of costs and benefits. In addition, this method ideally requires that quality of life be prospectively measured during a clinical trial, which is often not performed. In these cases, external estimates of quality of life must be applied to the trial population.

Decision analytical cost-effectiveness models have their own limitations. These analyses generally rely on 1 or more clinical trials for the input variables included in the model, including therapeutic efficacy and adverse event rates. This reliance may require that trial results from a short-term trial (often 1–5 years) be extrapolated to a much longer time horizon (often several decades). In addition, studies may show significantly different results, requiring meta-analysis to combine findings, which results in further uncertainty in the assessment of cost-effectiveness. The impact of the uncertainty in model input variables on cost-effectiveness can be tested using sensitivity analysis, in which the ICER is recalculated after systematically varying values of input parameters, allowing estimation of the variance in cost-effectiveness. However, poorly understood or poorly measured sources of uncertainty can persist. An additional source of uncertainty in a model is the structure and core assumptions used to create the model, often called structural uncertainty, which can be difficult or impossible to test in sensitivity analysis.[19,27]

COST-EFFECTIVENESS OF ICD THERAPY FOR PRIMARY PREVENTION OF SCD

Several studies have been published evaluating the cost-effectiveness of ICD therapy for primary prevention of SCD in patients with heart failure with decreased left ventricular ejection fraction, including studies affiliated with randomized trials and several decision analytical modeling studies (**Table 1**). Two seminal decision analytical studies, one in the United States and the other in Europe, have used the combined experience of the published randomized trials along with updated cost estimates to evaluate the cost-effectiveness of ICD therapy for primary prevention in these two settings.

Sanders and colleagues[33] published a comprehensive assessment of the cost-effectiveness of ICD therapy for the primary prevention of SCD in 2005. Their analysis used primary data from 8 clinical trials that had randomly assigned patients with left ventricular systolic dysfunction without a history of life-threatening ventricular arrhythmias to receive an ICD or an alternative medical therapy: DINAMIT, MADIT-I, MADIT-II, DEFINITE, COMPANION, MUSTT, SCD-HeFT, and CABG Patch.[1,3,5–7,39–41] They used a Markov decision model to estimate costs and quality-adjusted survival for a hypothetical cohort of patients who received either a prophylactic ICD or control medical therapy. They modeled the relative risk of death with ICD therapy compared with medical therapy based on the clinical efficacy reported for each clinical trial and then used health economic data to generate cost estimates. The health and economic outcomes varied greatly among the trial populations. In each population, prophylactic implantation of an ICD was more expensive than control therapy, with the increase in estimated lifetime discounted costs ranging from $55,700 in the CABG Patch trial to $101,500 in MUSTT (see **Table 1**). In 6 of the 8 populations, implantation of the ICD improved life expectancy relative to medical therapy, with the improvement in quality-adjusted survival ranging from 1.01 to 2.99 QALYs. The ICERs based on these trials ranged from $34,000 to $70,200 per QALY added. In 2 trials (DINAMIT and CABG Patch), the life expectancy of the patients who received an ICD was less than that of the patients who received control therapy, so the ICD was both more expensive and less effective than control therapy. However, the investigators concluded that with most assumptions, the prophylactic implantation of an ICD has a cost-effectiveness ratio less than $100,000 per QALY gained in patients at increased risk for SCD as the result of a reduced left ventricular ejection fraction. In sensitivity analyses, the investigators found that the ICERs improved with increasing effectiveness of ICDs, decreasing ICD cost, increasing interval between generator changes, increasing quality of life with ICDs, and increasing time with

an implanted ICD (ie, younger age at implant and fewer comorbidities).

In 2009, Cowie and colleagues[36] examined the quality-adjusted survival, costs, and cost-effectiveness of prophylactic implantation of an ICD in patients with left ventricular systolic dysfunction, adopting the perspective of the Belgian health care system to represent a typical European population. They based their analysis on the model of the cost-effectiveness of ICD therapy developed by Sanders and colleagues[33] in 2005. Prophylactic implantation of an ICD improved life expectancy relative to conventional therapy alone by 1.88 years (2.22 years undiscounted) on average for each patient. There were approximately 50% fewer SCD in those implanted with an ICD device compared with those on conventional medical therapy, with the benefit of ICD persisting throughout the lifetime of the patients modeled. Similarly, ICD implantation improved quality-adjusted life expectancy relative to conventional therapy, providing an additional 1.57 QALYs (1.86 undiscounted). Prophylactic implantation of an ICD cost an additional €46,413 (~$31,600 in 2009 US dollars) compared with conventional therapy. Most of the ICD cost was from the device and implant procedure costs (~70% per person) and the costs of ICD-related complications were small. For patients with a mean starting age of 61 years, the estimated ICER of ICD therapy compared with conventional medical therapy was €24,751 (~$16,800) per LY gained and €29,530 (~$20,080) per QALY gained. In sensitivity analyses, the investigators found that the ICER improved with increasing effectiveness of ICD therapy, increasing period between generator replacement, increasing quality of life with an ICD, and decreasing age at implant.

COST-EFFECTIVENESS OF ICD THERAPY FOR PRIMARY PREVENTION IN THE ELDERLY AND THOSE WITH MULTIPLE MEDICAL COMORBIDITIES

To examine the benefit of ICD therapy in patients at increased risk for mortality because of advanced age or multiple comorbidities, Chan and colleagues[37] evaluated the use of ICD therapy for primary prevention in patients with reduced left ventricular ejection fraction in a community-based setting of 7 outpatient cardiology clinics enrolled by the Ohio Heart and Vascular Center and the Lindner Clinical Trials Center between March 2001 and June 2005 and followed through March 2007. The study cohort comprised 965 patients (751 [77.8%] ischemic; 214 [22.2%] non-ischemic), of whom 494 (51.2%) received ICDs. Patients in this cohort were significantly older than those in primary prevention clinical trials; the median age was 67.3 years (interquartile range 57.7–74.5 years) in this cohort versus 60.1 years (interquartile range 51.6–68.4 years) in SCD-HeFT[6] (P<.001) and the mean age of ischemic heart failure patients in this cohort was 67.2 (±10) years in this cohort versus 64.4 (±10) years in MADIT-II[3] (P<.001). When adjusted for patient demographics and clinical characteristics, ICDs were associated with a 31% lower risk of death from all causes (adjusted hazard ratio [HR] 0.69; 95% confidence interval [CI] 0.50–0.96; P = .03). Subgroup analyses found that ICD therapy was associated with lower mortality regardless of age and cause or degree of left ventricular dysfunction. Similarly, ICD therapy was associated with lower mortality regardless of most comorbid medical conditions examined (symptomatic heart failure, diabetes mellitus, atrial fibrillation, peripheral vascular disease, prior stroke, and renal failure) and Holter study results. The investigators then used a Markov decision model, incorporating the mortality data from their analysis as well as cost data to generate cost-effectiveness estimates. Although older patients had higher mortalities, the investigators found that ICD therapy was associated with significant gains in quality-adjusted survival and was at least as cost-effective in patients 75 years of age or older as in younger patients, with an ICER of $82,531 per QALY for patients less than 65 years old, an ICER of $70,881 per QALY for patients 65 to 74 years old, and an ICER of $37,934 per QALY for patients 75 years and older. Among patients with major comorbid conditions, ICD therapy was associated with comparable or larger absolute mortality risk reductions annually than in patients without many of these major medical conditions. However, ICD therapy was found to be the most cost-effective for patients with 1 comorbidity (ICER of $49,677 per QALY) and least cost-effective for patients with 3 or more comorbidities (ICER of $93,485 per QALY).

Sanders and colleagues[38] further explored the effect of age on the cost-effectiveness of ICD therapy for the primary prevention of SCD in patients with heart failure with reduced left ventricular ejection fraction. They developed a Markov model to evaluate lifetime costs and benefits of ICD therapy compared with optimal medical therapy in patients greater than or equal to 65 years of age with left ventricular systolic dysfunction, with data derived from the literature and existing clinical trials of primary prevention of SCD. Estimated health and economic outcomes varied substantially among trial populations and with age. For 65-year-old patients in each trial population,

prophylactic implantation of an ICD was more expensive than control therapy. The increase in estimated lifetime discounted costs ranged from $69,620 (SCD-HeFT) to $118,284 (MADIT-I). In the 5 trials, ICD implantation improved life expectancy relative to control therapy, with the discounted increment ranging from 0.70 years in the SCD-HeFT trial to 4.44 years (MADIT-I trial) (undiscounted 0.98–6.30 years) or from 0.50 to 3.19 QALYs (undiscounted 0.71–4.52 QALYs). ICERs based on these trials ranged from $26,661/LY to $99,666/LY added and from $37,031/QALY to $138,458/QALY. For 75-year-old patients, findings were qualitatively similar to those seen in 65-year-old patients, although they showed reduced cost-effectiveness in all trial populations. They evaluated the overall impact of age on incremental cost-effectiveness of ICDs compared with control therapy in each trial and concluded that whether ICD therapy might be considered a good use of health care resources in an individual trial did not change dramatically based on age at implantation.

COST-EFFECTIVENESS OF ICD THERAPY FOR SECONDARY PREVENTION

Several studies have been performed to evaluate the cost-effectiveness of ICD therapy for secondary prevention in patients after ventricular arrhythmias or aborted SCD (**Table 2**). The most comprehensive and updated study was performed by Bryant and colleagues[48] for the United Kingdom National Health Service (NHS) Health Technology Assessment Program. The investigators undertook a systematic review and economic evaluation of ICDs in patients at risk of SCD from arrhythmias to inform the process for the National Institute for Clinical Excellence (NICE) to update its guidance in 2004 in the light of new evidence and in particular to incorporate relevant newly emerging UK data. Eleven electronic databases (including Medline, PubMed, Cochrane Database of Systematic Reviews, Cochrane Controlled Trials register, Embase) were searched from inception until January 2005. Studies of clinical effectiveness were combined through narrative synthesis with full tabulation of included studies. Meta-analysis was not considered appropriate because of heterogeneity in patient characteristics, comparative interventions, and duration of trials. A Markov decision analytical model with a 5-year time horizon was developed to examine the benefits and costs of ICDs compared with pharmacologic therapy. The economic evaluation adopted a UK NHS perspective for costs and benefits. It focused on hospital-based costs that were believed to represent the

Table 1
Cost-effectiveness of ICDs for primary prevention in published RCTs and decision analytical models

Title	Lead Author	Year	Model	Strategy	Cost	Effect (LYs)	Effect (QALY)	ICER (per LY Gained)	ICER (per QALY)	Comment
RCTs for ICD Primary Prevention										
The cost-effectiveness of automatic implantable cardiac defibrillators: results from MADIT[28]	Mushlin	1998	Based on MADIT-I	PT ICD	$75,980 $97,560	2.66 3.46	— —	— $27,000	— —	Time horizon for analysis of 4 y. Costs and survival rates discounted by 3% per annum.
Clinical and economic implications of the Multicenter Automatic Defibrillator Implantation Trial-II[29]	Al-Khatib	2005	Matched analysis based on cohort from Duke University Medical Center (1986–2001)	PT ICD	$40,661 $131,490	6.79 8.59	5.98[a] 7.56[a]	— $50,500	— $57,300	Matched analysis with lifetime projections of cost-effectiveness. Costs and survival discounted at 3% per annum
The cost-effectiveness of implantable cardioverter-defibrillators results from the Multicenter Automatic Defibrillator Implantation Trial (MADIT)-II[30]	Zwanziger	2006	Based on MADIT-II	PT ICD	$44,900 $84,100	2.725 2.892	— —	— $235,000	— —	Time horizon for analysis of 3.5 y. Costs and survival rates discounted by 3% per annum

Study	Author	Year	Based on	Group	Cost					Comments
Cost-effectiveness of defibrillator therapy or amiodarone in chronic stable heart failure: results from the Sudden Cardiac Death in Heart Failure Trial (SCD-HeFT)[31]	Mark	2006	Based on SCD-HeFT	Placebo	$42,971 (5 y)	—	—	—	—	Results of RCT with median 45.5 month follow-up used to project lifetime cost-effectiveness. Costs and survival rates discounted by 3% per annum
				PT	$49,338 (5 y)	8.41 (lifetime)	—	—	—	
				ICD	$61,938 (5 y)	10.87 (lifetime)	—	$38 389 (lifetime, $25,217–$80,160) (reference placebo)	$41,530 (lifetime) (reference placebo)	
Decision Analytical Models for ICD Primary Prevention										
Cost-effectiveness of primary implanted cardioverter-defibrillator for sudden death prevention in congestive heart failure[32]	Chen	2004	Based on patients with CHF	No ICD	$25,223	1.90	—	—	—	Lifetime cost-effectiveness. Costs and survival discounted at 3% per annum
				ICD	$122,947	2.90	—	—	$97,861	
Cost-effectiveness of implantable cardioverter-defibrillators[33]	Sanders	2005	Based on MADIT-I, MADIT-II, MUSTT, DEFINITE, COMPANION, and SCH-HeFT	PT	$37,800–$84,400	4.01–9.03	2.95–6.57	—	—	Lifetime cost-effectiveness. Costs and survival discounted at 3% per annum. Dominated strategies were more expensive and less effective.
				ICD	$106,100–$184,900	5.88–11.75	4.31–8.53	$25,300–$50,700	$34,000–$70,200	
			Based on CABG Patch and DINAMIT	PT	$78,600–$88,300	8.41–9.44	6.13–6.87	—	—	
				ICD	$134,400–$147,200	8.01–8.96	5.84–6.53	Dominated	Dominated	

(continued on next page)

Table 1
(*continued*)

Title	Lead Author	Year	Model	Strategy	Cost	Effect (LYs)	Effect (QALY)	ICER (per LY Gained)	ICER (per QALY)	Comment
Implantable or external defibrillators for individuals at increased risk of cardiac arrest: where cost-effectiveness hits fiscal reality[34]	Cram	2006	Based on patients who met MADIT-II criteria	EMS-D AED ICD	$75,305 $80,530 $189,965	6.59 6.66 7.73	5.76 5.81 6.66	— $74,643 $111,668 (reference EMS-D)	— $104,500 $127,400 (reference EMS-D)	Lifetime cost-effectiveness. Costs and survival discounted at 3% per annum
Cost-effectiveness of implantable cardioverter-defibrillators for primary prevention in a Belgian context[35]	Neyt	2008	Based on SCD-HeFT and Belgian cost data	PT ICD	— —	7.95 9.38	— —	— €59,989 (35,873–113,518)	— €71,428 (40,225–134,623)	Lifetime cost-effectiveness. Costs discounted at 3% and survival at 1.5% per annum
Lifetime cost-effectiveness of prophylactic implantation of a cardioverter defibrillator in patients with reduced left ventricular systolic function: results of Markov modelling in a European population[36]	Cowie	2009	Based on meta-analysis of 6 clinical trials	PT ICD and PT	€18,187 €64,600	6.71 8.58	5.70 7.27	— €24,751	— €29,530	Lifetime cost-effectiveness. Costs discounted at 3% and survival at 1.5% per annum

Decision Analytical Models for ICD Primary Prevention in Subpopulations

Study	Year	Subpopulation							Comments
Impact of age and medical comorbidity on the effectiveness of implantable cardioverter-defibrillators for primary prevention[37]	Chan	2009	Based on a subpopulation cohort, elderly patients 65 to 74 y old	No ICD	$84,527	6.43	5.68	—	—	Prospective cohort analysis with time horizon of 34 ± 16 mo with lifetime cost-effectiveness projected. Costs and survival discounted at 3% per annum
				ICD	$157,600	7.60	6.71	$62,456[a]	$70,881	
			Based on a subpopulation cohort, elderly patients 75 y or older	No ICD	$61,916	3.36	2.95	—	—	
				ICD	$138,813	5.66	4.98	$33,434[a]	$37,934	
			Based on a subpopulation cohort, patients with no comorbidities	No ICD	—	—	—	—	—	
				ICD	—	—	—	—	$62,060	
			Based on a subpopulation cohort, patients with 1 comorbid diagnosis	No ICD	—	—	—	—	—	
				ICD	—	—	—	—	$49,677	
			Based on a subpopulation cohort, patients with 2 comorbid diagnoses	No ICD	—	—	—	—	—	
				ICD	—	—	—	—	$71,274	
			Based on a subpopulation cohort, patients with 3 or more comorbid diagnoses	No ICD	—	—	—	—	—	
				ICD	—	—	—	—	$93,485	

(continued on next page)

Table 1
(continued)

Title	Lead Author	Year	Model	Strategy	Cost	Effect (LYs)	Effect (QALY)	ICER (per LY Gained)	ICER (per QALY)	Comment
Cost-effectiveness of implantable cardioverter defibrillators in patients ≥65 years of age[38]	Sanders	2010	Based on patients more than 65 y old from SCH-HeFT, MADIT-I, MADIT-II, MUSTT, and DEFINITE	PT	$42,366–$83,790	3.93–7.86	2.87–5.70	—	—	Lifetime cost-effectiveness. Costs and survival discounted at 3% per annum
				ICD	$130,880–$193,085	6.44–10.46	4.68–7.56	$26,661–$99,666	$37,031–$138,458	
			Based on patients more than 75 y of age from SCH-HeFT, MADIT-I, MADIT-II, MUSTT, & DEFINITE	PT	$41,369–$74,100	3.62–6.58	2.59–4.70	—	—	
				ICD	$122,505–$171,915	5.67–8.77	4.05–6.26	$28,200–$107,208	$ 39,564–$150,421	

Abbreviations: AED, automated external defibrillator; CHF, congestive heart failure; EMS-D, emergency medical services equipped with defibrillator; ICD, implantable cardioverter-defibrillator; ICER, incremental cost-effectiveness ratio; PT, pharmacologic therapy; QALY, quality-adjusted life year; €, euros; $, dollars (US); as of December 2009 $1 = €1.46.
a Values calculated based on published data.

most significant component in the provision of the service.

The investigators concluded that the evidence suggested that ICDs reduce mortality in patients with previous ventricular arrest or symptomatic sustained ventricular arrhythmias. Results suggested a 25% to 28% reduction in relative risk of death with an ICD that was largely caused by a 50% reduction in arrhythmic death.[49–51] The reduction in total mortality was estimated at 39% at 1 year, 27% at 2 years, and 31% at 3 years, with an average survival benefit associated with ICDs of 2.7 months at 3 years.[8–10]

The 2 secondary prevention trials[9,10] reporting quality of life had inconsistent findings using a range of measures. One reported that ICD and medical therapy were associated with similar self-perceived quality of life.[2] The development of adverse symptoms was associated with significant impairment in quality of life in both groups, as was the occurrence of sporadic shocks in ICD recipients.[2] The other reported better quality of life with ICD therapy than medical therapy, although this finding was not evident in patients who received numerous shocks from their device.[52]

The published economic evaluations report a variation in the cost per LY gained (LYG) and cost per QALY associated with ICD use. The cost per LYG ranged from CAD $17,100 to CAD $213,500 (USD $17,000 to $212,000) and the cost per QALY from CAD $37,000 to CAD $76,800 (USD $36,800 to $76,300). Because searches revealed that the cost-effectiveness evidence was lacking in internal validity and was of limited relevance to the United Kingdom, a new economic evaluation was conducted. Results showed that an improved survival can be achieved with ICDs compared with drug therapy, but with high additional cost. When assessing secondary prevention, the incremental cost per QALY ranged from GBP £88,000 to GBP £165,000 (USD $167,000 to $312,000), depending on mortality risk.

COST-EFFECTIVENESS OF CRT-P AND CRT-D

The cost-effectiveness of cardiac resynchronization therapy (CRT) has been evaluated using both RCT-based analysis as well as decision analytical modeling. The Cardiac Resynchronization in Heart Failure (CARE-HF) trial was an RCT conducted at 82 clinical centers in 12 European countries (**Table 3**).[13] Patients (n = 813) with NYHA class III or IV heart failure with decreased left ventricular ejection fraction (<35%) and cardiac dyssynchrony were randomized to CRT-P plus medical therapy (n = 409) versus medical therapy alone

(n = 404). The analysis of cost-effectiveness was specified a priori as a secondary outcome in the protocol and included data from all patients enrolled in the trial.[53] Health care costs were estimated from the use of substantial medical resources, with costs based on the UK NHS reference costs. Quality of life data were collected prospectively using validated questionnaires (the EQ-5D and Minnesota Living with Heart Failure questionnaires). During a mean follow-up of 29.4 months, patients assigned to CRT had significantly increased costs (EUR €4316 [USD $2900], 95% CI 1327–7485), as well as longer survival (0.10 years, 95% CI −0.01–0.21), and improved quality of life and QALYs (0.22, 95% CI 0.13–0.32). The ICER was EUR €43,596 (USD $29,600) per LY gained (95% CI −146,236–223,849) and EUR €19,319 (USD $13,100) per QALY gained (95% CI 5482–45,402). In sensitivity analysis, the results were sensitive to the cost of the device, implantation procedure, and hospitalization.

Multiple decision analytical studies have been performed to assess the cost-effectiveness of CRT devices for secondary prevention. Three recent decision analytical models have incorporated results from major RCTs (see **Table 3**).[55,56,58] These models have produced substantially disparate results because of differing model assumptions. The first of these studies was based on the results of the COMPANION trial with a time horizon of 7 years. The ICER was estimated to be $19,600 per QALY for CRT-P relative to medical therapy and $43,000 per QALY for CRT-D relative to medical therapy. However, the ICER for CRT-D compared with CRT-P was estimated at $160,000 per QALY.[7,55,59] Thus, the addition of the defibrillator component increased the costs substantially with a modest improvement in quality-adjusted survival, resulting in a high ICER.

Yao and colleagues[56] designed a model that combined the data from the COMPANION and CARE-HF trials (CARE-HF did not have a CRT-D arm). They estimated that, in a 65-year-old patient followed for the remainder of her lifetime, the ICER for CRT-P compared with medical therapy was EUR €7011 (USD $4800) (95% CI 5346–10,003) per LYG and EUR €7538 (USD $5100) (95% CI 5325–11,784) per QALY gained. The ICER for CRT-D compared with CRT-P was EUR €35,864 (USD $24,400) (95% CI 26,709–56,353) per LYG and EUR €47,909 (USD $32,600) (95% CI 35,703–79,438) per QALY gained. In sensitivity analysis, the ICER decreased significantly with increasing age.

The most recently published decision analytical model incorporated data from RCTs and used a UK health care perspective to evaluate the

Table 2
Cost-effectiveness of ICDs for secondary prevention in published RCTs and decision analytical models

Title	Author	Year	Model	Strategy	Cost	Effect (Life Years)	Effect (QALY)	ICER (per LY Gained)	ICER (per QALY)	Comment
RCTs for ICD Secondary Prevention										
Cost-effectiveness of implantable defibrillator as first-choice therapy versus electrophysiologically guided, tiered strategy in postinfarct sudden death survivors. A randomized study[42]	Wever	1996	Based on a randomized trial of 60 patients from the Netherlands	EPS-guided PT ICD	$63,032 $56,067	— —	— —	— $23,000	— —	Time horizon for analysis was 4 y with median follow-up of 729 d
Cost-effectiveness of the implantable cardioverter-defibrillator. Results from the Canadian Implantable Defibrillator Study (CIDS)[43]	O'Brien	2001	Based on CIDS	PT ICD	C$38,600 C$87,715	4.35 4.58	— —	— C$213,543	— —	Time horizon of 6.3 y
Cost-effectiveness of the implantable cardioverter-defibrillator versus antiarrhythmic drugs in survivors of serious ventricular tachyarrhythmias: results of the Antiarrhythmics Versus Implantable Defibrillators (AVID) economic analysis substudy[44]	Larsen	2002	Based on regression model for costs within the AVID trial	PT ICD	$71,421 $85,522	2.27 2.48	— —	— $66,677	— —	Time horizon of 3 y. Costs and survival discounted at 3% per annum

Study	Author	Year	Basis	Treatment	Cost	Life-years	ICER	ICER	Comments
Effectiveness and cost-effectiveness of implantable cardioverter defibrillators in the treatment of ventricular arrhythmias among Medicare beneficiaries[45]	Weiss	2002	Matched pair-analysis of Medicare patients	PT	$37,200	4.1	—	—	Time horizon for analysis of 8 y. Costs and survival discounted at 3% per annum
				ICD	$78,700	4.6	—	$78,400	
Analytical Decision Models for ICD Secondary Prevention									
An analysis of the cost-effectiveness of the implantable defibrillator[46]	Kuppermann	1990	Based on Medicare data	PT	$88,990	3.2	—	—	Lifetime cost-effectiveness
				ICD	$121,540	5.1	$17,100	—	
Cost-effectiveness of implantable cardioverter defibrillators relative to amiodarone for prevention of sudden cardiac death[47]	Owens	1997	Based on ongoing RCTs	PT	$71,400 (61,400–84,300)	7.8	—	—	Lifetime cost-effectiveness. Costs and survival discounted at 3% per annum. Data shown include intermediate-risk patients with an assumption that ICDs decrease mortality by 20%
				Sequential PT then ICD Treatment	$74,100 (63,700–88,000)	7.83	$101,900	$138,900	
				ICD	$110,500 (98,700–138,900)	8.49	$56,000 (reference Amiodarone)	$76,800 (reference Amiodarone)	
Decision economic model incorporating clinical effectiveness data from previous studies[48]	Bryant	2007	Based on RCTs and systematic reviews	PT	£25,816	1.85–1.97	—	—	Time horizon for analysis of 5 y. Costs discounted at 6% and survival at 1.5% per annum
				ICD	£48,339	2.11	—	£88,248–164,931	

Abbreviations: EPS, electrophysiology study; ICD, implantable cardioverter-defibrillator; ICER, incremental cost-effectiveness ratio; PT, pharmacologic therapy; QALY, quality-adjusted life year; $, dollars (US); C$, Canadian dollars; £, pounds sterling (as of December 2009, $1 = £1.62 = C$0.95).

Table 3
Cost-effectiveness of CRT in published RCTs and decision analytical models

Title and Reference	Lead Author	Year	Model	Strategy	Cost	Effect (LYs)	Effect (QALY)	ICER (per LY Gained)	ICER (per QALY)	Comments
RCTs for CRT										
Cost-effectiveness of cardiac resynchronization therapy: results from the CARE-HF trial[53]	Calvert	2005	Analysis based on CARE-HF	PT CRT-P	€15,795 €20,110	1.92 2.02	1.19 1.42	— €43,596 (-146, 236–223,849)	— €19,319 (5,482–45,402)	Time horizon for analysis of 29.4 mo. Costs and survival discounted at 3.5% per annum
Decision Analytical Models for CRT										
Cost-effectiveness of cardiac resynchronization therapy in patients with symptomatic heart failure[54]	Nichol	2004	Based on Early RCTs	PT CRT-P	$34,400 $64,400	— —	2.64 2.92	— —	$107,800 (79,800–156,500)	Lifetime cost-effectiveness. Costs and survival discounted at 3% per annum
Cost-effectiveness of cardiac resynchronization therapy in the Comparison of Medical Therapy, Pacing, and Defibrillation in Heart Failure (COMPANION) trial[55]	Feldman	2005	Based on COMPANION	PT CRT-P CRT-D	$46,000 $59,900 $82,200	3.37 3.87 4.15	2.30 3.01 3.15	— $28,100 $79,600[a] (reference CRT-P)	— $19,600 $159,300[a] (reference CRT-P)	Time horizon for analysis of 7 y. Costs and survival discounted at 3% per annum

Title	Author	Year	Basis	Therapy	Cost			ICER	ICER	Comments
The long-term cost-effectiveness of cardiac resynchronization therapy with or without an implantable cardioverter-defibrillator[56]	Yao	2007	Based on data from CARE-HF and COMPANION	PT	€39,060	6.1	4.08	—	—	Lifetime cost-effectiveness. Costs and survival discounted at 3.5% per annum
				CRT-P	€53,996	8.23	6.06	€7011 (5,346–10,003)	€7,538 (5,325–11,784)	
				CRT-D	€87,350	9.16	6.75	€35,874 (27,709–56,353) (reference CRT-P)	€47,909 (35,703–79,438) (reference CRT-P)	
The clinical effectiveness and cost-effectiveness of cardiac resynchronisation (biventricular pacing) for heart failure: systematic review and economic model[57]	Fox	2007	Based on a meta-analysis of all available RCTs	PT	£9,367	4.9	3.10	—	—	Lifetime cost-effectiveness. Costs and survival discounted at 3.5% per annum
				CRT-P	£20,997	5.8	3.80	—	£16,735 (14,630–20,333)	
				CRT-D	£32,687	6.2	4.09	—	£40,160 (£26,645–59,391) (reference CRT-P)	

Abbreviations: CRT-D, cardiac resynchronization therapy with defibrillator function; CRT-P, cardiac resynchronization therapy without defibrillator function; ICD, implantable cardioverter-defibrillator; ICER, incremental cost-effectiveness ratio; PT, pharmacologic therapy; QALY, quality-adjusted life year; €, euros; $, dollars (US); £, pounds sterling (as of December 2009, $1 = £1.62 = €1.46).

a Values calculated based on published data.

cost-effectiveness of CRT-P and CRT-D in a mixed age cohort (30–90 years) during a lifetime.[58] Compared with medical therapy, CRT-P conferred an additional 0.70 QALYs at a cost of GBP £11,630 (USD $7000). Thus, the investigators estimated an ICER of GBP £16,735 (USD $10,400) per QALY (range GBP £14,630–20,333) for CRT-P compared with pharmacologic therapy. CRT-D versus CRT-P conferred an additional 0.29 QALYs for an additional GBP £11,689 (USD $7200). Thus, the investigators estimated an ICER of GBP £40,160 per QALY (range GBP £26,645–59,391) for CRT-D compared with CRT-P.

Currently, no RCT-based or decision analytical cost-effectiveness studies have been undertaken including the results from the MADIT-CRT or RAFT trials.[11,12] The latter showed that, among patients with NYHA class II or III heart failure, a wide QRS complex, and decreased left ventricular ejection fraction, the addition of CRT to an ICD reduced rates of death (HR 0.75; 95% CI 0.62–0.91; $P = .003$) and hospitalization for heart failure (HR 0.68; 95% CI 0.56–0.83; $P<.001$). These finding may significantly affect effectiveness estimates for CRT-D and consequently estimates of cost-effectiveness.

FUTURE AREAS OF STUDY

There are several outstanding issues regarding ICDs and CRT devices that have not been well studied and that may significantly affect estimates of their cost-effectiveness. First, not all patients benefit from device implantation. For example, many patients who receive an ICD never have an appropriate discharge of the device and between one-third and one-half of patients who receive CRT do not respond with improved symptoms or cardiac function. When drugs are ineffective, they can be discontinued. However, implanted devices require a surgical procedure with higher up-front risk and costs than cardiovascular drugs. In addition, if a patient fails to benefit from the device, extraction or removal of the system itself would require a procedure. If the device is inactivated, then the patient is still exposed to the potential harms of device implantation, such as infection. Currently, there are no tests that can accurately predict which patients will benefit from these devices; however, if such diagnostic testing is developed, it may significantly narrow the target patient populations, improve the therapeutic efficacy, and consequently improve the cost-effectiveness of the devices.

Second, there are several unique features of ICDs and CRT devices that have not been well evaluated to this point and that may significantly affect cost-effectiveness. For example, the occurrence of shocks may be an independent predictor of poor outcome in patients with an ICD. In one series of 421 patients, the 4-year mortality after adjusting for left ventricular systolic dysfunction was greater in patients who received at least 1 shock (17% vs 11% for those receiving no shock); this difference in survival was significant only for patients with an left ventricular ejection fraction greater than or equal to 35%.[60] The 4-year mortality was also higher in patients who had multiple shocks (33% vs 20% for a single shock), with the difference in survival being significant only in those with an left ventricular ejection fraction less than 35%. The combination of a low left ventricular ejection fraction and multiple shocks identified a subgroup with a mortality 16-fold greater compared with those without these features. Other clinical issues that remain poorly elucidated and may affect cost-effectiveness are the need for single versus dual leads for ICDs, long-term rates of lead fractures and lead replacement procedures, generator replacement infection rates,[61] the frequency of hospitalizations and emergency evaluation because of inappropriate shocks, the use of CRT in right bundle branch block and NYHA I and II patients, and the use of ICDs and CRT devices in patients with chronic kidney disease.

Third, most cost-effectiveness studies have incorporated clinical efficacy data only from RCTs, and clinical effectiveness in community populations may significantly differ from trial populations. Currently, the Center for Medicare and Medicaid Services requires that its beneficiaries who receive an ICD for primary prevention be included in the National Cardiovascular Data ICD Registry, which is maintained by the American College of Cardiology in partnership with the Heart Rhythm Society. However, the current registry does not include CRT devices and, although many centers submit data on all patients who receive an ICD, it is not required for them to submit data on ICDs placed in patients for secondary prevention and in non–Medicare beneficiaries. In addition, the registry only includes in-hospital adverse events, so long-term follow-up data are not available. The importance of broader registries and other observational data from the community is highlighted by several recent ICD recalls and advisories,[62,63] and these data may have a significant impact on our future understanding of the cost-effectiveness of ICDs and CRT devices.[19]

Fourth, the cost-effectiveness of a therapy varies according to the willingness to pay of a given health care system. There is an increasing burden of coronary disease and heart failure in less developed health care settings such as China and India that will require cost-effectiveness analyses targeted at these more resource-limited settings.

SUMMARY

With the costs of health care increasing steadily, the need for rigorous evaluation of clinical effectiveness and costs is increasingly important. The number of patients eligible for ICD therapy has increased several fold based on recent trial results.[18] It is currently estimated that between 1% and 3% of all patients discharged alive after their index hospitalization for heart failure, and 15% to% 20 of patients seen in specialized heart failure clinics, meet criteria for CRT implantation,[64–67] and, of these patients, approximately one-half also meet trial eligibility criteria for an ICD.[19,68]

Multiple clinical trials have shown a significant increase in survival in patients with heart failure with decreased ejection fraction who receive an ICD for primary or secondary prevention of SCD. However, this benefit in clinical effectiveness comes at a significant economic cost. Nonetheless, multiple randomized trial-based analyses and decision analytical model studies have shown that ICD therapy is within a range generally considered cost-effective relative to medical therapy alone.

CRT-P improves both quality of life and survival in patients with symptomatic heart failure with decreased ejection fraction already treated with optimal medical management (NYHA functional class III and IV, and left ventricular ejection fraction <0.35), with a prolonged QRS complex (>120 milliseconds). Despite significant economic costs associated with CRT-P, in multiple studies it has been shown to be within a range generally considered cost-effective compared with medical therapy. CRT-D, which incorporates an ICD into the CRT system, reduces the risk of SCD in the same patient population. However, CRT-D is substantially more expensive than CRT-P, and it is unclear whether the improvement in survival is sufficient to justify the near doubling of costs.[19]

In conclusion, the weight of available evidence suggests that ICD therapy is safe, effective, and cost-effective for the primary and secondary prevention of SCD in patients with heart failure with decreased ejection fraction for health care systems in developed countries. Similarly, CRT-P has been shown to be safe, effective, and cost-effective in patients with advanced symptomatic systolic heart failure with a wide QRS complex. Early cost-effectiveness studies suggest that CRT-D modestly improves outcomes compared with optimal medical therapy, but it is uncertain whether the small clinical benefit of CRT-D compared with CRT-P justifies the substantial increase in costs. Cost-effectiveness studies incorporating the most recent CRT-D clinical trial results are currently lacking and may significantly change estimates of cost-effectiveness.

REFERENCES

1. Moss AJ, Hall WJ, Cannom DS, et al. Improved survival with an implanted defibrillator in patients with coronary disease at high risk for ventricular arrhythmia. Multicenter Automatic Defibrillator Implantation Trial Investigators. N Engl J Med 1996;335(26):1933–40.

2. Moss AJ, Fadl Y, Zareba W, et al. Survival benefit with an implanted defibrillator in relation to mortality risk in chronic coronary heart disease. Am J Cardiol 2001;88(5):516–20.

3. Moss AJ, Zareba W, Hall WJ, et al. Prophylactic implantation of a defibrillator in patients with myocardial infarction and reduced ejection fraction. N Engl J Med 2002;346(12):877–83.

4. Greenberg H, Case RB, Moss AJ, et al. Analysis of mortality events in the Multicenter Automatic Defibrillator Implantation Trial (MADIT-II). J Am Coll Cardiol 2004;43(8):1459–65.

5. Buxton AE, Lee KL, Fisher JD, et al. A randomized study of the prevention of sudden death in patients with coronary artery disease. Multicenter Unsustained Tachycardia Trial Investigators. N Engl J Med 1999;341(25):1882–90.

6. Bardy GH, Lee KL, Mark DB, et al. Amiodarone or an implantable cardioverter-defibrillator for congestive heart failure. N Engl J Med 2005;352(3):225–37.

7. Bristow MR, Saxon LA, Boehmer J, et al. Cardiac-resynchronization therapy with or without an implantable defibrillator in advanced chronic heart failure. N Engl J Med 2004;350(21):2140–50.

8. Kuck KH, Cappato R, Siebels J, et al. Randomized comparison of antiarrhythmic drug therapy with implantable defibrillators in patients resuscitated from cardiac arrest: the Cardiac Arrest Study Hamburg (CASH). Circulation 2000;102(7):748–54.

9. Connolly SJ, Gent M, Roberts RS, et al. Canadian Implantable Defibrillator Study (CIDS): a randomized trial of the implantable cardioverter defibrillator against amiodarone. Circulation 2000;101(11):1297–302.

10. A comparison of antiarrhythmic-drug therapy with implantable defibrillators in patients resuscitated from near-fatal ventricular arrhythmias. The Antiarrhythmics versus Implantable Defibrillators (AVID) Investigators. N Engl J Med 1997;337(22):1576–83.

11. Moss AJ, Hall WJ, Cannom DS, et al. Cardiac-resynchronization therapy for the prevention of heart-failure events. N Engl J Med 2009;361(14):1329–38.

12. Tang AS, Wells GA, Talajic M, et al. Cardiac-resynchronization therapy for mild-to-moderate heart failure. N Engl J Med 2010;363(25):2385–95.

13. Cleland JG, Daubert JC, Erdmann E, et al. The effect of cardiac resynchronization on morbidity and mortality in heart failure. N Engl J Med 2005;352(15):1539–49.

14. Saxon LA, Bristow MR, Boehmer J, et al. Predictors of sudden cardiac death and appropriate shock in the Comparison of Medical Therapy, Pacing, and Defibrillation in Heart Failure (COMPANION) Trial. Circulation 2006;114(25):2766–72.

15. Zipes DP, Camm AJ, Borggrefe M, et al. ACC/AHA/ESC 2006 guidelines for management of patients with ventricular arrhythmias and the prevention of sudden cardiac death–executive summary: a report of the American College of Cardiology/American Heart Association Task Force and the European Society of Cardiology Committee for Practice Guidelines (Writing Committee to Develop Guidelines for Management of Patients with Ventricular Arrhythmias and the Prevention of Sudden Cardiac Death) Developed in collaboration with the European Heart Rhythm Association and the Heart Rhythm Society. Eur Heart J 2006;27(17):2099–140.

16. Epstein AE, DiMarco JP, Ellenbogen KA, et al. ACC/AHA/HRS 2008 guidelines for device-based therapy of cardiac rhythm abnormalities: a report of the American College of Cardiology/American Heart Association Task Force on Practice Guidelines (Writing Committee to Revise the ACC/AHA/NASPE 2002 Guideline Update for Implantation of Cardiac Pacemakers and Antiarrhythmia Devices): developed in collaboration with the American Association for Thoracic Surgery and Society of Thoracic Surgeons. Circulation 2008;117(21):e350–408.

17. Seidl K, Senges J. Worldwide utilization of implantable cardioverter/defibrillators now and in the future. Card Electrophysiol Rev 2003;7(1):5–13.

18. McClellan MB, Tunis SR. Medicare coverage of ICDs. N Engl J Med 2005;352(3):222–4.

19. Dhruv K, Hlatky M. The cost effectiveness of cardiac resynchronization therapy. In: Abraham WT, Baliga RR, editors. Cardiac resynchronization therapy. Philadelphia: Wolters Kluwer Health, Lippincott Williams & Wilkins; 2010.

20. Neumann PJ, Rosen AB, Weinstein MC. Medicare and cost-effectiveness analysis. N Engl J Med 2005;353(14):1516–22.

21. Michael F, Drummond MJ, George WT, et al. Methods for the economic evaluation of health care programmes. 3rd edition. Oxford (United Kingdom): Oxford University Press; 2005.

22. Drummond MF, Sculpher MJ, Torrance GW, et al. Basic types of economic evaluation. In: Drummond MF, Sculpher MJ, Torrance GW, et al, editors. Methods for economic evaluation of health care programmes. 3rd edition. New York: Oxford University Press; 2005. p. 7–26.

23. Oliver A. At the end of the beginning: eliciting cardinal values for health states. Available at: http://www.lse.ac.uk/collections/LSEHealthAndSocialCare/pdf/DiscussionPaperSeries/DP2_2002.pdf. Accessed March 5, 2007. Last Updated 2-1-2002. LSE Health and Social Care Discussion Paper Number 2.2002.

24. CHOosing Interventions that are Cost Effective (WHO-CHOICE). World Health Organization. 2010. Available at: http://www.who.int/choice/costs/CER_levels/en/index.html. Accessed November 1, 2010.

25. Sonnenberg FA, Beck JR. Markov models in medical decision making: a practical guide. Med Decis Making 1993;13(4):322–38.

26. Beck JR, Pauker SG. The Markov process in medical prognosis. Med Decis Making 1983;3(4):419–58.

27. Drummond MF, Sculpher MJ, Torrance GW, et al. Critical assessment of economic evaluation. In: Methods for the economic evaluation of health care programmes. New York: Oxford University Press; 2005. p. 27–54.

28. Mushlin AI, Hall WJ, Zwanziger J, et al. The cost-effectiveness of automatic implantable cardiac defibrillators: results from MADIT. Multicenter Automatic Defibrillator Implantation Trial. Circulation 1998; 97(21):2129–35.

29. Al-Khatib SM, Anstrom KJ, Eisenstein EL, et al. Clinical and economic implications of the Multicenter Automatic Defibrillator Implantation Trial-II. Ann Intern Med 2005;142(8):593–600.

30. Zwanziger J, Hall WJ, Dick AW, et al. The cost effectiveness of implantable cardioverter-defibrillators: results from the Multicenter Automatic Defibrillator Implantation Trial (MADIT)-II. J Am Coll Cardiol 2006;47(11):2310–8.

31. Mark DB, Nelson CL, Anstrom KJ, et al. Cost-effectiveness of defibrillator therapy or amiodarone in chronic stable heart failure: results from the Sudden Cardiac Death in Heart Failure Trial (SCD-HeFT). Circulation 2006;114(2):135–42.

32. Chen L, Hay JW. Cost-effectiveness of primary implanted cardioverter defibrillator for sudden death prevention in congestive heart failure. Cardiovasc Drugs Ther 2004;18(2):161–70.

33. Sanders GD, Hlatky MA, Owens DK. Cost-effectiveness of implantable cardioverter-defibrillators. N Engl J Med 2005;353(14):1471–80.

34. Cram P, Katz D, Vijan S, et al. Implantable or external defibrillators for individuals at increased risk of cardiac arrest: where cost-effectiveness hits fiscal reality. Value Health 2006;9(5):292–302.

35. Neyt M, Thiry N, Ramaekers D, et al. Cost effectiveness of implantable cardioverter-defibrillators for primary prevention in a Belgian context. Appl Health Econ Health Policy 2008;6(1):67–80.

36. Cowie MR, Marshall D, Drummond M, et al. Lifetime cost-effectiveness of prophylactic implantation of a cardioverter defibrillator in patients with reduced left ventricular systolic function: results of Markov

modelling in a European population. Europace 2009;11(6):716–26.

37. Chan PS, Nallamothu BK, Spertus JA, et al. Impact of age and medical comorbidity on the effectiveness of implantable cardioverter-defibrillators for primary prevention. Circ Cardiovasc Qual Outcomes 2009; 2(1):16–24.

38. Sanders GD, Kong MH, Al-Khatib SM, et al. Cost-effectiveness of implantable cardioverter defibrillators in patients > or = 65 years of age. Am Heart J 2010;160(1):122–31.

39. Hohnloser SH, Kuck KH, Dorian P, et al. Prophylactic use of an implantable cardioverter-defibrillator after acute myocardial infarction. N Engl J Med 2004; 351(24):2481–8.

40. Kadish A, Dyer A, Daubert JP, et al. Prophylactic defibrillator implantation in patients with nonischemic dilated cardiomyopathy. N Engl J Med 2004; 350(21):2151–8.

41. Bigger JT Jr. Prophylactic use of implanted cardiac defibrillators in patients at high risk for ventricular arrhythmias after coronary-artery bypass graft surgery. Coronary Artery Bypass Graft (CABG) Patch Trial Investigators. N Engl J Med 1997; 337(22):1569–75.

42. Wever EF, Hauer RN, Schrijvers G, et al. Cost-effectiveness of implantable defibrillator as first-choice therapy versus electrophysiologically guided, tiered strategy in postinfarct sudden death survivors. A randomized study. Circulation 1996;93(3):489–96.

43. O'Brien BJ, Connolly SJ, Goeree R, et al. Cost-effectiveness of the implantable cardioverter-defibrillator: results from the Canadian Implantable Defibrillator Study (CIDS). Circulation 2001; 103(10):1416–21.

44. Larsen G, Hallstrom A, McAnulty J, et al. Cost-effectiveness of the implantable cardioverter-defibrillator versus antiarrhythmic drugs in survivors of serious ventricular tachyarrhythmias: results of the Antiarrhythmics Versus Implantable Defibrillators (AVID) economic analysis substudy. Circulation 2002; 105(17):2049–57.

45. Weiss JP, Saynina O, McDonald KM, et al. Effectiveness and cost-effectiveness of implantable cardioverter defibrillators in the treatment of ventricular arrhythmias among Medicare beneficiaries. Am J Med 2002;112(7):519–27.

46. Kuppermann M, Luce BR, McGovern B, et al. An analysis of the cost effectiveness of the implantable defibrillator. Circulation 1990;81(1):91–100.

47. Owens DK, Sanders GD, Harris RA, et al. Cost-effectiveness of implantable cardioverter defibrillators relative to amiodarone for prevention of sudden cardiac death. Ann Intern Med 1997;126(1):1–12.

48. Bryant J, Brodin H, Loveman E, et al. Clinical effectiveness and cost-effectiveness of implantable cardioverter defibrillators for arrhythmias: a systematic review and economic evaluation. Int J Technol Assess Health Care 2007;23(1):63–70.

49. Connolly SJ, Hallstrom AP, Cappato R, et al. Meta-analysis of the implantable cardioverter defibrillator secondary prevention trials. AVID, CASH and CIDS studies. Antiarrhythmics vs Implantable Defibrillator study. Cardiac Arrest Study Hamburg. Canadian Implantable Defibrillator Study. Eur Heart J 2000; 21(24):2071–8.

50. Ezekowitz JA, Armstrong PW, McAlister FA. Implantable cardioverter defibrillators in primary and secondary prevention: a systematic review of randomized, controlled trials. Ann Intern Med 2003; 138(6):445–52.

51. Lee DS, Green LD, Liu PP, et al. Effectiveness of implantable defibrillators for preventing arrhythmic events and death: a meta-analysis. J Am Coll Cardiol 2003;41(9):1573–82.

52. Schron EB, Exner DV, Yao Q, et al. Quality of life in the antiarrhythmics versus implantable defibrillators trial: impact of therapy and influence of adverse symptoms and defibrillator shocks. Circulation 2002;105(5):589–94.

53. Calvert MJ, Freemantle N, Yao G, et al. Cost-effectiveness of cardiac resynchronization therapy: results from the CARE-HF trial. Eur Heart J 2005; 26(24):2681–8.

54. Nichol G, Kaul P, Huszti E, et al. Cost-effectiveness of cardiac resynchronization therapy in patients with symptomatic heart failure. Ann Intern Med 2004;141(5):343–51.

55. Feldman AM, de Lissovoy G, Bristow MR, et al. Cost effectiveness of cardiac resynchronization therapy in the Comparison of Medical Therapy, Pacing, and Defibrillation in Heart Failure (COMPANION) trial. J Am Coll Cardiol 2005;46(12):2311–21.

56. Yao G, Freemantle N, Calvert MJ, et al. The long-term cost-effectiveness of cardiac resynchronization therapy with or without an implantable cardioverter-defibrillator. Eur Heart J 2007;28(1):42–51.

57. Fox M, Anderson R, Dean J. The clinical effectiveness and costeffectiveness of cardiac resynchronisation (biventricular pacing) for heart failure: systematic review and economic model. 2010. Available at: http://www.ncchta.org/fullmono/mon1147.pdf. Accessed November 16, 2010.

58. Fox M, Mealing S, Anderson R, et al. The clinical effectiveness and cost-effectiveness of cardiac resynchronisation (biventricular pacing) for heart failure: systematic review and economic model. Available at: http://www.ncchta.org/fullmono/mon1147.pdf. Accessed January 1, 2008 Health Technol Assess 2007; 11(47).

59. Hlatky MA. Cost effectiveness of cardiac resynchronization therapy. J Am Coll Cardiol 2005;46(12):2322–4.

60. Pacifico A, Ferlic LL, Cedillo-Salazar FR, et al. Shocks as predictors of survival in patients with implantable

cardioverter-defibrillators. J Am Coll Cardiol 1999; 34(1):204–10.

61. Wilson-Poole J. REPLACE registry. Paper presented at: American Heart Association Scientific Sessions. Orlando, FL, November 16, 2009.

62. HRS. Recommendations from the Heart Rhythm Society task force on device performance policies and guidelines. Endorsed by the American College of Cardiology Foundation (ACCF) and the American Heart Association (AHA) and the International Coalition of Pacing and Electrophysiology Organizations (COPE). 2007. Available at: http://www.hrsonline. org/uploadDocs/HRSTaskForceRecsFull.pdf. Accessed August 30, 2007.

63. Steinbrook R. The controversy over Guidant's implantable defibrillators. N Engl J Med 2005; 353(3):221–4.

64. Pedone C, Grigioni F, Boriani G, et al. Implications of cardiac resynchronization therapy and prophylactic defibrillator implantation among patients eligible for heart transplantation. Am J Cardiol 2004;93(3):371–3.

65. McAlister FA, Ezekowitz J, Dryden DM, et al. Cardiac resynchronization therapy and implantable cardiac defibrillators in left ventricular systolic dysfunction. Evidence report/technology assessment no. 152 (prepared by the University of Alberta Evidence-based Practice Center under contract no. 290-02-0023). 2007. Available at: http://www.ahrq.gov/clinic/tp/defibtp.htm. Accessed August 27, 2007.

66. McAlister FA, Tu JV, Newman A, et al. How many patients with heart failure are eligible for cardiac resynchronization? Insights from two prospective cohorts. Eur Heart J 2006;27(3):323–9.

67. Grimm W, Sharkova J, Funck R, et al. How many patients with dilated cardiomyopathy may potentially benefit from cardiac resynchronization therapy? Pacing Clin Electrophysiol 2003;26(1 Pt 2):155–7.

68. Toma M, McAlister FA, Ezekowitz J, et al. Proportion of patients followed in a specialized heart failure clinic needing an implantable cardioverter defibrillator as determined by applying different trial eligibility criteria. Am J Cardiol 2006;97(6):882–5.

Unusual ICD Access

Robert F. Rea, MD

KEYWORDS

- Implantable cardioverter-defibrillator
- Congenital heart disease • Venous occlusion
- Sudden cardiac death

Where there is a will, there is a way
—Anonymous

Placement of leads for pacemakers and defibrillators can be challenging, owing to congenital or acquired limitations to cardiac chamber access and congenital or acquired intracardiac anomalies that preclude typical lead placement. Such challenges have given rise to numerous novel approaches to lead placement, which are reviewed briefly in this article. Isolated case reports or small case series dominate the literature, reflecting the vagaries and infrequency of the surgical hurdles encountered and the variety of solutions developed, a testimony to the adage "where there is a will, there is a way." The belief that nearly any obstacle can be overcome underpins development of these novel approaches. This review is not encyclopedic but, it is hoped, will encourage creative thinking on the part of implanters when challenges arise.

AN ENTIRELY SUBCUTANEOUS CARDIOVERTER-DEFIBRILLATOR

The most definitive answer to difficulties in obtaining vascular access for placement of implantable cardioverter-defibrillator (ICD) leads is to eschew such placement altogether. In 2010, Bardy and colleagues[1] reported on initial experience with an entirely subcutaneous cardioverter-defibrillator. After experimenting with various subcutaneous electrode configurations, and after a pilot study of 6 patients, 55 patients were enrolled in a clinical trial using the device configuration shown in **Fig. 1**. Patients requiring antibradycardia pacing support were excluded, as were those with ventricular tachycardia known to be reliably terminable with antitachycardia pacing. Despite the absence of a sensing lead attached directly to the heart (endocardial or epicardial), detection of ventricular fibrillation was faithful in all patients and defibrillation was successful at 65 J (a requirement for proceeding to permanent implantation) in 98%, as exemplified in **Fig. 2**. While problems were encountered during the average of 10 months of follow-up (infection in 2 patients, lead dislodgement in 3, myopotential sensing in 3, inappropriate sensing in 1), 98% of patients were alive and 12 episodes of spontaneous ventricular tachycardia in 3 patients were successfully treated. This painstaking trial demonstrates the feasibility of ICD systems that altogether avoid endocardial/epicardial hardware in selected patients.

NOVEL TRANSVENOUS LEAD ACCESS TECHNIQUES

Owing to interruption or interdiction of typical venous access to the heart, due to vascular occlusion, presence of vascular anomalies, or intravascular hardware, several access techniques have been reported.

Femoral Vein Approach

This approach is attractive, owing to the caliber of the vessel and operator familiarity with anatomy and access techniques. While pacemaker lead placement from the femoral vein is mentioned in standard textbooks, ICD lead and pulse generator placement is more problematic owing to concerns regarding the adequacy of the shock vector in systems where a substantial portion of the hardware (leads and pulse generator) is not close to or apposed to the thoracic cage. Giudici and

The author has nothing to disclose.
Internal Medicine, Mayo Clinic and Foundation, 200 First Street South West, Rochester, MN 55905, USA
E-mail address: rfrea@mayo.edu

Card Electrophysiol Clin 3 (2011) 441–450
doi:10.1016/j.ccep.2011.05.009
1877-9182/11/$ – see front matter © 2011 Published by Elsevier Inc.

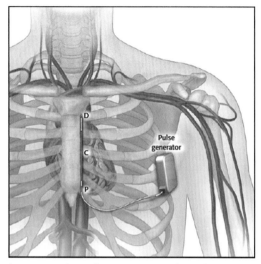

Fig. 1. Location of components of a subcutaneous implantable cardioverter-defibrillator (ICD) in situ. Distal (D) and proximal (P) ends of the LGen-S8 device are shown with the left lateral pulse generator and an 8-cm parasternal coil electrode (C). (*From* Bardy GH, Smith WM, Hood MA, et al. An entirely subcutaneous cardioverter-defibrillator. N Engl J Med 2010;363:39; with permission.)

colleagues[2] reported a patient with ventricular tachycardia and heart block in whom standard ICD implant was impossible, owing to interruption of vascular access from above by prior dialysis shunts/catheters. In addition to venous occlusions, this patient had extensive arterial vascular disease and had undergone bilateral above-the-knee amputations. The left femoral vein was

cannulated twice at the groin crease, and a pocket for the ICD pulse generator was made inferiorly in the anterior left thigh. With the use of standard tear-away sheaths, a long atrial pace/sense lead and a right ventricular ICD lead were placed at the interatrial septum and right ventricular outflow tract, respectively (**Fig. 3**). The pulse generator was placed in the left thigh. Defibrillation was successful at 23 J on two occasions. A slightly different approach was taken by Eldadah and Donahue[3] in a fully ambulatory patient; access was identical but the pulse generator was placed in the abdomen.

Traversing Chronic Total Venous Occlusions

Upper extremity venography showing occlusion of the subclavian/innominate/brachiocephalic veins does not necessarily completely preclude placement of ICD leads via these veins. As has been demonstrated with percutaneous coronary intervention, apparent chronic total vessel occlusions can be crossed with small guidewires, thus allowing recanalization. McCotter and colleagues[4] reported a series of 7 patients with chronic total venous occlusion in whom ICD or pacemaker lead placement was achieved. Apparently totally occluded veins were crossed with small hydrophilic guidewires, and angioplasty balloons were used to dilate the apparently occluded veins. In one case an occlusion could not be crossed antegradely. In this patient a loop snare was advanced retrogradely to the occlusions point and a micropuncture needle was placed into the loop from a subclavian approach. A 0.018-inch (0.46 mm)

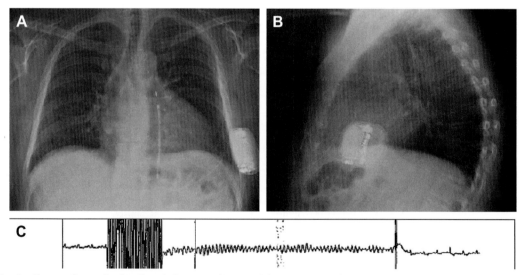

Fig. 2. Chest radiographs (*A, B*) and electrocardiogram (*C*) in a patient who underwent placement and testing of a subcutaneous ICD. (*From* Bardy GH, Smith WM, Hood MA, et al. An entirely subcutaneous cardioverter-defibrillator. N Engl J Med 2010;363:41; with permission.)

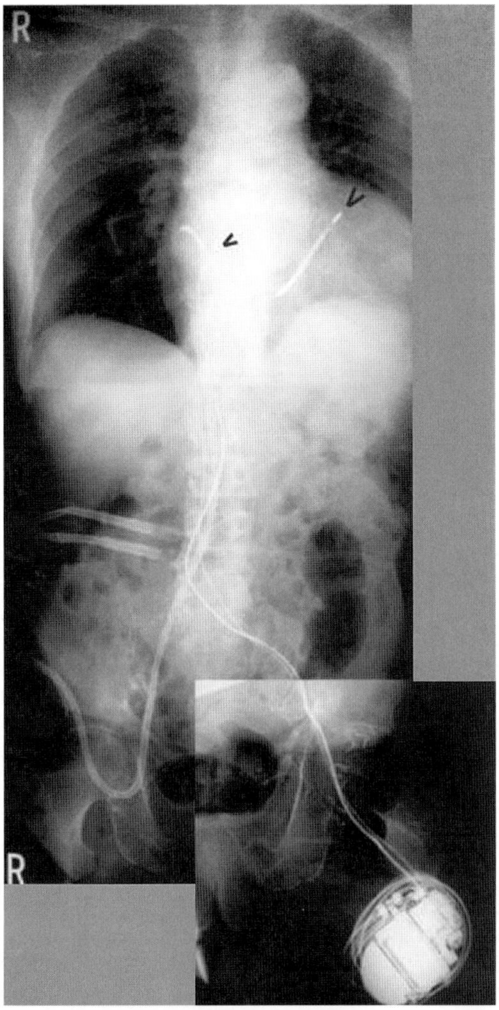

Fig. 3. Radiographs of ICD system showing lead placement in atrial septum and right ventricular outflow septum and device in the left thigh. (*From Giudici MC, Paul DL, Meierbachtol CJ. Active-can implantable cardioverter-defibrillator placement from a femoral approach. Pacing Clin Electrophysiol 2003; 26:1298; with permission.*)

diameter wire was advanced into the loop, grasped, and then pulled into the central circulation, thus permitting venoplasty and (in this case) placement of a pacemaker lead (**Fig. 4**). Whether such an approach would permit placement of a larger-diameter ICD lead is unclear.

In patients with occlusions due to indwelling leads that require device revision or upgrade, laser extraction of one or more of the indwelling leads can be performed, effectively recanalizing the occluded vessel.[5] Critical to success is retention of access to the central circulation with a guidewire after removal of leads and after placement of additional leads, when subsequent access will be required (retained guidewire technique).

Innominate Vein Access

Extraordinarily medial puncture of the subclavian vein can sometimes skirt more peripheral occlusions, likely a component of the procedure illustrated in **Fig. 4**. Planned, deliberate puncture of the right innominate vein was first reported by Aleksic and colleagues[6] in 2007, in 7 patients with otherwise limited venous access. Employing a "notch" technique, an 18-gauge locating needle was placed 1 cm above the right sternoclavicular joint and advanced at a 45° angle in the sagittal plane until venous blood return was encountered (**Fig. 5**). Both ICD and pacing leads were placed using standard sheaths/dilators and were tunneled to the pulse generator pocket. A review of the regional anatomy in **Fig. 5** shows the potential for serious complications, but in this series only one pneumothorax was seen. Adjunctive use of ultrasonography for vessel localization might facilitate this approach, but was not employed in this series.

NOVEL PLACEMENT OF INTRATHORACIC HARDWARE
Avoidance of Tricuspid Valve Prostheses

ICD or pacemaker lead interference with native[7] or bioprosthetic tricuspid valve function is well described, and mechanical tricuspid prostheses in general should not be crossed by leads at all. Whereas pacemaker leads may be placed relatively easily in coronary vein branches, ICD leads are more problematic owing to their bulk and the need for ventricular pacing and sensing, which cannot be effected from within the body of the coronary sinus proper. Grimard and colleagues[8] reported a patient with surgically repaired Ebstein's anomaly, a bioprosthetic tricuspid valve, and ventricular tachycardia who underwent ICD placement. To avoid crossing the prosthesis the ICD lead was placed in the inferior vena cava and a pace/sense lead was placed in a coronary vein, as shown in **Fig. 6**. Other investigators have used a similar approach, with placement of the ICD lead in the low atrium and the pace/sense lead in a coronary vein.[9]

Placement of ICD Shocking Coil in the Azygous Vein to Improve Defibrillation Threshold

The azygous vein carries deoxygenated blood from the abdomen and thorax back to the heart and empties into the superior vena cava. It is posterior and is rightward, at least at its origin.[10] During intracardiac lead placement from the left upper chest, this vein is often entered inadvertently if torque is

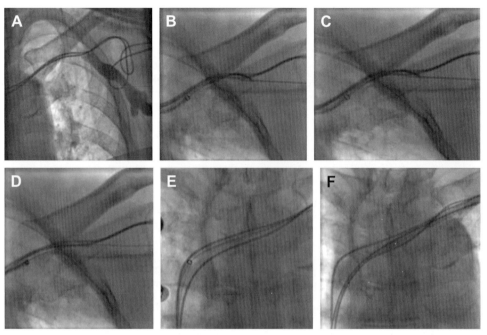

Fig. 4. Adjunctive use of a snare to traverse an occluded subclavian vein. (*A*) Occlusion of subclavian vein. (*B*) Long 5F sheath advanced to left brachiocephalic vein via the femoral vein. A 4-mm loop snare was advanced to the occluded site. A 21-gauge micropuncture needle was placed through the loop snare. (*C*) A 0.018-inch (0.46 mm) wire was advanced through the needle and loop snare. (*D*) Retraction of the loop snare pulling the 0.018-inch wire across the occlusion. (*E, F*) Serial dilation of the occluded site. (*From* McCotter CJ, Angle JF, Prudente LA, et al. Placement of transvenous pacemaker and ICD leads across total chronic occlusions. Pacing Clin Electrophysiol 2005;28:924; with permission.)

applied to a guidewire or lead at the superior vena cava right atrial junction. Its posterior location relative to the heart has been usurped by ICD implanters facing unacceptably high defibrillation thresholds; by placing an ICD lead in this vein the shock vector can be substantially altered. Cooper and colleagues[11] reported on 7 patients with unacceptably high defibrillation thresholds in whom an ICD lead was placed in the azygous vein. Addition of an azygous vein lead yielded an acceptable

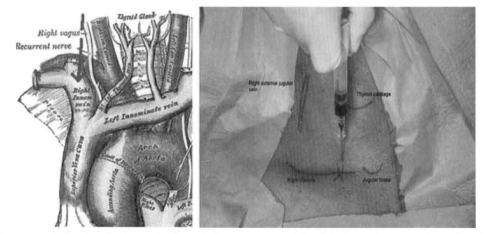

Fig. 5. Anatomic drawing (*left*) showing intended puncture site of the right innominate vein (*arrow*), and intraoperative photograph (*right*) showing the puncture technique and important anatomic landmarks. (*From* Aleksic I, Kottenberg-Assenmacher E, Kienbaum P, et al. The innominate vein as alternative venous access for complicated implantable cardioverter-defibrillator revisions. Pacing Clin Electrophysiol 2007;30:959; with permission.)

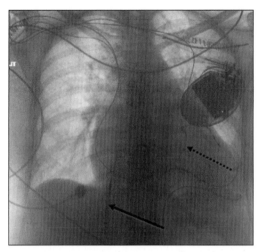

Fig. 6. Chest radiograph showing defibrillation coil in the inferior vena cava (*solid arrow*) and pace/sense lead in the coronary sinus (*dashed arrow*). (*From* Grimard C, May M, Babuty D. An original defibrillation lead implantation to avoid tricuspid prosthesis damage. Europace 2010;4:589; with permission.)

defibrillation threshold safety margin in 4 patients, and defibrillation success at the maximum device output in 2 patients. In one patient adequate defibrillation could not be achieved even with addition of a subcutaneous coil electrode. In **Fig. 7** the course of the azygous vein is shown, with a guidewire passing from the right side of the superior vena cava posteriorly and then medially. **Fig. 8** shows a chest radiograph in a patient who received an azygous vein coil.

One limitation of the azygous vein as a site for an ICD lead, however, is the lack of a convenient anatomic anchor for a lead helix. Bar-Cohen and colleagues[12] reported a patient with severe hypertrophic cardiomyopathy in whom an azygous vein

ICD lead migrated superiorly after an initially successful implant. A vascular plug was then deployed in the vein, and the ICD lead helix was fixed to the plug. **Figs. 9** and **10** show the reacted and the final lead azygous lead positions, and **Fig. 11** the extension of the lead helix into the vascular plug.

SURGICAL TECHNIQUES IN PEDIATRIC AND CONGENITAL HEART DISEASE PATIENTS

Smaller pediatric patients may not have venous caliber of sufficient size to accommodate bulky endovascular/endocardial hardware required for ICD systems such as is used in larger patients. In addition, owing to anticipated rapid axial skeletal growth in this age group, tensioning and potential dislodgment of endovascular leads is of some concern. Although indications for ICD therapy in this age group are uncommon, the increasing recognition of heritable conditions and their underlying genetic basis, such as long QT syndrome, have increased the use of ICDs in this group.

Pediatric Patients

The need for implantation of an ICD in a very small baby is rare. A 5-week-old child weighing 4.9 Kg with marked QT prolongation and recurrent ventricular arrhythmias underwent ICD implantation after attempts at medical therapy and cardiac denervation were unsuccessful. Two epicardial pace/sense electrodes were sutured to the left ventricle after opening of the pericardium. Next, a patch electrode was placed outside the thoracic cage just under the latissimus dorsi and serratus anterior muscles. The epicardial pace/sense electrodes and the patch electrodes were tunneled to the right upper quadrant pocket and connected

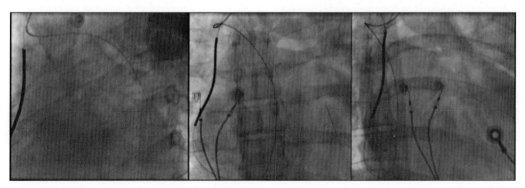

Fig. 7. Radiographs showing the course of a guidewire in the azygous vein in the left anterior oblique (*left*), anteroposterior (*center*), and right anterior oblique projections. (*From* Cooper JS, Latacha MP, Soto GE, et al. The azygous defibrillator lead for elevated defibrillation thresholds: implant technique, lead stability, and patient series. Pacing Clin Electrophysiol 2008;31:1407; with permission.)

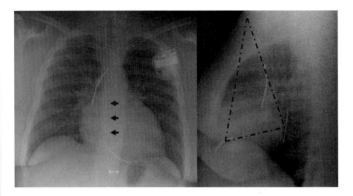

Fig. 8. (*Left*) Posteroanterior chest radiograph showing a single-lead defibrillator to which an azygous vein shock coil has been added (*arrows*). (*Right*) Lateral chest radiograph of the same patient showing the posterior location of the azygous vein coil and a shock vector between it, the active can, and the right ventricular coil. (*From* Cooper JS, Latacha MP, Soto GE, et al. The azygous defibrillator lead for elevated defibrillation thresholds: implant technique, lead stability, and patient series. Pacing Clin Electrophysiol 2008;31:1406; with permission.)

to the pulse generator (**Fig. 12**). The patient has been followed for nearly 5 years and to date has not required revision of his ICD system. **Fig. 13** is a current radiograph. There is a degree of tensioning of the leads compared with the prior radiograph shown in **Fig. 12**, raising concern that further growth may dictate a need for surgical revision. It is hoped that the current system may suffice until the patient is of sufficient size to permit placement of endocardial hardware or until a fully subcutaneous system is approved for pediatric use.

A similar case was reported by Berul and colleagues,[13] in which a subcutaneous array (rather than a subcutaneous patch) was combined with epicardial bipolar rate sense leads in a patient with repaired atrial and ventricular septal defects and aortic coarctation.

An alternative approach is to place an ICD lead in the pericardial space. A 5-year-old with long QT syndrome underwent placement of a single-coil ICD lead in the pericardial space combined with an extrapericardial patch electrode. Owing to migration of the pericardial ICD lead,

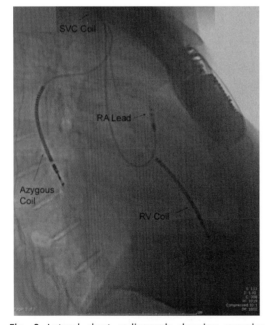

Fig. 9. Lateral chest radiograph showing superior retraction of an azygous ICD after initial implant. RA, right atrium; RV, right ventricle; SVC, superior vena cava. (*From* Bar-Cohen Y, Takao AM, Wells WJ, et al. Novel use of a vascular plug to anchor an azygous vein ICD lead. J Cardiovasc Electrophysiol 2010;21:100; with permission.)

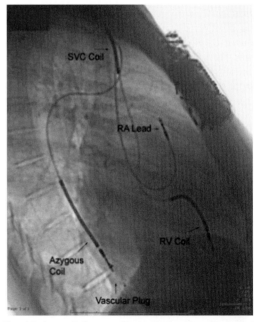

Fig. 10. Lateral chest radiograph showing final position of the azygous ICD lead after fixation. RA, right atrium; RV, right ventricle; SVC, superior vena cava. (*From* Bar-Cohen Y, Takao AM, Wells WJ, et al. Novel use of a vascular plug to anchor an azygous vein ICD lead. J Cardiovasc Electrophysiol 2010;21:100; with permission.)

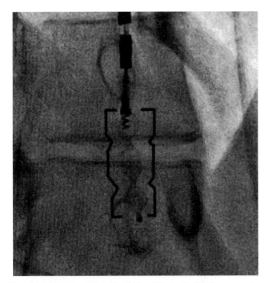

Fig. 11. Close-up detail of the ICD helix in the vascular plug. (*From* Bar-Cohen Y, Takao AM, Wells WJ, et al. Novel use of a vascular plug to anchor an azygous vein ICD lead. J Cardiovasc Electrophysiol 2010; 21:101; with permission.)

reoperation was required to fix the lead in place, and the resultant configuration is shown in **Fig. 14**.

To obviate the problem of migrating intrapericardial leads, others have used active fixation leads positioned in the transverse sinus. Hsia and coleagues[14] reported a series of 7 children, in which a single-coil ICD lead was placed in the transverse sinus via a subxiphoid pericardial window in patients with structural congenital heart disease circulation, poor venous access, or small size in the setting of heritable conditions

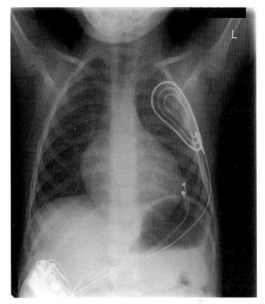

Fig. 13. Chest radiograph of the same patient shown in **Fig. 12** at 5 years of age.

associated with cardiac arrhythmias. Fluoroscopy was used intraoperatively to assist in lead placement. The ICD lead was actively fixed to the pericardium after its positioning in the transverse sinus. Epicardial pace/sense leads were placed via the same subxiphoid incision (**Fig. 15**).

The largest series of pediatric and congenital heart disease patients receiving ICDs was

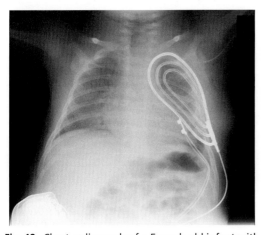

Fig. 12. Chest radiograph of a 5-week-old infant with long QT syndrome, with ICD subcutaneous patch electrode and epicardial pace/sense leads. See text for details.

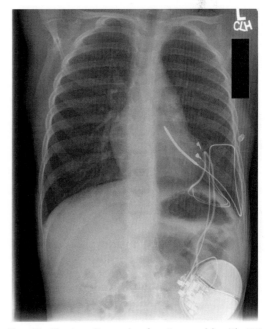

Fig. 14. Chest radiograph of a 5-year-old with ICD lead in the pericardial space. See text for details.

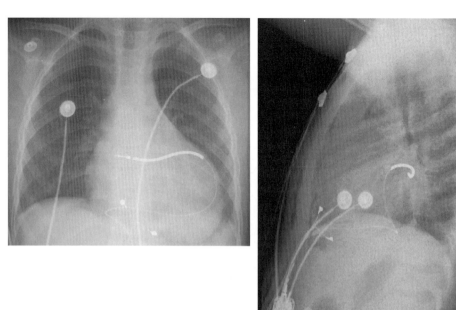

Fig. 15. Posteroanterior and lateral chest radiographs of a pediatric patient with ICD lead in the transverse pericardial sinus. See text for details. (*From* Hsia TY, Bradley SM, LaPage MJ, et al. Novel minimally invasive, intrapericardial implantable cardioverter-defibrillator coil system: a useful approach to arrhythmia therapy in children. Ann Thorac Surg 2009;87:1236; with permission.)

a multicenter collection of described surgical approaches in 22 patients reported from 11 pediatric centers in the United States and Europe.[15] The decision to use a nonconventional approach was based predominantly on patient size in 17 patients. The general approach was use of a subcutaneous array-based system as described by Berul, although 9 of the 22 configurations included a transvenous design lead placed on the epicardium. The small number of patients reported across a large number of centers illustrates the infrequency with which these approaches are used. And this infrequency, which indicates a tiny potential market, may help to explain why innovations in lead and pulse generator technology directed specifically at this patient group have been slow to emerge from industry.

Miscellaneous Approaches

An approach to intrapericardial lead placement in adult patients is to loop the ICD lead in the pericardial space around the heart, fixing it to the pericardium to prevent migration and maintain integrity of the loop (**Fig. 16**).[16] This approach is similar to the pericardial approach already described for pediatric patients, but with more generous anatomy in the adult there is sufficient territory to create a loop that may optimize the defibrillation shock vector.

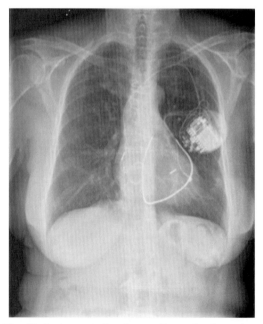

Fig. 16. Posteroanterior chest radiograph of a patient with ICD lead looped in the pericardial space. See text for details. (*From* Bhakta M, Obioha CC, Sorajja DA, et al. Nontraditional implantable cardioverter-defibrillator placement in adult patients with limited venous access: a case series. Pacing Clin Electrophysiol 2010;33:222; with permission.)

When venous access is severely limited but endocardial anatomy permits, pace/sense and ICD lead hardware can be placed transmyocardially, typically via an atriotomy and with the use of standard stylets, into the appropriate cardiac chambers. A 65-year-old patient with no venous access from the subclavian veins and with retroperitoneal fibrosis limiting access from the inferior vena cava underwent a limited right thoracotomy and intraoperative, fluoroscopically guided placement of right atrial and coronary sinus pacing leads and a right ventricular ICD lead.[17] In 2 pediatric patients with unfavorable anatomy for a percutaneous approach, a similar transatrial approach was taken.[18]

Many of the approaches described here seek to minimize the extent of tissue invasion with the use small incisions and clever lead delivery systems. Video-assisted pericardioscopy has been used experimentally for delivery of pacing leads to various epicardial sites.[19] It is likely that such an approach can be adapted for placement of bulkier ICD leads. This development raises the possibility that difficulties encountered during traditional or novel transvenous access attempts may be solved at the time such difficulties are encountered by changing to a minimally invasive pericardioscopic approach in the device implantation laboratory.

SUMMARY

Implantation of cardioverter-defibrillator systems in patients with compromised central venous access, patients with acquired or iatrogenic barriers to standard lead positioning, and patients with congenital heart disease requires careful assessment of patient anatomy and use of lead delivery systems in novel, unorthodox ways. Novel transvenous placement of intrathoracic hardware, as well as use of the pericardial space and subcutaneous tissue compartments can allow safe and effective use of this therapy in this group of patients.

REFERENCES

1. Bardy GH, Smith WM, Hood MA, et al. An entirely subcutaneous cardioverter-defibrillator. N Engl J Med 2010;363:36–44.
2. Giudici MC, Paul DL, Meierbachtol CJ. Active-can implantable cardioverter defibrillator placement from a femoral approach. Pacing Clin Electrophysiol 2003;26:1297–8.
3. Eldadah ZA, Donahue K. Successful implantable cardioverter defibrillator placement in an ambulatory patient without thoracic vein access. J Cardiovasc Electrophysiol 2004;15:716–8.
4. McCotter CJ, Angle JF, Prudente LA, et al. Placement of transvenous pacemaker and ICD leads across total chronic occlusions. Pacing Clin Electrophysiol 2005;28:921–5.
5. Gula LJ, Ames A, Woodburn A, et al. Central venous occlusion is not an obstacle to device upgrade with the assistance of laser extraction. Pacing Clin Electrophysiol 2005;28:661–8.
6. Aleksic I, Kottenberg-Assenmacher E, Kienbaum P, et al. The innominate vein as alternative venous access for complicated implantable cardioverter defibrillator revisions. Pacing Clin Electrophysiol 2007;30:957–60.
7. Lin G, Nishimura R, Connolly H, et al. Severe symptomatic tricuspid valve regurgitation due to permanent pacemaker or implantable cardioverter-defibrillator leads. J Am Coll Cardiol 2005;45:1672–5.
8. Grimard C, May M, Babuty D. An original defibrillation lead implantation to avoid tricuspid prosthesis damage. Europace 2010;4:589–90.
9. Biffi M, Bertini M, Ziacchi M, et al. Transvenous cardioverter-defibrillator implantation in a patient with tricuspid mechanical prosthesis. J Cardiovasc Electrophysiol 2007;18:329–31.
10. Available at: http://en.wikipedia.org/wiki/Azygos_vein. Accessed October 14, 2010.
11. Cooper JS, Latacha MP, Soto GE, et al. The azygous defibrillator lead for elevated defibrillation thresholds: implant technique, lead stability, and patient series. Pacing Clin Electrophysiol 2008; 31:1405–10.
12. Bar-Cohen Y, Takao AM, Wells WJ, et al. Novel use of a vascular plug to anchor an azygous vein ICD lead. J Cardiovasc Electrophysiol 2010;21:99–102.
13. Berul CI, Triedman JK, Forbess J, et al. Minimally invasive cardioverter defibrillator implantation for children. Pacing Clin Electrophysiol 2001;24: 1789–94.
14. Hsia TY, Bradley SM, LaPage MJ, et al. Novel minimally invasive, intrapericardial implantable cardioverter defibrillator coil system: a useful approach to arrhythmia therapy in children. Ann Thorac Surg 2009;87:1234–9.
15. Stephenson EA, Batra AS, Knilans TK, et al. A multicenter experience with novel implantable cardioverter defibrillator configurations in the pediatric and congenital heart disease population. J Cardiovasc Electrophysiol 2006;17:1–6.
16. Bhakta M, Obioha CC, Sorajja DA, et al. Nontraditional implantable cardioverter defibrillator placement in adult patients with limited venous access: a case series. Pacing Clin Electrophysiol 2010;33: 217–25.
17. Giudici M, Augelli NV, Longo CA, et al. Endovascular bi-ventricular pacing-defibrillator placement using a transatrial approach. J Interv Card Electrophysiol 2010;27:143–5.

18. Cannon BC, Friedman RA, Fenrich AL, et al. Innovative techniques for placement of implantable cardioverter-defibrillator leads in patients with limited venous access to the heart. Pacing Clin Electrophysiol 2006;29:181–7.

19. Hatam N, Amerini AL, Stenier F, et al. Video-assisted pericardioscopic surgery: refinement of a new technique for implanting epimyocardial pacemaker leads. Eur J Cardiothorac Surg 2010. DOI:10.1016/j.ejcts.06.016.

Caring for the Heart and Mind in ICD Patients

Jessica Ford, MA[a], Katherine E. Cutitta, BA[a],
Lawrence K. Woodrow, MA[a], Kari Kirian, MA[a],
Samuel F. Sears, PhD[a,b,*]

KEYWORDS

- Implantable cardioverter-defibrillator
- Psychosocial functioning • Quality of life

The implantable cardioverter-defibrillator (ICD) is the premier treatment for patients at risk for sudden cardiac arrest. The successes of clinical trials in reducing mortality allow a greater focus on the psychological and patient-centered outcomes following implantation with an ICD. Anxiety and/or depressive symptoms are common (ranging from 13% to 48% of patients). This psychological morbidity is often related to coping with a chronic cardiac condition, implantation of the ICD, experience or anticipation of defibrillation, and mortality concerns.[1] At present, a major focus of patient-centered ICD research is to reduce these negative psychological effects by employing educational, supportive, and cognitive-behavioral interventions.[2–4] ICD-specific education provided in face-to face settings or electronically on such topics as managing arrhythmias, review of medications, ICD purpose and function, return to activities, and symptom and device monitoring have helped patients understand and accept their condition.[3] Providing social support in the form of nursing contact, patient calls, and support groups can reduce psychological distress and improve physiologic functioning.[3] Finally, cognitive-behavioral therapy (CBT) has demonstrated effectiveness in decreasing anxiety and depression in patients who fear their ICD, instead of embracing it as a source of protection.[2,4] Through systematic interventions, the risk of psychological morbidity can be reduced in ICD patients. This article discusses the psychosocial impact of ICD implantation and shock, risk and resiliency factors of psychosocial distress, recent advances in psychosocial treatment of patients with ICDs, and clinical management strategies that can be used by electrophysiologists and cardiologists in managing patients with ICDs and psychological comorbidities.

PSYCHOSOCIAL OUTCOMES POST-ICD IMPLANT AND SHOCK

Psychological adjustment to cardiac conditions and the implantation of a biomedical device can represent a significant stressor that can tax an individual's or a family's coping abilities. Both the recognition of the seriousness of the disease state and the reliance on the ICD prompt some psychological accommodation of its meaning and impact. Despite advances in ICD technology, patients may still have difficulty adjusting to life with an ICD. In fact, as many as 24% of patients with an ICD report low treatment satisfaction,[5] prompting

Disclosures: Dr Sears serves as a consultant to Medtronic and has or has had research grants from Medtronic and St Jude Medical. All funds are directed to East Carolina University. Dr Sears also has received speaker honorarium from Medtronic, Boston Scientific, St Jude Medical, and Biotronik. No other authors have disclosures to report.
[a] Department of Psychology, East Carolina University, East Fifth Street, Greenville, NC 27858, USA
[b] Department of Cardiovascular Sciences, East Carolina University, East Carolina Heart Institute, Heart Drive, Greenville, NC 27834, USA
* Corresponding author. 104 Rawl Building, East Carolina University, Greenville, NC 27858.
E-mail address: searss@ecu.edu

Card Electrophysiol Clin 3 (2011) 451–462
doi:10.1016/j.ccep.2011.05.010

further investigations of patient-centric outcomes. Normative concerns of ICD patients often addressed in cardiac clinics are wide ranging but can include reliance and acceptance of living with technology,[6–8] coping with shock and storm,[8,9] body image concerns,[10] dealing with recall,[11,12] and sexual dysfunction.[13–15] These concerns may affect device acceptance, which can be defined as understanding and psychologically accommodating the advantages and disadvantages of having an ICD, in addition to deriving biomedical, psychological, and social functioning benefits from the ICD.[7] Device acceptance is important because those ICD patients with high device acceptance are also more likely to have greater quality of life (QOL) than ICD patients with low device acceptance.[6] Patients with lower device acceptance are also more likely to have symptomatic heart failure, type D personality, anxiety symptoms, or depressive symptoms. Device acceptance is also lower in the elderly and in patients without partners.[16] These concerns or low device acceptance may result in feelings of distress or anger. Even these normative emotional responses have been shown to induce arrhythmogenic T-wave alternans.[17,18] Above and beyond normative concerns and emotional experience are more acute psychological comorbidities such as anxiety and depression. Methods of addressing normative concerns and prophylaxis of psychological comorbidity are discussed in further detail in the section "Clinical management of critical events."

Anxiety

General or ICD-specific anxiety as a psychological morbidity presents itself in 13% to 38% of ICD recipients.[19–21] Recent longitudinal assessment of anxiety over the course of the first year of ICD implant indicated that approximately 35% of patients at baseline reported significant anxiety, while approximately 15% of patients reported anxiety at 6-month and 12-month follow-up without any specific treatment.[22] In another longitudinal study, the chronicity of anxiety in defibrillator patients was further supported, with 54% of patients anxious at implantation still clinically anxious at 12 months.[23] Anxiety is associated with avoidance of activities as means of "playing it safe," which can reduce the ICD patient's engagement and enjoyment in life. At some level, anxiety is a reaction to the "threat of loss" of functional independence or QOL, and that description fits well here. Self-reported anxiety has also been linked to self-reported general health in ICD patients.[24] Anxiety has been found to increase

the likelihood of mortality and cardiovascular events in patients with heart disease.[25,26] For the ICD patient, anxiety may also be particularly focused on shock anxiety rather than on more generalized anxiety foci.[27]

Anxiety reactions are understandable given that ICD patients have perhaps already faced a near-death experience or have certainly had to face news of their high risk for sudden cardiac death. Recently, the posttraumatic stress disorder (PTSD)-ICD connection was demonstrated to be prevalent, distressing, and potentially deadly. Ladwig and colleagues[28] found that 20% of ICD patients reported significant PTSD symptoms, which summated to a 3.2-times greater likelihood of mortality within 5 years compared with ICD patients with no to moderate symptom levels of PTSD, even after controlling for cardiac disease burden, age, and sex. These data provide further support for expanding the cardiac clinic focus to psychosocial functioning in ICD patients.

Depression

Significant depressive symptoms manifest across all cardiac patient populations and affect between 18% and 33% of ICD patients.[29,30] Some have even noted this prevalence to be as high as 41%.[19] The shock experience has been compared with "learned helplessness." Repeatedly experiencing negative events (eg, cardiac arrest, myocardial infarction, heart failure diagnosis, defibrillations, ICD storm, recall) creates a reduction in patients' belief in their ability to cope and attempts to manage illness.[31,32] Depressive symptoms may also mark risk for increased shock. The Triggers of Ventricular Arrhythmias (TOVA) study examined baseline depressive scores and their prospective clinical impact (N = 645). Rates of depression were approximately 18%, and the depressed group was more likely to receive shock and receive a shock sooner in the follow-up period.[30]

Depressive personality features have also been explored and posited as the type D personality. Individuals with type D personality traits have a tendency toward worry, gloominess, and social inhibition, which are associated with higher rates of depression.[33] In a set of 371 ICD patients, type D personality was found in 22.4% of the sample.[34] In addition to being associated with depression in patients with ICDs, type D personality is also associated with chronic anxiety in these patients.[23] Those patients with anxiety and type D personality traits are at greater risk of ventricular arrhythmia (hazard ratio [HR]: 1.89) than other ICD patients.[24] Furthermore, patients with type D personality traits prior to implantation with ICD are also at greater risk of mortality at 2-year follow-up (HR: 2.79) than patients who did not endorse these personality traits.[34]

In summary, the psychosocial functioning of ICD patients is increasingly well studied and has demonstrated significant impact in key medical and patient-centric outcomes such as shock.[30] This aspect is especially important given that appropriate and inappropriate shock have been associated with increased mortality.[35]

RISK AND RESILIENCY FACTORS FOR PSYCHOSOCIAL DISTRESS

Stratification of psychosocial risk has been a research focus because access to specialty mental health services such as a cardiac psychologist is not common. This section reviews risk factors that can be used to help identify patients who may be in need of specialty services.

Demographic Factors Predicting Adjustment to ICD Implantation

Demographically, women and patients younger than 50 years tend to be at greatest risk for developing psychological problems following ICD implantation or shock.[16,36] Young ICD patients may view their cardiac condition as "age inappropriate" and disruptive to more aspects of daily life including key periods of developmental, social, and familial processes.[37] For example, among patients younger than 40 years with ICDs 63% have concerns about clothing fit, 75% have concerns about their ability to socialize with the ICD, and 50% have concerns about the ICD's impact on sexual activity.[38] In addition, younger patients tend to have the greatest decrease in social support following ICD implantation.[39,40] Lower social support is also a predictor of anxiety development in ICD patients.[41]

Women, specifically those younger than 50 years, also have greater difficulty adjusting to ICD implantation.[36] In women, body image is a significant concern due to the visibility of the implant and scar. Some electrophysiologists have attempted to reduce these concerns with submammary implantation of the device.[10] Also, somatosensory amplification, or a tendency to focus on bodily sensations and appraise them as abnormal, tends to be higher in women and has been found to mediate the sex differences in anxiety levels of patients with defibrillators.[42] Additional concerns facing women with ICDs are role reentry, concerns about child bearing and routine mammograms, and sensitivity of breast tissue during recovery.[43] Collectively, women have specific needs related to coping with their device. Women have benefited from customized psychosocial treatment.[44]

Device-Triggered Factors Predicting Adjustment to ICD Implantation

Multiple reviews on the QOL outcomes of ICD patients are now available.[45–48] The results generally suggest that ICD patients have QOL reports at least equal to, if not better than patients treated with antiarrhythmic medications. In addition, patients receiving biventricular pacing or cardiac resynchronization therapy via their ICD have also been shown to have improvements in attention and information processing.[49] However, these discussions have generally focused on the impact of shock on QOL. Recently, Pedersen and colleagues[50] reviewed the sizeable 7 primary or secondary prevention trials that assessed QOL and suggested that the existing evidence does not universally implicate ICD shock as a QOL spoiler. In short, they suggest that the research evidence of the negative impact is mixed when measured with generic QOL instruments, and instead point toward the need for greater attention to individual factors such as personality, psychological distress, and device-specific QOL measurement. In an accompanying editorial, Sears and Kirian[51] suggested that ICD shocks remain a "critical" event, because they are a significant "clinical" event that warrants expert handling to make adjustments medically and psychologically. Regardless, shock remains a focus for patients and providers and was the subject of recent American and European articles suggesting comprehensive management spanning medical and psychological care.[52,53] Despite questions regarding the impact of one defibrillation, there is a substantial amount of evidence that patients who experience greater than 5 shocks or a shock storm have lower QOL and greater emotional distress.[54–59] In addition to pain, following defibrillation many patients become hypervigilant to internal physiology, avoid activities they associate with the shock experience, and catastrophize the meaning of the defibrillation (eg, associating defibrillation with increased potential for future defibrillations or worsening of cardiac condition), resulting in a cycle of diminishing QOL.[4]

Factors Predicting Resiliency Following ICD Implantation

Beyond the characteristics predicting maladjustment, resiliency factors have also been identified that are likely to increase the ability to cope with the demands of living with an ICD. Specifically, optimism has been found to buffer against reductions in QOL.[60] In fact, among 88 patients implanted with ICDs, those with more optimism prior to surgery had greater subsequent mental health and social functioning at 8-month and 14-month follow-up than those lower on the personality trait. In addition, ICD patients with greater levels of positive health expectations before the surgery reported greater satisfaction with their overall health than those with lower positive health expectations. Characteristics specifically targeted in most CBTs have also been found to buffer against psychological distress, including coping style and the patients' appraisal of their ability to cope with the challenges of living with an ICD.[61] Specifically, problem-focused coping style and low threat and challenge appraisal were significantly predictive of having less total mood disturbance. Mood was significantly predictive of functional status at 3 months after surgery. Appraisal of control over cardiac condition, coping resources, and the effects of the ICD on the patient's social world are also predictors of resilience.[61]

Overall, patients who are young (<50 years old), are female, have a premorbid psychiatric diagnosis, have inadequate social support, or have a history of receiving greater than 5 defibrillations are most likely to experience psychological distress. For quick reference, **Table 1** presents the research-indicated risk and resiliency factors for developing psychological sequelae following ICD implantation or shock.

Although these general risk factors for psychosocial distress may be helpful in identifying patients in need, they are neither sensitive nor specific enough to rely on completely. Knowledge of the symptoms of anxiety, depression, and PTSD, and the way these symptoms present in ICD patients, can be applied to assist in clinical decision making. **Table 2** shows symptoms of anxiety, depression, and PTSD according to the *Diagnostic and Statistical Manual of Mental Disorders* (Fourth Edition, Text Revised) (DSM IV-TR)[62] and ways these symptoms may present in an ICD patient. Assessment using ICD-specific measures of device acceptance, adjustment, QOL, and psychological distress can provide additional data points from which to determine the best course of action in ICD patient care.[43]

CLINICAL MANAGEMENT OF CRITICAL EVENTS TO IMPROVE QUALITY OF LIFE IN PATIENTS

Psychosocial functioning ICD patients can be addressed in clinical encounters. Following implantation, after the experience of defibrillation, in case of recall, and at the end of life are all time points when impactful discussion can reduce the likelihood of future distress.

Perioperative

Following implantation with an ICD, patients may have a variety of questions. In addition to curiosities about the device and its function, it is likely that questions about activity restrictions and change of social role will arise. Dunbar[63] suggests that providers deliver information about the implantation, the device itself, defibrillation, expected psychological responses, and behavioral methods of preventing arrhythmias to patients with ICDs and their families in efforts to reduce normative distress related to receiving a device. It is important that early in the patient-provider relationship a dialog begins in which feeling safe, becoming a survivor rather than a victim, reengaging in activities, and bolstering relationship support are emphasized as key components of physical and psychological recovery.[64]

The first goal of communication following implantation should be engendering feelings of safety. Patients can be reassured that every effort to reduce the potential of defibrillation is being made.[65] For example, understanding the purpose of antitachycardia pacing, medication usage and adherence, and programming specificities may be particularly reassuring for patients. Further, taking active steps to help the patient manage the behavioral components of cardiovascular disease can go a long way in promoting feelings of control and safety (eg, medication adherence,

---

Table 1
Risk and resiliency factors in patients with implantable cardioverter-defibrillators

Risk Factors	Resiliency Factors

• Age <50 years
• Female gender
• Shocks, especially if >5
• Premorbid psychological difficulties
• Low social support
• Poor understanding of condition and device
• More severe medical condition
	• Optimism/positive health expectations
	• Problem focused coping orientation
	• Low appraisal of threat of the ICD
	• Social Support
	  ○ Patient-provider relationship
	  ○ Family/caregivers
	• Faith in ICD and doctor
	• Informed about cardiac condition and device
	• Active lifestyle of work/recreation

Table 2
Presentation of psychological distress in patients with implantable cardioverter-defibrillators

Psychological Disorder	Main DSM IV-TR Criteria	Examples of Presentation in ICD Patients
Depression	• Depressed mood • Loss of interest or pleasure • Significant weight loss or gain • Insomnia or hypersomnia • Psychomotor agitation or retardation • Fatigue or loss of energy • Feelings of worthlessness or excessive guilt • Difficulty concentrating • Recurrent thoughts of death	• Feelings of sadness that they must rely on the ICD or related to severity of cardiac condition • Patient reports he or she no longer desires to participate in recreational or work activities, due to the ICD "getting in the way" or fear that others will ask about/be concerned about the ICD
Anxiety	• Excessive anxiety or worry that is difficult to control • Restlessness • Difficulty concentrating • Irritability • Muscle tension • Sleep disturbance	• Frequent worry about cardiac condition or potential for defibrillation • Fidgeting in clinic • Chest pain related to tension in intercostals

Posttraumatic stress	• Exposure to a traumatic event
	  ○ With perceived threat of death/ serious injury
	  ○ Feelings of fear, helplessness, or horror
	• Reexperiencing
	• Avoidance
	• Increased arousal
	• Duration >1 month
		• Trauma event:
		  ○ Sudden cardiac arrest
		  ○ Surgery
		  ○ Defibrillation
		• Nightmares about defibrillation, phantom shocks, ruminates about the shock
		• Avoids places or stimuli associated with the shock
		• Constantly monitoring bodily functions: always aware of heart rate, periventricular contractions, or any sense of chest pain

improving dietary habits, increasing physical activity, and reducing tobacco use).[64]

Psychological adjustment can include encouraging a sense of survivorship. Patients with heart disease may feel like victims of the disease. It is helpful to communicate to patients that their decision to protect themselves from sudden cardiac arrest with an ICD indicates strength. Reinforce that living with an ICD has challenges, but as survivors they are well equipped to handle these challenges. Providing patients with tools will help elicit genuine feelings of survivorship and safety. One such tool is a "shock plan." The gold-standard plan has 3 recommendations: if the patient feels fine following a single defibrillation he or she is encouraged to call the clinic during business hours; however, if the patient experiences a single shock and does not feel well or if he/she experiences multiple shocks, he or she is encouraged to seek emergency care.[65] Shock plans can be discussed and given as a handout for quick reference.

Promoting reengagement in activities can be paramount to patients with ICDs.[66] Following implantation with an ICD, patients may feel fearful of overworking their hearts. Substantial evidence supports referral to cardiac rehabilitation programs as an effective method of engagement.[66] Cardiac rehabilitation provides a safe place where patients can improve not only their cardiac functioning but also confidence in their remaining physical abilities. In addition, it is important to provide accurate information and dispel myths regarding what patients are and are not able to do (eg, arc welding).

Patients can also be encouraged to discuss the ICD with their family members and caregivers. Enlisting social support is not only beneficial to the patient, but can reduce the psychological distress of family members. Marx and colleagues found in a sample of 82 family members of ICD patients that emotional distress was highest at time of implant. Stress during these times of recovery and adjustment may be assuaged with education and open discussion.[67] "Coping with my partner's

ICD and cardiac disease" from the *Cardiology Patient Page* may be a good resource that can be provided to patients' caregivers. In this article, 16 strategies are suggested for adjusting to the ICD, managing psychological distress, and maintaining relationships.[68]

Following Defibrillation

The experience of shock can reawaken anxieties that had been assuaged following implantation. Following defibrillation, patients often believe that they are at greater risk for future shocks. Clinicians can explain that defibrillation does not always mean a worsening cardiac condition or that there is greater risk of future shock. It can be helpful to describe why the patient received the shock (eg, hypokalemia, ventricular fibrillation) and that this is unrelated to the activity they were engaged in at the time. Often, defibrillation reduces patients' faith in the device and their future. Patients may need help to refocus on the fact that living with an ICD shows their commitment to living. Clinicians can accentuate a survivorship mentality and remind patients about their tools of coping.

Perhaps the most QOL-reducing behavior following defibrillation is avoidance of activity. Following defibrillation, a classic conditioning response is common in patients with ICDs. A variety of stimuli may be associated with the event; including physiologic arousal (eg, increased heart rate) or external cues (eg, the couch where the patient was sitting). Some patients begin avoiding these stimuli altogether, slowly reducing the number of activities in which they feel safe. Educating patients about the normalcy of this reaction, and reassuring them that physical activity or other stimuli that preceded shock are safe, are crucial.[64] Cardiac rehabilitation or repeated stress test exposures are also helpful in patients who fear that physical activity will induce a cardiac event.

In the Case of Recall

Device recall is a reality many patients must face. All of the major device companies have had recalls in the last decade.[69] Under the threat of recall, many patients overestimate the likelihood that their device could fail. In fact, Gibson and colleagues[69] found that 71% of patients undergoing recall overestimate the probability that the device will fail. In this sample, patients also reported feelings of anxiety (36%), anger (13%), sadness (13%), and frustration (23%). Studies examining the effect of device recall on general and device-specific QOL, clinical anxiety, and depressive symptoms have been inconclusive.[11,70,71] However, there is evidence that patients experience anxiety related to device recall, regardless of whether or not the recall is for their device.[12]

Patients with ICDs reported significantly more confidence in device recall information when the source was their physician or a manufacturer rather than the media.[12] Keren and colleagues[71] conducted a survey of 416 ICD patients. Patients in the advisory group for a recall of Fidelis leads did not have increased depression, anxiety, shock anxiety, or lower device acceptance than nonadvisory patients; unless they experienced inappropriate shock or lead fracture. Thirty-seven percent of patients with a fractured lead had significant anxiety. This number jumped to nearly 50% if they also had inappropriate shock. Depression was similarly elevated (43.7%) in patients who experienced inappropriate shock. Device acceptance was also negatively affected by lead fracture and inappropriate shock related to recall.

Perhaps the most obvious way to help patients experiencing recall of a device is clarification of the risk associated with recall and generator change. As stated before, patients regularly overestimate their risk.[70] Overall, risk of device failure ranges from 0.009% to 2.6%, with an average of a 0.44% risk.[72] However, a study of 732 generator change outs at the Mayo Clinic in Rochester found the risk of complication following surgery to be 1.24%. Overall, risk of device failure and surgical complications of replacement are very low.[72] In a study examining the effect of recall, in which participants and their families were debriefed regarding the risk related to recall and given an opportunity to ask questions in addition to individual meetings with their electrophysiologist, device acceptance was not lower in ICD patients experiencing recall.[70] In addition, an intervention study examined the effects of brief nurse-delivered counseling intended to reduce overestimation of risk following recall in 100 patients.[73] Worry significantly dropped following intervention, and this reduction in worry was maintained at a 6-month follow-up.

End of Life

Taking care of patients during end of life can be difficult for patients, families, and physicians. According to family members, only 27 of a sample of 100 patients at end of life had conversations about deactivating their ICD as they neared death.[74] In addition, these conversations were often the result of acute crisis rather than planned discussion. Recently, an expert consensus statement was published that centered on managing requests for withdrawal of ICD therapy near the end of life.[75] The statement provides some clarification regarding ethical and religious issues of defibrillator deactivation in various populations. Key discussions about end of life should be had at various time points in care for patients with ICDs. Points of discussion regarding end of life throughout the continuum of care are integrated in **Table 3**. It is highly recommended that discussions regarding end of life include patients' families and caregivers, as they may potentially become legal surrogates or proxies in the case that patients are no longer competent to make their own decisions. Discussion with family members and caregivers about end of life, the patient's illness, the device, goals of care, and desired outcomes are also likely to reduce distress in family members that may adversely affect the patient.

Methods of reducing psychological distress vary depending on the time at which the patient expresses concerns (ranging from before implantation to after electrical storm) and extent of psychological distress. For this reason, a continuum of care providing different forms of support at different stages should be in place for patients who require this technology. **Table 3** shows the ICD time-point spectrum with associated education and discussion suggestions.

Using Mental Health Professionals

Should psychosocial adjustment remain difficult for a patient following discussion of these strategies for coping, referral to a mental health professional is the best practice. In a review of psychosocial treatments for ICD patients by Salmoirago-Blotcher and Ockene,[76] the investigators concluded that overall, CBT is most effective in reducing anxiety and depression.

Most CBT interventions for ICD patients include ICD-specific education, shock planning, relaxation and stress management techniques, as well as cognitive and behavioral techniques.[2,4,77–79] Some of the newer CBT interventions also include symptom management,[80] exercise or cardiac rehabilitation components,[81–83] social or group support,[4,82–85] coverage of female-specific ICD concerns,[44] and more technological computer-based intervention.[85] The majority of these interventions focus on ICD patients, but lack a component specifically tailored to the anxiety response following defibrillation. Sears' "Shock and Stress Management Protocol" is one intervention, including a specific focus on helping patients who have experienced shock to regain QOL and device acceptance as well as on reducing anxiety about future shocks.[4] Among studies that found reduction of depression, the majority include an exercise or cardiac rehabilitation component.[76]

These studies were also shown to significantly increase physical functioning. However, small sample size is a significant limitation of the majority of these studies. Recently, Lewin and colleagues[83] demonstrated that providing patients with information before and after surgery in addition to 3 brief telephone contacts with a trained allied health professional reduced anxiety, depression, limitations in physical activity, and health care costs in a large randomized control trial (N = 192). Collectively, there are a variety of evidence-based interventions that have been shown to help a variety of different groups of ICD patients across the continuum of experience related to living with an ICD.

Support Groups

Support groups give patients an opportunity to obtain practical information about life with an ICD, meet others with ICDs, and secure emotional support.[79] Themes of helpful support groups include the exploration of patient perspectives through story telling; triggers that encourage help-seeking in the group; provision of meaningful information about what to expect, what's normal, how and why the device works, and what to do after shock; group camaraderie; use of an empowering expert facilitator; and inclusion of caregivers and support persons.[86]

Studies examining the effects of patient support groups on psychosocial and health outcomes are few in number, have small sample sizes, and regularly lack randomized controls.[87–89] However, there has been one randomized control trial examining an intervention including 2 meetings with a support group, telehealth, and in-person individual meetings with a psychiatric nurse.[90] Both the intervention and control group benefited over time and the investigators concluded that there is limited additional benefit of support groups for ICD patients. These conclusions may be premature because of the relatively small sample size (N = 34) and small dose of support group treatment. Although there is a paucity of evidence that support groups improve psychosocial or health outcomes as yet, the venue of a social support group can be maintained for little cost or effort and can provide benefit to patients in distress. In fact, Myers and James[91] found that those with greater anxiety and lower social support self-selected to participate in a support group. Unfortunately, the effect of the group itself was not measured. Taken together, the research regarding support groups is inconclusive. However, there is likely clinical utility in providing these inexpensive group services.

Table 3
The continuum of care: impactful discussion with ICD patients about critical events

Time Point	Perioperative	Following Defibrillation	In the Case of Recall	End of Life
Discussion points	Thoroughly cover patients' cardiac condition Clarify the purpose of the device Explain how the device works (eg, pacing, defibrillation) Create shock plan Emphasize safety of activities while clarifying activities to avoid (eg, arc welding) Attempt to include family/caregivers Encourage patients to create an advanced directive/living will Inform of potential future deactivation if desired at end of life	Emphasize that defibrillation is not indicative of worsening cardiac condition Stress steps taken to prevent future arrhythmias and defibrillations Review shock plan Encourage reengagement in activities/situations associated with shock Discuss experience with caregivers and family members if possible Assess for excessive shock anxiety, lowered device acceptance, or trauma reaction	Inform patients of recall If their device is included in the recall, discuss risk of device failure and risk of surgical intervention Try to reassure and reestablish faith in the device Attempt to include families and caregivers	Explore the patient's understanding of the device and his or her conceptualization of resuscitation Assist patient in reevaluating the benefits and burdens of the ICD Discuss patient's continued needs (eg, continued use of the ICD at full capacity, continued pacing without defibrillation capabilities, complete deactivation) Assess patient's quality of life, functional status, and need to refer to palliative care or supportive services Encourage inclusion of family members/caregivers

SUMMARY

Achieving the full value of the ICD by receiving protection from sudden cardiac arrest and achieving optimal QOL requires increased systematic assessment and care-of-patient perspectives. ICD patients are unique because they require medical care to control the progression of cardiac disease as well as psychosocial care aimed at addressing adjustment issues of living with biomedical technology. Patients with ICDs have a greater prevalence of anxiety and depression than the general public.[1] Many, even those who do not develop a psychological disorder, have concerns about living with an ICD that requires attention and care. Normative concerns across the continuum of care can be addressed in the context of a series of empathic and thorough discussions.[64] Additional screening of patients for the risk and resiliency factors of psychosocial distress (eg, age <50, female gender, shock experience),[16,36] the use of validated disease-specific measures,[43] and evaluating patients for the signs and symptoms of psychological distress can help identify patients who need more support. At present, the best option for these patients is a cognitive-behavioral intervention provided by a qualified mental health provider.[76] Support groups may also be helpful for patients learning to cope with life after device implantation.[89] Patients with ICDs have the best medical treatment available. However, this is only half of the picture. Electrophysiologists and cardiologists who work with these patients face the challenge of providing therapeutic care of both the heart and the mind.

REFERENCES

1. Sears S, Conti J. Understanding implantable cardioverter defibrillator shocks and storms: medical and psychosocial considerations for research and clinical care. Clin Cardiol 2003;26:107–11.
2. Kohn C, Petrucci R, Baessler C, et al. The effect of psychological intervention on patients' long-term adjustment to the ICD: a prospective study. Pacing Clin Electrophysiol 2000;23:450–6.
3. Matchett M, Kirian K, Hazelton G, et al. Common presenting psychosocial problems for implantable cardioverter defibrillator patients: a primer for consulting professionals. In: Sher L, editor. Psychological factors and cardiovascular disorders. Hauppauge (NY): Nova Sciences Publishers, Inc; 2009. p. 331–49.
4. Sears S, Sowell L, Kuhl E, et al. The ICD shock and stress management program: a randomized trial of psychosocial treatment to optimize quality of life in ICD patients. Pacing Clin Electrophysiol 2007;30: 858–64.
5. Ladwig K-H, Deisenhofer I, Simon H, et al. Characteristics associated with low treatment satisfaction in patients with implanted cardioverter defibrillators: results from the LICAD study. Pacing Clin Electrophysiol 2005;28:506–13.
6. Burns J, Sears S, Sotile R, et al. Do patients accept implantable atrial defibrillation therapy? Results from the Patient Atrial Shock Survey of Acceptance and Tolerance (PASSAT) Study. J Cardiovasc Electrophysiol 2004;15:286–92.
7. Burns J, Serber E, Keim S, et al. Measuring patient acceptance of implantable cardiac device therapy: initial psychometric investigation of the Florida Patient Acceptance Survey. J Cardiovasc Electrophysiol 2005;16:384–90.
8. Sears S, Conti J. Psychological aspects of cardiac devices and recalls in patients with implantable cardioverter defibrillators. Am J Cardiol 2006;98: 565–7.
9. Kuijpers P, Honig A, Wellens H. Effect of treatment of panic disorder in patients with frequent ICD discharges: a pilot study. Gen Hosp Psychiatry 2002;24:181–4.
10. Sowell L, Kuhl E, Sears S, et al. Device implant technique and consideration of body image: specific procedures for implantable cardioverter defibrillators in female patients. J Womens Health (Larchmt) 2006;15:830–5.
11. Cuculi F, Herzig W, Kobza R, et al. Psychological distress in patients with ICD recall. Pacing Clin Electrophysiol 2006;29:1261–5.
12. Stutts L, Conti J, Aranda J, et al. Patient evaluation of ICD recall communication strategies: a vignette study. Pacing Clin Electrophysiol 2007;30:1105–11.
13. Steinke E. Sexual concerns of patients and partners after an implantable cardioverter defibrillator. Dimens Crit Care Nurs 2003;22:89–96.
14. Steinke E, Gill-Hopple K, Valdez D, et al. Sexual concerns and educational needs after an implantable cardioverter defibrillator. Heart Lung 2005;34: 299–308.
15. Vazquez L, Sears S, Shea J, et al. Sexual health for patients with an implantable cardioverter defibrillator. Circulation 2010;122:465–7.
16. Pedersen S, Spindler H, Johansen J, et al. Correlates of patient acceptance of the cardioverter defibrillator: cross-validation of the Florida Patient Acceptance Survey in Danish patients. Pacing Clin Electrophysiol 2008;31:1168–77.
17. Lampert R. Anger and ventricular arrhythmias. Curr Opin Cardiol 2010;25:46–52.
18. Lampert R, Shusterman V, Burg M, et al. Anger-induced T-wave alternans predicts future ventricular arrhythmias in patients with implantable cardioverter-defibrillators. J Am Coll Cardiol 2009;53:774–8.

19. Bilge A, Ozben B, Demircan S, et al. Depression and anxiety status of patients with implantable cardioverter defibrillator and precipitating factors. Pacing Clin Electrophysiol 2006;29:619–26.

20. Griegel L, Black C, Goulden L, et al. Anxiety and depression in patients receiving implanted cardioverter-defibrillators: a longitudinal investigation. Int J Psychiatry Med 1997;27:57–69.

21. Sears S, Todaro J. Electrophysiology, pacing, and arrhythmia. Examining the psychosocial impact of implantable cardioverter defibrillators: a literature review. Science 1999;489:481–9.

22. Kapa S, Rotondi-Trevisan D, Mariano Z, et al. Psychopathology in patients with ICDs over time: results of a prospective study. Pacing Clin Electrophysiol 2010;33:198–208.

23. Pedersen S, Broek K, Theuns D, et al. Risk of chronic anxiety in implantable defibrillator patients: a multicenter study. Int J Cardiol 2009. Available at: http://dx.doi.org/10.1016/j.ijcard.2009.09.549. Accessed August 21, 2010.

24. Broek K, Nyklícek I, Denollet J. Anxiety predicts poor perceived health in patients with an implantable defibrillator. Psychosomatics 2009;50:483–92.

25. Martens E, Jonge P, Na B, et al. Scared to death? Generalized anxiety disorder and cardiovascular events in patients with stable coronary heart disease: the Heart and Soul Study. Arch Gen Psychiatry 2010;67:750–8.

26. Shibeshi W, Young-Xu Y, Blatt C. Anxiety worsens prognosis in patients with coronary artery disease. J Am Coll Cardiol 2007;49:2021–7.

27. Kuhl E, Dixit N, Walker R, et al. Measurement of patient fears about implantable cardioverter defibrillator shock: an initial evaluation of the Florida Shock Anxiety Scale. Pacing Clin Electrophysiol 2006;29:614–8.

28. Ladwig K-H, Baumert J, Marten-Mittag B, et al. Posttraumatic stress symptoms and predicted mortality in patients with implantable cardioverter-defibrillators: results from the prospective living with an implanted cardioverter-defibrillator study. Arch Gen Psychiatry 2008;65:1324–30.

29. Sears S, Todaro J, Urizar G, et al. Assessing the psychosocial impact of the ICD: a national survey of implantable cardioverter defibrillator health care providers. Pacing Clin Electrophysiol 2000;23:939–45.

30. Whang W, Albert C, Sears S, et al. Depression as a predictor for appropriate shocks among patients with implantable cardioverter-defibrillators: results from the Triggers of Ventricular Arrhythmias (TOVA) study. J Am Coll Cardiol 2005;45:1090–5.

31. Goodman M, Hess B. Provide a human model supporting the learned helplessness theory of depression? Gen Hosp Psychiatry 1999;8343:382–5.

32. Sears S, Conti J, Curtis A, et al. Affective distress and implantable cardioverter defibrillators: cases for psychological and behavioral interventions. Pacing Clin Electrophysiol 1999;22:1831–4.

33. Pedersen S, Domburg R, Theuns D, et al. Type D personality is associated with increased anxiety and depressive symptoms in patients with an implantable cardioverter defibrillator and their partners. Psychosom Med 2004;66:714–9.

34. Pedersen S, Broek K, Erdman R, et al. Pre-implantation implantable cardioverter defibrillator concerns and Type D personality increase the risk of mortality in patients with an implantable cardioverter defibrillator. Europace 2010;12:1446–52.

35. Sweeney M, Sherfesee L, DeGroot P, et al. Differences in effects of electrical therapy type for ventricular arrhythmias on mortality in implantable cardioverter-defibrillator patients. Heart Rhythm 2010;7:353–60.

36. Vazquez L, Kuhl E, Shea J, et al. Age-specific differences in women with implantable cardioverter defibrillators: an international multi center study. Pacing Clin Electrophysiol 2008;31:1528–34.

37. Sears S, Burns J, Handberg E, et al. Young at heart: understanding the unique psychosocial adjustment of young implantable cardioverter defibrillator recipients. Pacing Clin Electrophysiol 2001;24:1113–7.

38. Dubin A, Batsford W, Lewis R, et al. Quality-of-life in patients receiving implantable cardioverter defibrillators at or before age 40. Pacing Clin Electrophysiol 1996;19:1555–9.

39. Hallas C, Burke J, White D, et al. Pre-ICD illness beliefs affect postimplant perceptions of control and patient quality of life. Pacing Clin Electrophysiol 2010;33:256–65.

40. Thomas S, Friedmann E, Gottlieb S, et al. Changes in psychosocial distress in outpatients with heart failure with implantable cardioverter defibrillators. Heart Lung 2009;38:109–20.

41. Pedersen S, Theuns D, Jordaens L, et al. Course of anxiety and device-related concerns in implantable cardioverter defibrillator patients the first year post implantation. Europace 2010;12:1119–26.

42. Versteeg H, Baumert J, Kolb C, et al. Somatosensory amplification mediates sex differences in psychological distress among cardioverter-defibrillator patients. Health Psychol 2010;29:477–83.

43. Natale A, Davidson T, Geiger M, et al. Implantable cardioverter-defibrillators and pregnancy: a safe combination? Circulation 1997;96:2808–12.

44. Vazquez L, Conti J, Sears S. Female-specific education, management, and lifestyle enhancement for implantable cardioverter defibrillator patients: the FEMALE-ICD study. Pacing Clin Electrophysiol 2010;33:1131–40.

45. Bostwick J, Sola C. An updated review of implantable cardioverter/defibrillators, induced anxiety, and quality of life. Psychiatr Clin North Am 2007;30:677–88.

46. Pedersen S, Sears S, Burg M, et al. Does ICD indication affect quality of life and levels of distress? Pacing Clin Electrophysiol 2009;32:153–6.

47. Sears S, Conti J. Quality of life and psychological functioning of ICD patients. Heart 2002;87:488–93.

48. Sears S, Matchett M, Conti J. Effective management of ICD patient psychosocial issues and patient critical events. J Cardiovasc Electrophysiol 2009;20: 1297–304.

49. Dixit N, Vazquez L, Cross N, et al. Cardiac resynchronization therapy: a pilot study examining cognitive change in patients before and after treatment. Clin Cardiol 2010;33:84–8.

50. Pedersen S, Broek K, Berg M, et al. Shock as a determinant of poor patient-centered outcomes in implantable cardioverter defibrillator patients: is there more to it than meets the eye? Pacing Clin Electrophysiol 2010;33:1430–6.

51. Sears S, Kirian K. Shock and patient-centered outcomes research: is an ICD shock still a critical event? Pacing Clin Electrophysiol 2010;33:1437–41.

52. Braunschweig F, Boriani G, Bauer A, et al. Management of patients receiving implantable cardiac defibrillator shocks: recommendations for acute and long-term patient management. Europace 2010;12: 1673–90.

53. Mishkin J, Saxonhouse S, Woo G, et al. Appropriate evaluation and treatment of heart failure patients after implantable cardioverter-defibrillator discharge: time to go beyond the initial shock. J Am Coll Cardiol 2009; 54:1993–2000.

54. Heller S, Ormont M, Lidagoster L, et al. Psychosocial outcome after ICD implantation: a current perspective. Pacing Clin Electrophysiol 1998;21:1207–15.

55. Herrmann C, Mühen F, Schaumann A, et al. Standardized assessment of psychological well-being and quality-of-life in patients with implanted defibrillators. Pacing Clin Electrophysiol 1997;20:95–103.

56. Irvine J, Dorian P, Baker B, et al. Quality of life in the Canadian Implantable Defibrillator Study (CIDS). Am Heart J 2002;144:282–9.

57. Lüderitz B, Jung W, Deister A, et al. Patient acceptance of the implantable cardioverter defibrillator in ventricular tachyarrhythmias. Pacing Clin Electrophysiol 1993;16:1815–21.

58. Passman R, Subacius H, Ruo B, et al. Implantable cardioverter defibrillators and quality of life: results from the defibrillators in nonischemic cardiomyopathy treatment evaluation study. Arch Intern Med 2007;167:2226–32.

59. Redhead A, Turkington D, Rao S, et al. Psychopathology in postinfarction patients implanted with cardioverter-defibrillators for secondary prevention. A cross-sectional, case-controlled study. J Psychosom Res 2010;69:555–63.

60. Sears S, Serber E, Lewis T, et al. Do positive health expectations and optimism relate to quality-of-life outcomes for the patient with an implantable cardioverter defibrillator? J Cardiopulm Rehabil 2004; 24:324–31.

61. Dunbar S, Jenkins L, Hawthorne M, et al. Factors associated with outcomes 3 months after implantable cardioverter defibrillator insertion. Heart Lung 1999;28:303–15.

62. American Psychiatric Association. Diagnostic and statistical manual of mental disorders. Text revision. 4th edition. Washington, DC: American Psychiatric Association; 2000.

63. Dunbar S. Psychosocial issues of patients with implantable cardioverter defibrillators. Am J Crit Care 2005;14:294–303.

64. Sears S, Sowell L, Cross N, et al. Clinical management of key concerns for patients with implantable cardioverter defibrillators. In: Lu F, Benditt D, editors. Cardiac pacing and defibrillation: principle and practice. P.R. China: People's Medical Publishing House; 2008. p. 586–94.

65. Sears S, Shea J, Conti J. Cardiology patient page. How to respond to an implantable cardioverter-defibrillator shock. Circulation 2005;111:380–2.

66. Shea J. Quality of life issues in patients with implantable cardioverter defibrillators: driving, occupation, and recreation. AACN Clin Issues 2004;15:478–89.

67. Marx A, Bollman A, Dunbar SB, et al. Psychological reactions among family members of patients with implantable defibrillators. Int J Psychiatry Med 2001;31:375–87.

68. Hazelton G, Sears S, Kirian K, et al. Cardiology patient page. coping with my partner's ICD and cardiac disease. Circulation 2009;120:73–6.

69. Gibson D, Kuntz K, Levenson J, et al. Decision-making, emotional distress, and quality of life in patients affected by the recall of their implantable cardioverter defibrillator. Europace 2008;10:540–4.

70. Birnie D, Sears S, Green M, et al. No long-term psychological morbidity living with an implantable cardioverter defibrillator under advisory: the Medtronic Marquis experience. Europace 2009;11:26–30.

71. Keren A, Sears S, Nery P, et al. Psychological adjustment in ICD patients living with advisory fidelis leads. J Cardiovasc Electrophysiol 2011;22:57–63.

72. Kapa S, Hyberger L, Rea R, et al. Complication risk with pulse generator change: implications when reacting to a device advisory or recall. Pacing Clin Electrophysiol 2007;30:730–3.

73. Fisher J, Koulogiannis K, Lewallen L, et al. The psychological impact of implantable cardioverter-defibrillator recalls and the durable positive effects of counseling. Pacing Clin Electrophysiol 2009;32: 1012–6.

74. Goldstein N, Lampert R, Bradley E, et al. Management of implantable cardioverter defibrillators in end-of-life care. Ann Intern Med 2004;141:835–8.

75. Lampert R, Hayes D, Annas G, et al. HRS Expert Consensus Statement on the Management of Cardiovascular Implantable Electronic Devices (CIEDs) in patients nearing end of life or requesting withdrawal of therapy this document was developed in collaboration with the American College of Cardiol. Heart Rhythm 2010;7:1008–26.

76. Salmoirago-Blotcher E, Ockene I. Methodological limitations of psychosocial interventions in patients with an implantable cardioverter-defibrillator (ICD) a systematic review. BMC Cardiovasc Disord 2009;9:56.

77. Chevalier P, Cottraux J, Mollard E, et al. Prevention of implantable defibrillator shocks by cognitive behavioral therapy: a pilot trial. Am Heart J 2006;151:191.

78. Dougherty C, Lewis F, Thompson E, et al. Short-term efficacy of a telephone intervention by expert nurses after an implantable cardioverter defibrillator. Pacing Clin Electrophysiol 2004;27:1594–602.

79. Edelman S, Lemon J, Kidman A. Psychological therapies for recipients of implantable cardioverter defibrillators. Heart Lung 2003;32:234–40.

80. Dunbar S, Langberg J, Reilly C, et al. Effect of a psychoeducational intervention on depression, anxiety, and health resource use in implantable cardioverter defibrillator patients. Pacing Clin Electrophysiol 2009;32:1259–71.

81. Fitchet A, Doherty P, Bundy C, et al. Comprehensive cardiac rehabilitation programme for implantable cardioverter-defibrillator patients: a randomised controlled trial. Heart 2003;89:155–60.

82. Frizelle D, Lewin R, Kaye G, et al. Cognitive-behavioural rehabilitation programme for patients with an implanted cardioverter defibrillator: a pilot study. Br J Health Psychol 2004;9:381–92.

83. Lewin R, Coulton S, Frizelle D, et al. A brief cognitive behavioural preimplantation and rehabilitation programme for patients receiving an implantable cardioverter-defibrillator improves physical health and reduces psychological morbidity and unplanned readmissions. Heart 2009;95:63–9.

84. Carlsson E, Olsson S, Hertervig E. The role of the nurse in enhancing quality of life in patients with an implantable cardioverter-defibrillator: the Swedish experience. Prog Cardiovasc Nurs 2002;17:18–25.

85. Kuhl E, Sears S, Conti J. Using computers to improve the psychosocial care of implantable cardioverter defibrillator recipients. Pacing Clin Electrophysiol 2006;29:1426–33.

86. Dickerson S, Posluszny M, Kennedy M. Help seeking in a support group for recipients of implantable cardioverter defibrillators and their support persons. Heart Lung 2000;29:87–96.

87. Badger J, Morris J. Observations of a support group intervention for automatic implantable cardioverter defibrillator recipients and their spouses. Heart Lung 1989;18:238–43.

88. Dickerson SS, Wu YW, Kennedy MC. A CNS-facilitated ICD support group: a clinical project evaluation. Clin Nurse Spec 2006;20:146–53.

89. Molchany C, Peterson K. The psychosocial effects of support group intervention on AICD recipients and their significant others. Prog Cardiovasc Nurs 1994;9:23–9.

90. Sneed N, Finch N, Michel Y. The effect of psychosocial nursing intervention on the mood state of patients with implantable cardioverter defibrillators and their caregivers. Prog Cardiovasc Nurs 1997;12:4–14.

91. Myers G, James G. Social support, anxiety, and support group participation in patients with an implantable cardioverter defibrillator. Prog Cardiovasc Nurs 2008;23:160–7.

Advances in Remote Monitoring of Implantable Cardiac Devices

Niraj Varma, MA, DM, FRCP*, Bruce L. Wilkoff, MD

KEYWORDS

- Cardiac implantable electronic devices • ICD
- Remote monitoring • Follow-up • Recall management
- Early detection

The implantation of cardiac electronic devices has increased substantially over the past decade in response to widening indications. Subsequent monitoring is an integral part of both device and patient care but remains unguided by any prospectively derived data. Current practice generally follows an in-clinic follow-up protocol by physicians or device specialists to retrieve stored diagnostic data. For implantable cardioverter defibrillators (ICDs) and cardiac resynchronization therapy (CRT) devices, this is performed at short intervals because of safety concerns.[1] Consensus suggests that patients with ICDs should be evaluated routinely every 3 to 6 months either in person during clinic checks or through remote mechanisms. This recommendation represents a significant clinical burden that may increase further when devices reach elective replacement indicator (ERI) or in response to product advisories and recalls.[1–3] Additional challenges are the ability for early problem detection, management of unscheduled encounters, and management of data downloaded from increasingly complex devices. Recently developed remote monitoring technologies may provide mechanisms for performing intensive device surveillance without overburdening device clinics.

REMOTE MONITORING

Technologies available operate differently. Mode of operation and level of patient involvement during transmission vary among monitoring systems. Wand-based systems require patient-driven downloads relayed via telephone connections to following facilities.[4,5] This process may be time-consuming, could challenge compliance, and remains vulnerable to overlooking asymptomatic events. This form of remote monitoring essentially substitutes for conventional in-person evaluation and is likely to yield similar data transfer and problem discovery rates. Thus, when used to follow-up a pacemaker population, clinically actionable events took several months for discovery and only 66% of the data were transmitted.[6] This technology may fail to reduce cardiac-related resource use.[7] In contrast, an automatic transmission mechanism fully independent of patient or physician interaction has considerable advantages. It uses automatic (cellular- or landline-based) data transmissions, which may be reviewed securely via the Internet (**Fig. 1**). This form of technology was pioneered by Biotronik (Home Monitoring; Berlin, Germany; approved by the U.S. Food and Drug Administration [FDA] in 2002). Reliability and early notification ability

Disclosures: Dr Varma was Consultant to Biotronik for and Principal Investigator of the TRUST Trial. Dr Wilkoff is an unpaid advisor for Medtronic, St Jude Medical, Boston Scientific, Inner Pulse, and Spectranetics.
Cardiac Pacing and Electrophysiology, HVI 9500 Euclid Avenue Desk J2-2, Cleveland Clinic, Cleveland, OH 44195, USA
* Corresponding author.
E-mail address: varman@ccf.org

Card Electrophysiol Clin 3 (2011) 463–472
doi:10.1016/j.ccep.2011.05.011
1877-9182/11/$ – see front matter © 2011 Elsevier Inc. All rights reserved.

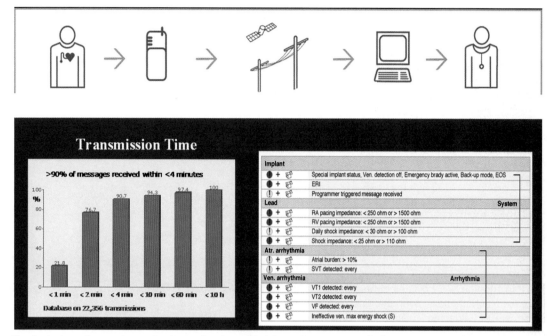

Fig. 1. Automatic remote monitoring technology. (*Top*) A very low-power radiofrequency transmitter circuitry integrated within the pulse generator wirelessly transmits stored data on a daily basis to a mobile communicator (typically placed bedside at night). The data are relayed wirelessly or via landline (automatically seeking the first path available) to a service center. The wireless transmission ability is especially useful since almost 20% (and increasing) of United States households are currently estimated to have no landline facility. The service center receives incoming data and generates a customized summary available to the physician online via secure Internet access. Thus, daily patient monitoring occurs with trend analysis information of typical follow-up data (eg, battery status, lead impedance, sensing function). Service center processing and data upload on the remote Web page are automatic, bypassing potential delays (and errors) associated with manual processing. Critical event data may be transmitted immediately and flagged for attention on the remote Web page. Automatic alerts occur for silent but potentially dangerous events and include transmission of intracardiac electrograms similar to those available during office device interrogations, providing the ability for early detection and enabling prompt clinical intervention, if necessary. (*Bottom, left*) A feasibility study with Home Monitoring showed that more than 90% of transmissions were received in less than 5 minutes with 100% preservation of data integrity. (*Bottom, right*) Example of clinician alerts. Although an event notification may be potentially triggered every day, in practice these messages occurred infrequently. ((*Bottom, left*) *From* Varma N, Stambler B, Chun S. Detection of atrial fibrillation by implanted devices with wireless data transmission capability. Pacing Clin Electrophysiol 2005;28(Suppl 1):S133–6; with permission.)

of this communication system were excellent,[8] and system operation is not energy costly. Other manufacturers have followed with the development of similar automatic technologies (ie, CareLink Network; Medtronic Inc, Minneapolis, MN, USA), Latitude Patient Management System (Boston Scientific, St Paul, MN, USA), and the Merlin (St Jude Medical, Sylmar, Los Angeles). Each system is proprietary and works only with compatible devices from the same manufacturer. The ability for automatic remote monitoring to maintain surveillance, supplement and often supplant "routine" in-clinic evaluations, and rapidly bring to attention significant data to enable clinical intervention was tested in the TRUST (Home Monitoring) and CONNECT (CareLink) trials.

TRUST Trial

TRUST was a prospective multicenter clinical study comparing conventional and remote interrogation.[9,10] This trial enrolled 1450 patients at 102 sites in the United States and randomized them to either remote monitoring or conventional care groups (**Fig. 2**). Results showed that remote monitoring reduced health care use by approximately 50%, as measured by the sum of all 3 monthly scheduled and unscheduled (eg, emergency room visits, patient- or physician-initiated checks) hospital evaluations that occurred. This decrease resulted predominantly from the reduction in scheduled encounters, the bulk of which involve collection of routine measurements only

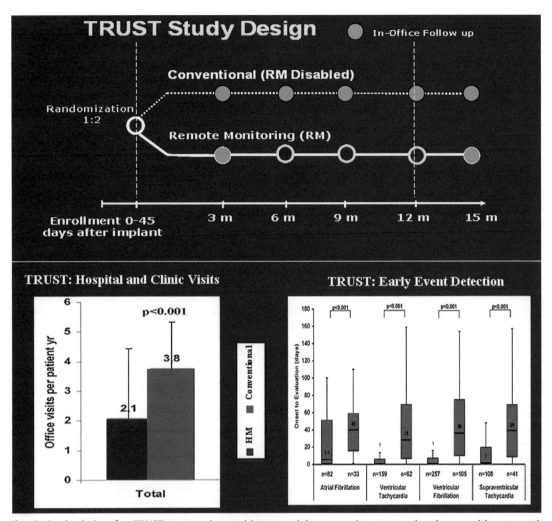

Fig. 2. Study design for TRUST prospective multicenter trials, comparing conventional care with automatic remote monitoring in clinical management of a large ICD population. (*Top*) After randomization, all patients with an ICD had scheduled follow-ups at 3, 6, 9, 12, and 15 months postimplant, and unscheduled (interim) evaluations as needed. Patients in conventional care were evaluated in-hospital only. Patients assigned to remote management had office visits at 3 and 15 months. At 6, 9, and 12 months and for interim visits, data were remotely retrieved and evaluated. Between these periodic checks, automatic event notifications were evaluated online and patients brought in for office visits if deemed necessary by the investigator. (*Bottom left*) In the TRUST study, remote interrogation reduced cardiac resource (ie, scheduled and unscheduled clinic and hospital visits), including responses to heart monitoring event notifications, by 45% in 1 year.[10] (*Bottom right*) Time to physician evaluation of arrhythmias was within less than 48 hours with remote monitoring (including silent events). Similar results were reported in the CONNECT study.[11] ((*Top*) From Varma N. Rationale and design of a prospective study of the efficacy of a remote monitoring system used in implantable cardioverter defibrillator follow-up: the Lumos-T Reduces Routine Office Device Follow-Up Study (TRUST) study. Am Heart J 2007;154:1029–34; with permission; and (*Bottom, right*) Varma N, Epstein A, Irimpen A, et al. Efficacy and safety of automatic remote monitoring for ICD Follow-Up: the TRUST trial. Circulation 2010;122:325–32; with permission.)

(eg, battery status, lead impedance, sensing function), requiring no clinical intervention (eg, reprogramming, alteration of antiarrhythmic medications), and could be performed through online data review. The reduction in face-to-face visits was accomplished safely, because no difference was seen between the study arms in mortality, incidence of strokes, and events requiring surgical interventions (eg, device explants, lead revision).

Remote monitoring also permitted earlier detection and physician evaluation of cardiac or device problems despite fewer face-to-face encounters (median <3 days compared with >1 month with conventional care). Furthermore, remote monitoring was associated with greater follow-up adherence to 3 monthly calender-based checks. This greater adherence is presumably because patient data may be monitored remotely anytime and from anywhere, as opposed to conventional care, which relies on patients to present themselves physically in their physician's office.

The CONNECT trial used a similar study design in a separate patient group with a different wireless remote technology. Results confirmed that remote interrogation effectively substituted for in-office visits and reduced time from clinical event to clinical decision. A significant shortening of hospital length of stay was observed, possibly because of a positive impact on patient health. Overall hospital costs were reduced by use of remote technology.[11]

Implementation

TRUST results indicate that remote monitoring may be used for device management to substitute for in-office follow-up and also provide a mechanism for early detection. This application gained FDA approval in May 2009.[12] Remote management does not supplant the important in-person follow-up at 2 to 12 weeks postimplant and yearly as indicated by the Heart Rhythm Society (HRS) guidance document.[1] The in-person evaluations allow assessment of wound healing, determination of chronic thresholds, and setting of final pacing parameters.[13,14] Problems such as lead perforations or failures requiring revision and symptomatic reactions to implantation (eg, pacemaker syndrome, diaphragmatic pacing, pocket infection) cluster in this early postimplant period and occur more frequently with dual-chamber or resynchronization units.[13–15] At the 3-month encounter, continuation of postimplant follow-up must be emphasized. Patients or their family must appreciate that ICDs and CRTs require careful surveillance, gain familiarity with remote monitoring, and understand their responsibility in adhering to the follow-up schedule.

After the in-person 3-month postimplant assessment, face-to-face checks may be scheduled once yearly with interim 3-monthly checks via remote monitoring. If an actionable (or questionable) event is detected, the patient may be asked to report for formal assessment. However, this occurs infrequently, because TRUST showed that approximately 90% of these 3-monthly checks did not require an intervention. Current systems provide an opportunity for patient notification via the receiver (call-back function, third-party arrhythmia service, or live interaction) that may be reassuring for patients during remote follow-up.

However, remote manual testing or reprogramming of devices, although feasible from an engineering perspective, is not currently available because of safety and security concerns. Hence, actionable events, even if straightforward and easily resolved with simple reprogramming, require in-person assessment. Management of unscheduled checks may be also facilitated. For example, with patient inquiries, online data and electrogram evaluation may be used to determine the best management, such as with either a hospital visit or reassurance only. The capacity for early detection is exceptionally valuable for detecting silent events and directing clinical intervention (**Figs 3** and **4**).[8,16,17]

Conventional monitoring methods demand increased frequency of scheduled visits to allow for events such as generators approaching ERI, deviations in lead behavior (impedance, sensing, or threshold), and for ICD components under advisory, which also tend to manifest with battery, high-voltage circuitry, or lead failure.[18] In contrast, physicians following these patients with remote monitoring may perform accelerated follow-up online and wait for affected devices to self-declare an issue rapidly,[19] thus avoiding overloading device clinics with nonactionable inpatient encounters.

Device clinic

Remote management has been adopted by several large-volume centers, where it plays an essential and dominant role (**Fig. 5**). (Remote care pertains to device management and is not intended to replace consultations with internists, cardiologists, or heart failure specialists that may otherwise occur). Implementation requires a change in workflow patterns to maintain consistent scheduled device interrogations, with daily attention to remote Web sites to evaluate event notifications. Web site review may be conducted rapidly compared with in-person follow-up, thus improving clinic efficiencies and delivering prompt communication to patients when necessary (especially valuable for potentially dangerous asymptomatic events). This process is likely to commit fewer hospital personnel while maintaining greater patient surveillance. Thus, use of remote monitoring reduced both physician and patient time compared with conventional care.[20] In another study, a nurse expert in cardiac pacing consulted the remote Web site daily and reviewed problematic transmissions with a physician. During a mean follow-up of 227 ± 128 days, 23,545 daily messages and 1665 alert events were received. The nurse and physician spent an average of 1 and 0.2 hours per week, respectively, analyzing the data. The mean connection time per patient was 2 minutes, and had decreased to 1.65 minutes

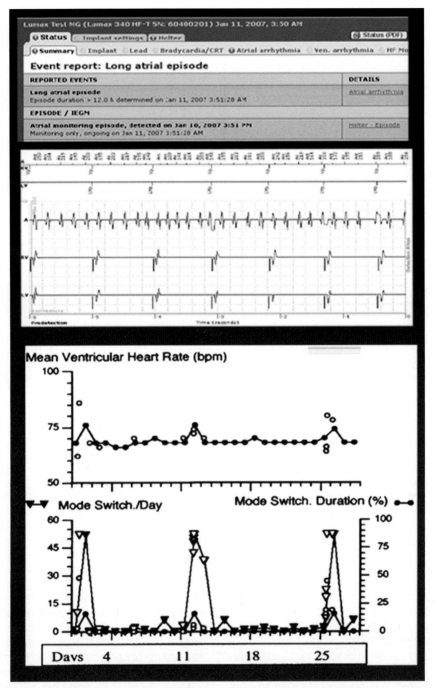

Fig. 3. Examples of Web site review of event notification data. (*Top*) Event notification of atrial fibrillation (*top*) with accompanying wirelessly transmitted intracardiac electrograms. (*Bottom*) A patient's atrial fibrillation history may be reviewed on the Web page (*bottom*). Frequency and duration of mode switches and simultaneous mean ventricular rate data are presented as graphic trends over time. Three paroxysmal atrial fibrillation episodes occurring over 29 days are illustrated. Although more than 50 mode switches (*triangles*) are recorded during each episode, the mode switch duration (*circles*) is less than 20%, indicating a light overall atrial fibrillation burden for these particular events. The three paroxysmal atrial fibrillation episodes are each accompanied by simultaneous increases in mean ventricular heart rates. ((*Bottom*) From Varma N, Stambler B, Chun S. Detection of atrial fibrillation by implanted devices with wireless data transmission capability. Pacing Clin Electrophysiol 2005;28(Suppl 1):S133–6; with permission.)

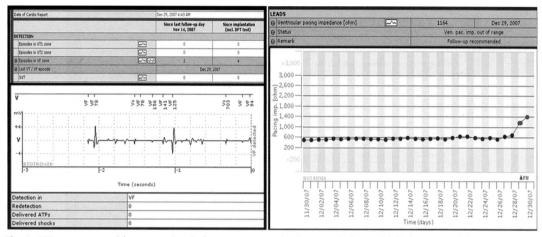

Fig. 4. ICD generator with automatic wireless remote monitoring coupled to a Fidelis (MDT 6949) lead. Two event notifications that were transmitted immediately on occurrence of lead fracture, occurring silently during sleep at 4:43 AM, 6 weeks after last clinic follow-up on November 14. (*Left panel*) Two occurrences of detection in the ventricular fibrillation (VF) zone are noted (*top*) and flagged (*red exclamation mark on yellow background*). The accompanying wirelessly transmitted electrogram showed irregular sensed events (markers indicate coupling intervals as short as 78 ms) with VF detection (*marked the green lettering*). No therapy was delivered, indicating spontaneous event termination. (*Right panel*) The second event report is a separate notification in response to the same event, indicating a lead impedance alert. Lead impedance trend was stable at less than 600 Ω in prior weeks, but then suddenly increased more than 500 Ω, triggering an event notification (*red*), although this absolute value was still within specifications. Electrogram definition is modest in first-generation device with wireless intracardiac electrogram transmission (Lumos). Current-generation devices transmit electrograms with improved resolution (1/128 seconds) and longer duration, including postdetection sequences (eg, see **Fig. 2**). The clinic received these notices and informed the patient, who was then reviewed urgently within 24 hours and treated with lead extraction and replacement. The case shows the value of remote monitoring with daily automatic surveillance and rapid, automatic (ie, without patient participation) event notification to the clinic of fault detection, which enabled prompt intervention. The addition of nonsustained ventricular tachycardia events to the impedance deviation improves the specificity of detection of lead failure. Without automatic wireless remote monitoring, presentation may have occurred later with inappropriate shocks, or catastrophically with failure of pacing or VF sensing. (*From* Varma N. Remote monitoring for advisories: automatic early detection of silent lead failure. Pacing Clin Electrophysiol 2009;32:525–7; with permission; and *Data from* Gunderson BD, Swerdlow CD, Wilcox JM, et al. Causes of ventricular oversensing in implantable cardioverter-defibrillators: implications for diagnosis of lead fracture. Heart Rhythm 2010;7:626–33.)

per patient for the last 50 connections. The nurse submitted 133 transmissions from 56 patients to the physician. Thus, remote interrogation optimized medical treatment and device programming, at low cost for the health care system.[21] Patients have expressed confidence in their remote management. Recent evaluations show an excellent level (>95%) of acceptance and satisfaction with remote interrogation.[22] In TRUST, no patients assigned to remote interrogation crossed over during the study, and 98% elected to retain this follow-up mode on trial conclusion.[23]

Reimbursement guidelines for remote interrogation and in-person programming evaluations were established in the United States in January 2009. The remote follow-up provides a single fee for all interrogations performed within a 90-day period. Although most patients experience no events during the 90 days, some may have several transmissions, and the physician and device clinic are paid for

monitoring these transmissions and creating a report. However, if a remote interrogation prompts an in-person evaluation, called a *programming evaluation*, this is billable in addition. The programming evaluation, which can also be performed at least yearly, includes an interrogation and evaluation of capture, sensing, sensor, rhythms, and overall function through the programmer. There is no need to permanently alter the programmed parameters to consider this a programming evaluation.

Emerging Applications

Lead and device performance
Monitoring hardware performance is a physician responsibility expressed in recent HRS position statements and often demanded by patients.[23] The task is challenging in view of increasing volume, device complexity, and advisory notices. Intensive monitoring through increasing office visits

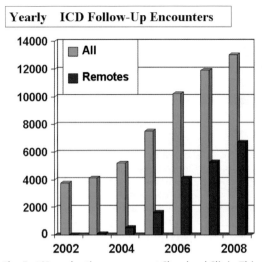

Fig. 5. ICD evaluations per year at Cleveland Clinic. This shows the steadily increasing volume of encounters and the increasing proportion performed remotely. (*Courtesy of* E. Ching RN, Cleveland Clinic Foundation, Cleveland, OH.)

(eg, monthly) is impractical, onerous, and inefficient (because problem incidence is very low) and is likely to fail to detect potentially catastrophic problems occurring between interrogations.[24,25] Remote monitoring systems relying on patient-driven communication may have similar limitations for detecting asymptomatic failure.

In contrast, remote technology that provides constant surveillance of system integrity with automatic alerts of significant problems (as they occur) eliminates the burden of patients having to monitor their own devices frequently and coordinate with clinic services. Remote interrogation follow-up systems enhanced the discovery of system issues (even when asymptomatic) and enabled prompt clinical decisions regarding conservative versus surgical management.[26] Performance problems were often asymptomatic. In contrast, conventional monitoring methods underreported device-related problems. **Fig. 4** illustrates the benefit of remote monitoring in the management of recalled components.[2,17] Nonsustained arrhythmia notification triggered not only by arrhythmias but also by events such as lead noise/T-wave oversensing may cause battery depletion and also presage shock delivery, causing patient morbidity.[15,26] Shock burden reduction, especially if inappropriate, is a major current concern. Remote interrogation's early detection of these asymptomatic problems provides an opportunity for early preventative action.[27] The ability to collect detailed device-specific data, with component function assessed daily and automatic archiving, sets

a precedent for longitudinal evaluation of lead and generator performance.

Monitoring disease progression

Patients undergoing ICD therapy commonly have heart failure, which is a dynamic condition. The development of acute decompensation is complex, involving several processes (eg, hemodynamic, neurohumoral, electrophysiologic, and vascular abnormalities) that converge to manifest with fluid congestion. After hospitalization, management is directed to identification and correction of precipitating factors and comorbidities, and management of fluid overload, arrhythmias, and any conduction system problems. Therapeutic strategies aimed at interrupting this series of events are potentially valuable, and may be possible because, in most cases, pathophysiologic processes progress over days to weeks before clinical presentation with a fluid-overloaded state. Retrieved records from implanted devices, which record multiple patient parameters, further support this strategy. A typical example is illustrated in **Fig. 6** (top). However, the initial inciting events are varied and their early detection is challenging because they are generally asymptomatic. Therefore, early detection through remote monitoring technology is potentially important. For example, atrial fibrillation[28,29] may increase risk of heart failure and stroke and possibly facilitate ventricular arrhythmias. Atrial fibrillation may be associated with periods of rapid conduction, which is important because the benefit of CRT may be reduced when pacing is diminished to less than 92%.[30] Both the advent of atrial fibrillation and the withdrawal of ventricular pacing in CRT defibrillation may be immediately detected through remote interrogation monitoring (see **Figs. 4** and **6**, bottom). Action taken based on these notifications may prevent hospitalizations.[31] In the future, incorporation of sensor technology may provide sentinel notification of conditions, leading to decompensation and prompt rapid preemptive therapy. This concept may form the basis of stand-alone implantable cardiac monitors.[32–34] Remote monitoring provides the mechanism for accessing and delivering prioritized data collected by these increasingly sophisticated implantable units.

FUTURE

Automatic longitudinal data collection with remote interrogation lays a foundation for clinical outcomes studies that are especially important for heart failure, for which a variety of implantable sensors are under development. The ability to process several parameters and notify deviation

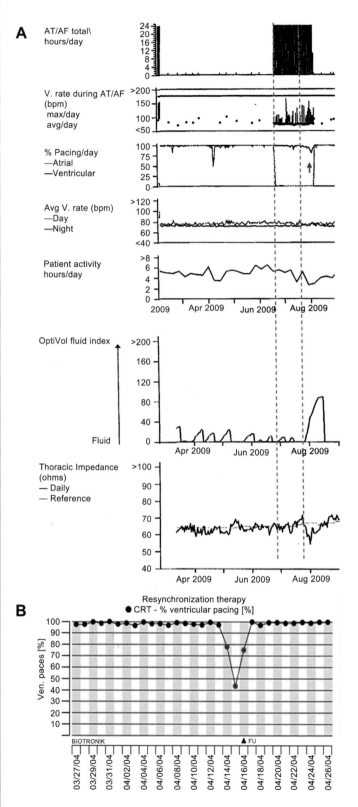

Fig. 6. (*A*) Middle-aged man with ischemic cardiomyopathy and left bundle branch lock treated with cardiac resynchronization therapy defibrillator He had several bouts of atrial fibrillation requiring cardioversion and was maintained on dofetilide. The patient experienced lassitude and worsening shortness of breath in the face of unchanged daily weights or worsening edema for several weeks. However, he contacted providers late, only when fluid congestion started to occur. At outpatient evaluation, he was found to have both atrial fibrillation and congestive heart failure and was admitted for treatment with diuretics. Device interrogation revealed several notable features. The patient had developed persistent atrial fibrillation (atrial fibrillation hours/day) before development of heart failure symptoms. Note initiation toward the end of June (*first vertical blue dashed line*) marked by withdrawal of atrial pacing, although presentation with clinical decompensation occurred 6 weeks later in August. A steeper rate of deterioration in parameters is marked by the second vertical blue dashed line in the 2 to 3 weeks preceding hospitalization. These episodes were characterized by longer bursts of accelerated ventricular rates, greater loss of biventricular pacing to approximately 80% (*arrow*), diminished patient activity, and progressively increasing intrathoracic impedance (Optivol fluid index). This index is derived from the difference between the daily and reference intrathoracic impedance (*bottom graph*) and may reflect accumulation of fluid in the thorax. Prompt resolution in all of these parameters occurred after treatment of atrial fibrillation. He was treated with diuretics and cardioverted. He later experienced relapse, with similar episodes precipitated by atrial fibrillation, and underwent ablative therapy for atrial fibrillation. His condition stabilized. (*B*) Trend of CRT pacing. Loss of pacing is event notified (*red dots*), resulting in a clinic evaluation (FU) and therapy. CRT pacing resumes at greater than 95% (*black dots*). ([*A*] From Varma N. Automatic remote monitoring of implantable cardiac devices in heart failure, 2010 cardiac devices in heart failure: the TRUST trial. Journal of Innovations in Cardiac Rhythm Management 2010;1:22–9; with permission.)

in a prespecified combination may improve the specificity of disease detection, as illustrated in the recent PARTNERS HF study.[35] Access to Internet-based information systems provides a framework for multidisciplinary communication and collaboration. Examination of large consolidated databases derived from remote access allows the effects of diseases or device programming on patient morbidity and mortality to be assessed.[36]

REFERENCES

1. Wilkoff BL, Auricchio A, Brugada J, et al. HRS/EHRA expert consensus on the monitoring of cardiovascular implantable electronic devices (CIEDs): description of techniques, indications, personnel, frequency and ethical considerations. Heart Rhythm 2008;5:907–25.
2. Carlson MD, Wilkoff BL, Maisel WH, et al. Recommendations from the Heart Rhythm Society Task Force on Device Performance Policies and Guidelines Endorsed by the American College of Cardiology Foundation (ACCF) and the American Heart Association (AHA) and the International Coalition of Pacing and Electrophysiology Organizations (COPE). Heart Rhythm 2006;3:1250–73.
3. Maisel WH, Hauser RG, Hammill SC, et al. Recommendations from the Heart Rhythm Society Task Force on Lead Performance Policies and Guidelines: developed in collaboration with the American College of Cardiology (ACC) and the American Heart Association (AHA). Heart Rhythm 2009;6:869–85.
4. Schoenfeld MH, Compton SJ, Mead RH, et al. Remote monitoring of implantable cardioverter defibrillators: a prospective analysis. Pacing Clin Electrophysiol 2004;27:757–63.
5. Joseph GK, Wilkoff BL, Dresing T, et al. Remote interrogation and monitoring of implantable cardioverter defibrillators. J Interv Card Electrophysiol 2004;11:161–6.
6. Crossley GH, Chen J, Choucair W, et al. Clinical benefits of remote versus transtelephonic monitoring of implanted pacemakers. J Am Coll Cardiol 2009;54:2012–9.
7. Al-Khatib SM, Piccini JP, Knight D, et al. Remote monitoring of implantable cardioverter defibrillators versus quarterly device interrogations in clinic: results from a randomized pilot clinical trial. J Cardiovasc Electrophysiol 2010;21:545–50.
8. Varma N, Stambler B, Chun S. Detection of atrial fibrillation by implanted devices with wireless data transmission capability. Pacing Clin Electrophysiol 2005;28(Suppl 1):S133–6.
9. Varma N. Rationale and design of a prospective study of the efficacy of a remote monitoring system used in implantable cardioverter defibrillator follow-up: the Lumos-T Reduces Routine Office Device Follow-Up Study (TRUST) study. Am Heart J 2007;154:1029–34.
10. Varma N, Epstein A, Irimpen A, et al. Efficacy and safety of automatic remote monitoring for ICD Follow-Up: the TRUST trial. Circulation 2010;122:325–32.
11. Crossley G, Boyle A, Vitense H, et al. The clinical evaluation of remote notification to reduce time to clinical decision (CONNECT) trial: the value of wireless remote monitoring with automatic clinician alerts. J Am Coll Cardiol 2011;57(10):1181–9.
12. FDA. Home monitoring. Available at: http://www.fda.gov/MedicalDevices/ProductsandMedicalProcedures/DeviceApprovalsandClearances/PMAApprovals/ucm166550.htm2009;P050023/S020. Accessed June 6, 2011.
13. Brugada P. What evidence do we have to replace in-hospital implantable cardioverter defibrillator follow-up? Clin Res Cardiol 2006;95(Suppl 3):III3–9.
14. Senges-Becker JC, Klostermann M, Becker R, et al. What is the "optimal" follow-up schedule for ICD patients? Europace 2005;7:319–26.
15. Lee DS, Krahn AD, Healey JS, et al. Evaluation of early complications related to De Novo cardioverter defibrillator implantation insights from the Ontario ICD database. J Am Coll Cardiol 2010;55:774–82.
16. Varma N, Johnson MA. Prevalence of cancelled shock therapy and relationship to shock delivery in recipients of implantable cardioverter-defibrillators assessed by remote monitoring. Pacing Clin Electrophysiol 2009;32(Suppl 1):S42–6.
17. Varma N. Remote monitoring for advisories: automatic early detection of silent lead failure. Pacing Clin Electrophysiol 2009;32:525–7.
18. Hauser RG, Kallinen L. Deaths associated with implantable cardioverter defibrillator failure and deactivation reported in the United States food and drug administration manufacturer and user facility device experience database. Heart Rhythm 2004;1:399–405.
19. Varma N, Epstein A, Irimpen A, et al. TRUST Investigators. Early detection of ICD events using remote monitoring: the TRUST trial. Heart Rhythm J 2009;6:S73.
20. Raatikainen MJ, Uusimaa P, van Ginneken MM, et al. Remote monitoring of implantable cardioverter defibrillator patients: a safe, time-saving, and cost-effective means for follow-up. Europace 2008;10:1145–51.
21. Ricci RP, Morichelli L, Santini M. Home monitoring remote control of pacemaker and implantable cardioverter defibrillator patients in clinical practice: impact on medical management and health-care resource utilization. Europace 2008;10:164–70.
22. Ricci RP, Morichelli L, Quarta L, et al. Long-term patient acceptance of and satisfaction with implanted device remote monitoring. Europace 2010;12:674–9.

23. Varma N, Stambler B. Patient aspects of remote home monitoring of ICDs—the TRUST trial. Circulation 2011;123(7):e247.

24. Medtronic. Physician advisory letter: urgent medical device information Sprint Fidelis® lead patient management recommendations. 2007. Available at: http://www.medtronicheartleadrecall.com/20071015-physician-letter.htm. Accessed June 6, 2011.

25. Kallinen LM, Hauser RG, Lee KW, et al. Failure of impedance monitoring to prevent adverse clinical events caused by fracture of a recalled high-voltage implantable cardioverter-defibrillator lead. Heart Rhythm 2008;5:775–9.

26. Varma N. Monitoring performance of cardiac implantable electronic devices using automatic remote monitoring: results from the TRUST Trial. Heart Rhythm 2010;7(5S):S365.

27. Varma N, Michalski J, Epstein A, et al. Automatic remote monitoring of ICD lead and generator performance: the TRUST trial. Circ Arrhythm Electrophysiol 2010;3(5):428–36.

28. Ehrlich JR, Hohnloser SH. Milestones in the management of atrial fibrillation. Heart Rhythm 2009;6:S62–7.

29. Bunch TJ, Day JD, Olshansky B, et al. Newly detected atrial fibrillation in patients with an implantable cardioverter-defibrillator is a strong risk marker of increased mortality. Heart Rhythm 2009;6:2–8.

30. Koplan BA, Kaplan AJ, Weiner S, et al. Heart failure decompensation and all-cause mortality in relation to percent biventricular pacing in patients with heart failure: is a goal of 100% biventricular pacing necessary? J Am Coll Cardiol 2009;53:355–60.

31. Arya A, Block M, Kautzner J, et al. Influence of home monitoring on the clinical status of heart failure patients: design and rationale of the IN-TIME study. Eur J Heart Fail 2008;10:1143–8.

32. Hoppe UC, Vanderheyden M, Sievert H, et al. Chronic monitoring of pulmonary artery pressure in patients with severe heart failure: multicentre experience of the monitoring Pulmonary Artery Pressure by Implantable device Responding to Ultrasonic Signal (PAPIRUS) II study. Heart 2009;95:1091–7.

33. Ritzema J, Melton IC, Richards AM, et al. Direct left atrial pressure monitoring in ambulatory heart failure patients: initial experience with a new permanent implantable device. Circulation 2007;116:2952–9.

34. Khoury DS, Naware M, Siou J, et al. Ambulatory monitoring of congestive heart failure by multiple bioelectric impedance vectors. J Am Coll Cardiol 2009;53:1075–81.

35. Whellan DJ, Ousdigian KT, Al-Khatib SM, et al. Combined heart failure device diagnostics identify patients at higher risk of subsequent heart failure hospitalizations: results from PARTNERS HF (Program to Access and Review Trending Information and Evaluate Correlation to Symptoms in Patients With Heart Failure) study. J Am Coll Cardiol 2010;55:1803–10.

36. Borek P, Koehler J, Ziegler P, et al. Impact of AF on mortality in 44,104 patients with CRT-D. Heart Rhythm 2010;7:S26.

Defibrillation Threshold: Testing, Upper Limit of Vulnerability, and Methods for Reduction

Henry H. Hsia, MD, FHRS[a],*, Karin K.M. Chia, MBBS[b],
John C. Evans, MD[c]

KEYWORDS
• Defibrillation • Threshold • ULV • Testing

DEFINITIONS

The term defibrillation threshold (DFT) is commonly used as a measure of defibrillation efficacy, often associated with the testing procedures at the time of defibrillator implantation. DFT represents the effective shock energies required to successful terminate ventricular fibrillation (VF). The term defibrillation threshold is often vaguely defined and poorly understood. The defibrillation requirements, expressed in terms of energy, voltage, or current, are best described by a probabilistic dose-response curve and not a single threshold (**Fig. 1**).[1–4]

The defibrillation success curve represents the probability for successful defibrillation versus shock energies. The probabilistic nature of the DFT may be caused by random variation of multiple factors that are not yet fully understood. These factors include myocardial mass,[5] metabolic variables, ischemia, antiarrhythmic drugs, duration of fibrillation,[6] current vectors and waveforms,[7] distributions of current/voltage gradient, and the cellular/tissue electrophysiologic characteristics at the time of shock delivery across the heart.[8] To truly define the DFT curve, repeated fibrillation induction and defibrillation attempts at various shock energies are required to plot such a dose-response curve, which is impractical and potentially hazardous in the clinical setting.

Because the sigmoidal dose-response curve lacks the abrupt transition from effectiveness to ineffectiveness, energy margins are measured during DFT determinations (see **Fig. 1**). The efficacy margin represents the increase in energy required to move from the measured DFT up the probability curve to achieve consistent, greater than 99% likelihood of successful defibrillation (E_{99}). The safety margin is defined as the difference in energy between the implantable cardioverter-defibrillator (ICD) output (E_{ICD}) and the minimum shock energy requirement for consistent defibrillation (E_{99}). The safety margin is a measure of the width of the plateau between the ICD output and the energies that fail to effect successful defibrillation. The safety margin should be large enough to accommodate shifts in the defibrillation requirements to higher energies, which may arise as a result of prolonged fibrillation duration, metabolic abnormalities, ischemia, antiarrhythmic drug use, or progression of the underlying disease.

[a] Cardiac Electrophysiology and Arrhythmia Service, Stanford University Medical Center, 300 Pasteur Drive, H2146, Stanford, CA 94305-5233, USA
[b] Department of Cardiology, Royal Brisbane and Women's Hospital, Herston, QLD 4029, Australia
[c] Pacific Heart Associates, 300 North Graham, Suite 320, Portland, OR 97227, USA
* Corresponding author.
E-mail address: hhsia@cvmed.stanford.edu

Card Electrophysiol Clin 3 (2011) 473–492
doi:10.1016/j.ccep.2011.05.012

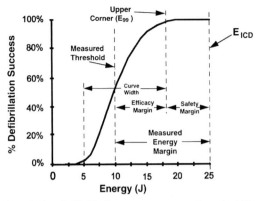

Fig. 1. The defibrillation success curve: % probability for successful defibrillation versus shock energies. The energy margin measured during the DFT testing (E_{ICD}-DFT) includes a safety margin and an efficacy margin. The safety margin of the device is defined as the difference between the ICD output (E_{ICD}) and the upper corner of the defibrillation success curve with greater than or equal to 99% likelihood of achieving defibrillation (E_{99}). The efficacy margin represents the increase in energy required to move from the measured DFT up the curve to energies that consistently defibrillate (E_{99}). (*Modified from* Singer I, Lang D. Defibrillation threshold: clinical utility and therapeutic implications. Pacing Clin Electrophysiol 1992;15:933; with permission.)

METHODS OF EVALUATING SAFETY MARGIN

The goal of DFT testing is to ensure that the energy required for defibrillation is always less than the energy that the device is able to deliver. The energy margin measured during the DFT testing (E_{ICD}-DFT) includes both safety margin and efficacy margin. The accuracy of such DFT determination is therefore dependent on the width of the curve.[2–4] In general, techniques for assessing the energy margins are threshold methods or verification methods.

Threshold Method

The threshold methods test a sequence of repeated fibrillation induction-defibrillation episodes at various shock intensities until a threshold is reached, notably, 1 energy level successfully defibrillated, whereas a slightly different shock strength (higher or lower) failed. Such DFT assessment is best viewed as a method for finding the general location of the defibrillation success curve (**Fig. 2**). However, for any given algorithm, the measured DFT value and the accuracy of the method are influenced by the initial shock energy tested and the direction in which energies are changed during testing.[2] If the initial shock is successful, subsequent defibrillation shocks are decreased in successive trials until a failure is

encountered (**Fig. 3**A). Such decreasing-step DFTs (DFT-decrement) using ~20% reduction in energies distribute asymmetrically toward the upper end (right side) of the dose-response curve. The measured DFT is defined as the minimum energy capable of defibrillate; the lowest energy of defibrillation (LED). Based on both probability analysis and animal studies, the measured DFT/LED is most probably located near the ~70% to 75% defibrillation success curve.[1,2,9]

Increasing-step DFTs (DFT-increment) start at lower shock energy, using incremental steps of higher strength until successful defibrillation is achieved (see **Fig. 3**A). This protocol's test energies distribute asymmetrically toward the lower end (left side) of the dose-response curve, with the most probable DFT location near the ~25% of the defibrillation success curve. Such step-down or step-up DFT protocols only yield gross estimation of the DFT curve location. Smaller energy steps reduce variation but do not necessarily improve the accuracy.[2]

Enhanced DFT

Various system-specific, or patient-specific (such as ischemia or antiarrhythmic drug use) factors may result in a rightward (unfavorable) shift of the defibrillation success curve and reduce the safety margin (see **Fig. 2**). Additional defibrillation trials at the measured DFT energy have been proposed to help to clarify the efficacy and safety margins. Such enhanced DFT protocols include DFT+ and DFT++.[3,4] If the first additional VF conversion test is successful at the DFT energy, it is described as DFT+, whereas 2 additional conversion tests that are successful at the DFT are depicted as DFT++. These enhanced DFT protocols deliver repeated shocks at the measured DFT and improve the accuracy of locating the dose-response curve. If repeated defibrillation shocks are successful, there is a greater chance that DFT is high on the curve (curve A see **Fig. 2**). The efficacy margin needed to reach ~100% success is thus small, and the measured safety margin represents the actual margin of safety. If the additional testing fails (DFT+) or results in a mixed outcome (1 success and 1 failure, DFT++), there is high probability that the measured DFT is on the sloping portion of the curve (curve C, see **Fig. 2**).

Verification Method

The verification methods do not require the patient to be tested with energy levels that fail to defibrillate. These methods include step-down success (SDS) testing and the single-energy success protocols.[1,3,4] These techniques are abbreviated

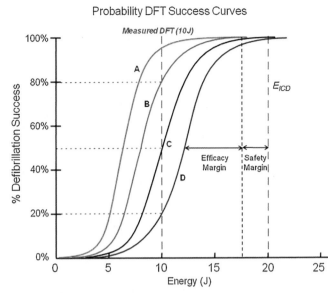

Fig. 2. Four possible defibrillation success curves, with a measured DFT of 10 J. Curve A represents a patient with low defibrillation energy requirement with a measured DFT (10 J) located at the top of the defibrillation success curve (>90% efficacy). Curve D represents a patient who requires high shock strength to ensure defibrillation success with a measured DFT located at the bottom of the defibrillation success curve (10 J associated with $\leq$20% success). A device output (E_{ICD}) of 20 J translates to a safety margin of greater than 10 J for curve A but only 2.5 J for curve D. Curves B and C represent patients with intermediate shock efficacy with DFTs located between 50% and 80% probability of successful defibrillation, with smaller safety margins. Curves B to D also may represent a rightward (unfavorable) shift of the defibrillation success curve with reduced safety margin (see text for details).

and do not estimate the defibrillation success curve but establish the upper boundary of its location.

In the single-energy success protocols, the shock strength that provided successful defibrillation is tested multiple times (1S, 2S, 3S) to verify a consistent margin of safety. The 1-episode, single-energy testing (1S protocol) has limited accuracy because the single shock energy that yielded successful

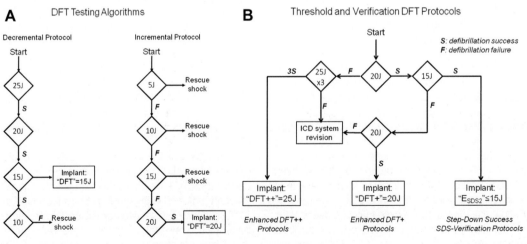

Fig. 3. DFT testing algorithms: (*A*) Examples of decreasing-step (decrement) and increasing-step (increment) DFT threshold method to determine safety margins of defibrillation. The measured DFT is defined as the minimum energy resulting in successful defibrillation. (*B*) Example of a DFT protocol that incorporates both verification and threshold methods for assessing the safety margins (see text for details). (*Adapted from* Singer I, Lang D. The defibrillation threshold. In: Kroll M, Lehmann M, editors. Implantable cardioverter defibrillator therapy. Norwell (MA): Kluwer Academic Publishers; 1996. p. 89–130; with permission.)

defibrillation may lie anywhere along the defibrillation probability curve (5%–95%). Assuming the worst-case scenario, with the 1S energy located at the bottom of the curve ($\leq$5%), the efficacy and safety margins have to be adjusted to accommodate the full width of the defibrillation success curve, which translates to a minimal shock energy requirement of more than 3.5 times the 1S test energy (see **Figs. 1** and **2**).

Statistically, if the defibrillation efficacy is tested by requiring 2 successful conversions at a single energy (E_{2S}), this 2S protocol predicts a DFT value that is higher on the defibrillation success curve ($\geq$25%). In the worst-case scenario, the energy associated with 25% success forms the lower boundary of the 2S confidence interval. The efficacy margin needed to reach 100% success for the 2S protocol would be similar to the margin needed for increasing-step DFTs with the programmed ICD output (E_{ICD}) $\geq$2.0 $\times$ measured DFT (E_{2S}) (see earlier). If the first defibrillation attempt in the 2S protocol is successful but the second trail failed, the test energy is somewhere on the defibrillation curve between E_5 and E_{95}. Either provision for a larger energy margin or revision of the ICD system is required.

Alternatively, further testing to define the DFT is performed. The 3S protocol provides greater precision with 3 test shocks at 1 energy. Because more VF conversions are observed at a test energy, the upper boundary for the defibrillation curve is more accurately established. The possible location on the defibrillation curve yielding 3 successful conversions (3S) ranges from 40% to 100% success. Again, the worst-case scenario predicts E3S ~E40, and the minimum shock energy of 1.7 times the measured DFT (E_{3S}) for 100% conversion success.

The SDS verification protocol is similar to the threshold method (see **Fig. 3**B). It tests the defibrillation efficacy using step-down energies (not necessarily to failure) and defines the upper limit for the decreasing-steps DFT ($DFT_{decr\ step} \leq DFT_{SDS2}$) (**Table 1**). Fig. 3B shows an example of defibrillation testing protocol that uses both verification and threshold methods for assessing the safety margins. The procedure begins at 20 J using a SDS protocol. If the initial SDS energy results in successful conversion of VF, the next lower energy (E_{SDS2}) of 15 J is tested. If both trials are successful, the E_{SDS2} is 15 J and the minimum ICD output for implant equals 2.0$\times E_{SDS2}$ = 30 J. If the second shock energy (15 J) fails to defibrillate, reconfirmation of the safety margin using the enhanced DFT protocol with an additional VF conversion at the higher energy (20 J) is tested (DFT+). If high DFT is encountered (>20 J), the ICD system should be revised and testing repeated. Alternatively, a higher energy (25 J) may be tested with double confirmation using the DFT++ protocol, provided that the ICD can deliver the minimum energy requirement of 1.7$\times DFT_{3S}$ to ensure defibrillation success.

Despite the inherent variability and limitations, the measured DFT provides a quantitative estimate of the ability to defibrillate with a predictable relationship to the dose-response curve (see **Table 1**). Energy delivered at 1.5 times average measured DFT was predicted to achieve ~100% defibrillation success for a single shock in animal studies. Clinically, a margin of greater than or equal to 10 J between the ICD energy output and the measured DFT should be sought to ensure defibrillation efficacy.[10]

MECHANISMS OF DEFIBRILLATION AND ELECTROPHYSIOLOGIC EFFECTS OF SHOCKS

Understanding the mechanisms of fibrillation and defibrillation provides insight into DFT and the upper limit of vulnerability (ULV). VF has been described since the turn of the century.[11,12] The development of modern electrical and optical mapping techniques has allowed direct recording and imaging of ventricular fibrillatory activities. Multiple spiral waves with dynamic instabilities have been observed during VF. These random reentries are continuously colliding, and fractionating with wave breaks and rotor formation (**Fig. 4**).[13–17]

The cellular membrane responses to shocks are critically dependent on the local electrical field intensity/voltage gradient (V/cm) and refractory state, but are independent of the rhythm itself (sinus, paced, or VF).[18,19] At subthreshold shock strengths with weak voltage gradients, shocks behave similarly to pacing stimuli and myocardium is only excitable beyond the refractory period.[19,20] However, myocardium is rarely absolutely refractory to a sufficiently strong stimulus, and the ability of a shock to further depolarize refractory myocardium has a progressive dependence on the local effective shock strength with a linear response (**Fig. 5**).[8,17,20]

Such shock-induced refractory period extension measured by ADT beyond the normal action potential duration (APD) is also a function of shock timing (coupling interval [CI]) (see **Fig. 5**). At long CIs, the ADT is nearly the same for all shock strengths because they all evoke an action potential of nearly the same duration (weak or strong shocks). The strong shock strengths produce ADT at all CIs, reflecting its ability to depolarize the myocardium at any point during the cardiac cycle.

During fibrillation, multiple random reentry waves exist, with constantly changing depolarization and

Table 1
Minimum energy margins for various threshold and verification DFT protocols

Test Methods	Worst-case Location on the Defibrillation Success Curve	Minimum Energy Requirement for >99% Defibrillation Success
$DFT_{decr\ step}$	E_{25}	$2.0 \times DFT$
DFT+	E_{50}	$1.5 \times DFT+$
DFT++	E_{75}	$1.2 \times DFT++$
SDS	E_{25}	$2.0 \times DFT_{SDS2}$
Single energy 2S	E_{25}	$2.0 \times DFT_{2S}$
Single energy 3S	E_{40}	$1.7 \times DFT_{3S}$

Values derived from mathematical extrapolations of data reported by Davy and colleagues.[1]
Abbreviations: E, energy; S, success.
Adapted from Singer I, Lang D. The defibrillation threshold. In: Kroll M, Lehmann M, editors. Implantable cardioverter defibrillator therapy. Norwell (MA): Kluwer Academic Publishers; 1996. p. 99; with permission.

repolarization. At the instant of shock delivery, it encounters myocardium at various states of refractoriness across the heart (**Fig. 6**, **Box 1**). With sufficiently strong shock strengths, the amount of refractory period extension (ADT) is a linearly related to the shock CI and the local cellular refractory state. That is, a shock delivered near diastole (tracings f and g in **Fig. 6**) induces additional depolarization equal to a full action potential response, whereas a shock delivered near the upstroke (tracings a and b in **Fig. 6**) produces minimal further depolarization. Myocardium at intermediate refractory states (tracings c–e in **Fig. 6**) responds with moderate ADT. In addition to refractory extension, such suprathreshold shock (shock strength ≥DFT) synchronizes the postshock repolarization phase that results in a uniform myocardial excitability across the heart after successful defibrillation.[21–23]

Critical Mass Hypothesis

The critical mass hypothesis states that a critical mass of myocardium is required for continuation of multiple random reentries that sustain fibrillation.[5,13] For successful defibrillation, depolarization of all cardiac cells and eliminating 100% of the fibrillation waves are not necessary because some residual fibrillatory activity terminates spontaneously.[22] If defibrillation of the critical mass is not achieved, fibrillation persists because postshock residual wavefronts exist, often located in the region of minimum voltage gradient, which continues and propagates the fibrillation activations.[11]

ULV Hypothesis

When a weak shock is delivered during fibrillation, immediate reinitiation of reentry and arrhythmia occur, consistent with the critical mass concept.

However, a postshock isoelectric window of electrical quiescence was observed in experimental studies after near-threshold failed defibrillation shocks (**Fig. 7**). These findings suggest that a near-threshold defibrillation shock terminates all activation wavefronts but fails to terminate fibrillation because the same shock reinitiates arrhythmia after an isoelectric window.[19,24,25]

Mechanisms of Fibrillation Induction

Commotio cordis describes sudden death in young sports participants without structural heart disease, caused by low-energy impact to the chest wall.[26] When the impact was delivered within a narrow vulnerable window during cardiac repolarization, often just before the peak of the T wave, fibrillation can be consistently induced; this is the mechanical correlate of the electrical phenomenon of the ULV.[27] A low-energy electrical stimulus delivered during the myocardial vulnerable refractory period induces reentry/fibrillation in both ventricle and atrium.[28] This method of VF induction is so effective that the T wave shock is a standard induction protocol for intraoperative implant evaluation of ICD defibrillation efficacy.

Shock-induced fibrillation is related to both shock intensity and its timing to tissue refractoriness.[18,19,28,29] When the shock field strength is less than a critical strength (−5 V/cm) that interacts with refractory tissue, unidirectional block and reentry may occur around a critical point even in the absence of nonuniform anisotropy (**Fig. 8**). When the local shock voltage is more than the critical value, the intracellular potential is increased such that the sodium current is inactivated and differences in potential gradients among cells during repolarization is minimized. There is no a propagation wavefront, and no VF can be induced regardless of the myocardial refractoriness.

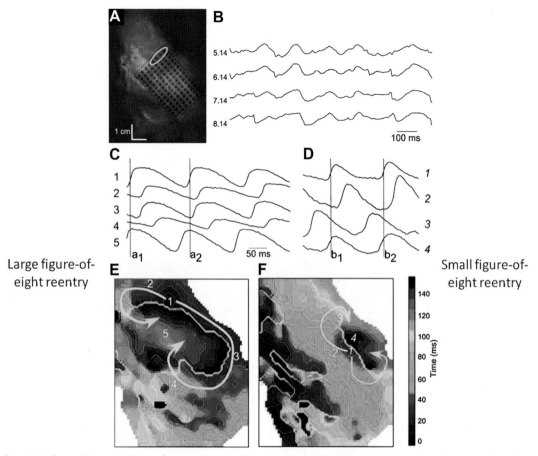

Fig. 4. Explanted human hearts from patients with cardiomyopathy who underwent cardiac transplantation. (*A*) The rectangular high-density epicardial multielectrode mapping array is placed over the interventricular septum. The yellow oval depicts the area where local electrograms were recorded from the multielectrode mapping plaque during VF. (*B*) Local electrograms from the multielectrode contact mapping array show VF waveforms in unipolar configuration. (*C*) Optical signals recorded during a large figure-of-eight activation sequence as shown in (*E*). Signals 1 to 5 correspond to sites 1 to 5 on the optical map indicated in (*E*). The time interval a_1 to a_2 indicates the 140-millisecond activation sequence (cycle length of the reentry) as depicted in (*E*). (*D*) Optical signals recorded during a small figure-of-eight activation sequence seen in (*F*). Signals 1 to 4 correspond to sites 1 to 4 in (*F*). The time interval b_1 to b_2 indicates the period depicted by the isochrone map shown in (*F*). (*E*) Ten-millisecond isochrone maps derived from optical signals during VF within time interval a_1 to a_2 shown in (*C*). A large figure-of-eight activation sequence is clearly visible starting at site 1. (*F*) Isochronal activation map with 10-millisecond isochrones obtained during VF 3 seconds after the map seen in (*E*). A smaller figure-of-eight sequence starting at a different location can be seen. (*From* Nanthakumar K, Jalife J, Massé S, et al. Optical mapping of Langendorff-perfused human hearts: establishing a model for the study of ventricular fibrillation in humans. Am J Physiol Heart Circ Physiol 2007;293:H877; with permission.)

As described earlier, although the near-threshold defibrillation shock eliminates most/all of the VF activation wavefronts, the same shock encounters some part of the myocardium at its vulnerable states and reentry can be induced. However, if the shock strength is sufficiently strong ($\geq$ULV) and achieves a local voltage gradient of more than 5 V/cm across the whole heart, successful defibrillation results without reinitiation of VF. In reality, the critical mass hypothesis and the ULV hypothesis are not mutually

exclusive. They provide a framework and unified scheme for linking the processes of defibrillation and shock-induced fibrillation.[8,17,23,24]

THE ULV

Although there is no doubt that the ICD therapy improves survival in high-risk patients, mortality in patients with ICDs is influenced by the type of therapy delivered.[30] Shock is associated with an increased mortality risk because both appropriate

Effects of Coupling Interval and Shock Field Strength on
Additional Depolarization Time (ADT)

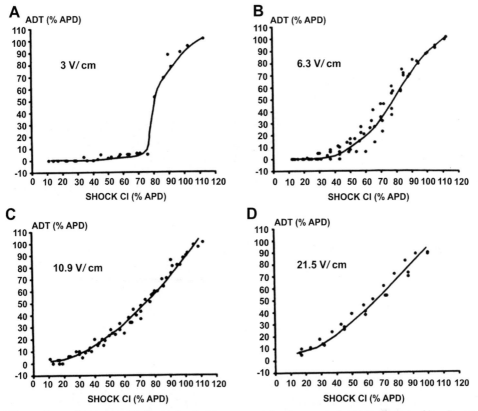

Fig. 5. Effects of coupling interval (CI) and shock strength on refractory periods. Prolongation of local myocardial refractory period measured by the shock-induced ADT as a percentage of the control action potential duration (APD) is dependent on the shock CI. Myocardium is rarely absolutely refractory to a sufficiently strong stimulus. At a low shock voltage gradients (*A*: 3 V/cm), shocks behave like pacing stimuli and myocardium is only excitable beyond it refractory period (>70% of APD); an all-or-none response was observed. However, at a high shock voltage gradients (*D*: 21.5 V/cm), a linear response of the ADT to shock strength was observed. At the intermediate shock strengths (*B*, *C*), intermediate, or graded, responses were noted. (*From* Dillon S, Mehra R. Prolongation of ventricular refractoriness by defibrillation shocks may be due to additional depolarization of the action potential. J Cardiovasc Electrophysiol 1992;3(5):453; with permission.)

and inappropriate ICD shocks are significant predictors of death compared with antitachycardia pacing (ATP). A positive correlation exists between the number of shocks and risk of death.[31,32] High-energy shocks with strengths sufficient to terminate VF cause myocardial damage, manifesting as local injury current and biomarker release.[33–35] These may be associated with postresuscitation myocardial depression and electromechanical dissociation (EMD).[36]

The risk of myocardial dysfunction resulting from exposure to multiple fibrillation-defibrillation episodes often limits the amount of defibrillation testing and, hence, the accuracy of assessing the safety margins. It would be ideal if these margins could be determined quickly and

accurately without repeated exposure to fibrillation events. The ULV has recently gain recognition as an alternative method to assess the defibrillation efficacy for ICDs without inducing VF.[37,38] The ULV is the shock strength more than which electrical stimulation cannot induce ventricular fibrillation even when the stimulus occurs during the vulnerable period of the cardiac cycle. Clinically, it is defined as the weakest T wave shock that does not induce fibrillation.

The ULV has been closely correlated with the DFT in humans, both in sinus rhythm and during ventricular pacing (**Fig. 9**).[39–42] It is more reproducible than a single-point DFT measurement, and temporal changes in the ULV predict temporal changes in the DFT.[42,43] The ULV represents

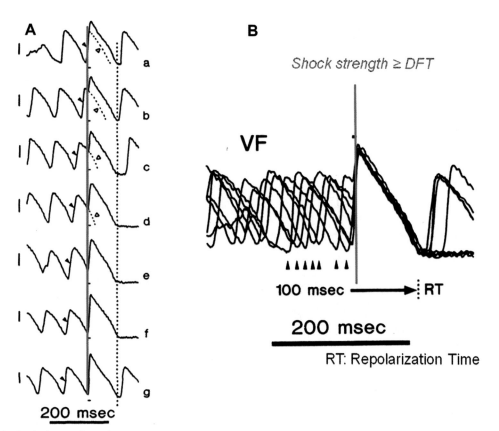

Fig. 6. Optical recordings during VF showing a constant repolarization time after a successful defibrillating shock delivered during VF. (*A*) Seven simultaneous recordings (a–g) were performed across a rabbit ventricle during an episode of VF. Each tracing represents a separate recording at a single site on the ventricle. The traces are aligned with respect to the time of the shock (indicated by the red line). The dashed curve indicated by the unfilled arrowheads in traces a to d indicate an extrapolation of the time course of the action potential had the shock not been applied. The filled arrowheads indicate the preshock upstrokes of the action potential just before shock delivery. The vertical dashed line intercepts all of the traces at the point of maximum membrane repolarization and shows a constant postshock repolarization time (see text for details). (*B*) Same tracings are superimposed and aligned with respect to the shock (*red line*). Upstrokes of preshock local action potentials are indicated by filled arrowheads. A suprathreshold shock (shock strength ≥DFT) results in a constant repolarization time (RT) of 100 milliseconds. (*From* Dillon S. Synchronized repolarization after defibrillation shocks: a possible component of the defibrillation process demonstrated by optical recordings in rabbit heart. Circulation 1992;85(5):1865–78; with permission.)

a simple, clinically applicable method to determine the defibrillation efficacy, both in the acute defibrillator implantation setting as well during chronic device follow-up.[43–45] Shock strengths of 3 to 5 J more than the defined ULV are associated with greater than 90% probability of successful defibrillation, and represent a good estimate of the minimal acute safety margin for implantable defibrillator first shocks.[41,43,44] The relationship between ULV and DFT is independent of shock waveform.[46] However, discrepancies between ULV and DFT may occur in 5% of patients. Absence of coronary disease or previously documented ventricular arrhythmias predicts such a discrepancy.[47]

Box 1
Defibrillation shock effects

1. Encounters myocardium at various states of refractoriness

2. Similar to pacing outputs, but the local myocardium is never absolutely refract to sufficient shock strength

3. Causes additional depolarization time (ADT) with refractory extension

4. The delay in repolarization is dependent on shock strength and timing

5. Promotes homogeneous repolarization

6. Suppression of propagating wavefronts

Activation Patterns in Failed Defibrillation

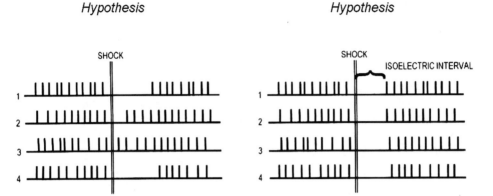

Fig. 7. Activation patterns in failed defibrillation. The left panel depicts local electrical recordings from 4 (tracings 1–4) different myocardial regions across the heart. After delivery of a weak shock that fails to defibrillate, fibrillation persists because postshock residual wavefronts exist, and continue to propagate, consistent with the critical mass hypothesis. The right panel illustrates the ULV hypothesis. After delivery of a near-threshold failed defibrillation shock, a postshock isoelectric interval of electrical quiescence is noted before reinitiation of fibrillation, which suggests that the shock terminates electrical activations but reinduces arrhythmia when the shock energy is less than the ULV.

Many different protocols have been described to determine the ULV. The vulnerability safety margin (VSM) test consists of 3 or 4 shocks of 14 to 18 J delivered at multiple CIs relative to the peak T wave (from −30 to −50 milliseconds before to +10 to +20 milliseconds after) after a paced drivetrain at a cycle length of 500 milliseconds.[37,38] If VF is not induced, the VSM screening is considered adequate with the ULV and DFT less than the shock energy. The alternative ULV testing consists of a step-down protocol.[48] The T wave shock is delivered near (at or −20 millisecond earlier) the peak of the latest-peaking monophasic T wave after a pacing train from the right ventricular apical lead at a cycle length of 400 to 500 milliseconds. The rescue defibrillating shock is programmed at 3 to 5 J more than the induction shock. Decrementing energies are delivered with an attempt to bracket the ULV/DFT. When VF is induced, the ULV is defined as the last induction shock that did not induce VF. The lowest-energy rescue shock that successfully terminates VF defines the DFT (**Fig. 10**).

DEFIBRILLATION WAVEFORMS

In addition to the defibrillator electrode placement and subsequent current vectors, the shape of the defibrillation waveform also plays an important role in determining the efficacy of the defibrillation

shocks.[49] All standard defibrillators have charge-capacitor systems for the delivery of high-energy shocks, and the waveforms describe the shape of the capacitive discharges. Analogous to fluids, electrons (charges) are stored in a complaint vessel (capacitor) that discharges into a low-resistance cardiac tissue and results in flow (current). The capacitor charges dissipate exponentially according to Ohm's law until it is truncated. Such truncated exponential capacitive discharge represents the classic monophasic shock waveform and can be described by the tilt (**Fig. 11**). Tilt is the initial leading edge voltage on the capacitor (Vi), minus the final trailing edge voltage (Vf), divided by the initial leading edge voltage (Vi). This formula is also correct for the first phase of the biphasic waveform.

Theoretically, the initial positive phase (P1) of the biphasic waveform charges the cellular membrane, identical to that of a standard monophasic waveform. The second negative phase (P2) prevents refibrillation by removing or burping the charges deposited on myocardial cells by phase 1, the so-called charge-burping theory.[50] Such biphasic waveform minimizes postshock arrhythmias and ventricular dysfunction, and improves the safety of defibrillation.[7]

Multiple studies using different lead configurations in animals and humans have consistently shown superior defibrillating efficacy of the

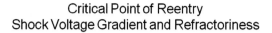

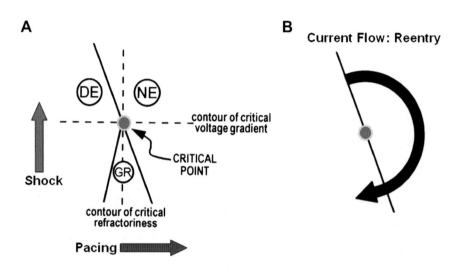

DE: Direct Excitation   GR: Graded Response   NE: No Effect

Fig. 8. The left panel depicts the activation pattern as the result of interaction between the shock voltage gradient and tissue refractoriness in canine experimental data. A shock stimulus (*red arrow*) is delivered along the bottom with the voltage gradient strongest near the bottom and weakest near the top. Pacing (*blue arrow*) was performed perpendicular to the shock strength orientation; depolarization wavefront propagates from left to right. Tissue recovery (repolarization) follows a similar direction to that of depolarization, with most recovered tissue near the left and more refractory tissue near the right. A critical point of reentry exists when a critical local shock strength (~5 V/cm) interacts with refractory tissue. When strong shock gradient interacts with recovered tissue, direct cellular excitation (DE) results. When weak shock gradient interacts with more refractory tissue, no cellular depolarization (NE) occurs. A region of graded response (GR) is observed that causes a temporary prolongation of refractoriness during stimulation of refractory tissue. The right panel illustrates the induction of current flow and subsequent reentry. Tissue in the DE region has an increased positive cellular membrane potential, whereas cellular membrane potential remains negative in the NE regions. A large intracellular potential gradient exists at the boundary between the DE and NE regions, and the GR region represents areas of prolonged refractoriness that constitute unidirectional block, and reentry can occur around a critical point. (Part (*A*) *from* Frazier D, Wolf P, Wharton J, et al. Stimulus-induced critical point: mechanism for electrical initiation of reentry in normal canine myocardium. J Clin Invest 1989;83(3):1039–52; with permission; and part (*B*) *from* Knisley S, Smith W, Ideker R. Effect of field stimulation on cellular repolarization in rabbit myocardium: implications for reentry induction. Circ Res 1992;70(4): 707–15; with permission.)

biphasic waveform compared with that of the monophasic waveform.[50–53] Although monophasic shocks produced greater magnitude of refractory period extension than biphasic shocks, the biphasic waveform limits the postshock spatial heterogeneity of refractoriness, supporting the hypothesis that tissue homogeneity is a more likely predictor of defibrillation efficacy than the magnitude of refractoriness.[54] These results indicate that biphasic shocks, with the initial positive P1 phase longer than the terminal negative P2 phase, markedly reduce energy requirements for defibrillation.[50]

DEFIBRILLATION POLARITY AND CURRENT PATHWAY

In addition to the defibrillation waveforms, current polarity and pathway also influence the efficacy of the defibrillation shocks. Historically, the right ventricular (RV) ICD electrode is designated as the cathode (−) and the term reversed polarity denotes an anodal (RV+) configuration. Comparing the cathodal (RV−) with the anodal (RV+) polarities, RV+ has lower measured DFTs in 46% of the patients, and higher DFTs in 12% of the patients. No difference in DFTs was observed in

Correlation of ULV and DFT

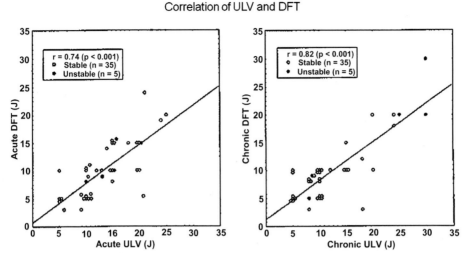

Fig. 9. Scatter plots with regression line show the correlation between ULV on the abscissa and DFT on the ordinate. Good correlations exist between the ULV and DFT for both acute (*left panel*) and chronic measurements (*right panel*). Open circles denote stable patients and closed circles denote unstable patients. *r*, Pearson correlation coefficient. (*Adapted from* Martin D, Chen P, Hwang C, et al. Upper limit of vulnerability predicts chronic defibrillation threshold for transvenous implantable defibrillators. J Cardiovasc Electrophysiol 1997;8(3):245; with permission.)

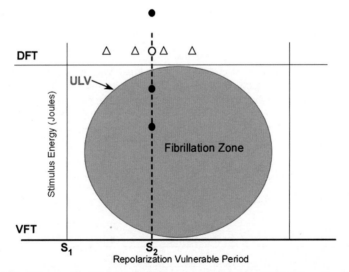

Fig. 10. The relationship between the ULV and the DFT is described by the CI (S1–S2) on the abscissa and the stimulus energy on the ordinate axis. When critically timed stimuli encounter partially refractory tissues in the vulnerable repolarization period (*pink circle*), fibrillation can be induced. When the stimulus is delivered too early (short S1–S2), the tissue is too refractory to be depolarized. A late-coupled (long S1–S2) stimulus behaves like a pacing output and the critical point for reentry cannot be generated. If the shock strength is weaker than the Ventricular fibrillation threshold (<VFT), or when the shock strength is sufficiently strong that achieves a high local voltage gradient (>5 V/cm) across the myocardium (>DFT), no VF can be induced. The VSM test consists of delivery of fixed energy T wave induction attempts at multiple CIs across the repolarization period (*open triangles*). If VF was not induced, the VSM is considered adequate and more than the DFT. The step-down ULV protocol uses decrementing T wave shocks delivered near the peak of the latest-peaking T wave (*circles*). VF is induced when a critically timed stimulus encounters tissues in the vulnerable repolarization period (fibrillation zone). ULV is defined as the last induction shock that did not induce VF (*open circles*).

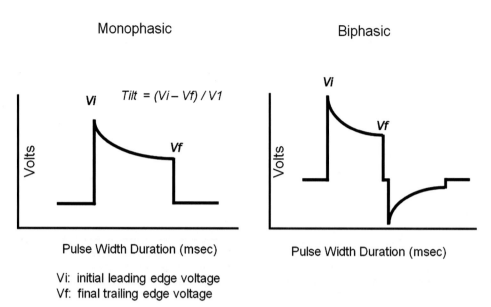

Capacitor Shock Waveforms

Monophasic · **Biphasic**

$Tilt = (Vi - Vf) / V1$

Vi: initial leading edge voltage
Vf: final trailing edge voltage

Fig. 11. Capacitor shock waveforms. The figure depicts the classic monophasic and biphasic waveforms. The tilt of the shock waveform is also illustrated (see text for details).

42% of the subjects. Although the magnitude of DFT reduction with RV+ polarity is only modest at ~17%, anodal RV is preferable most of the time because measured DFTs are better or the same in 88% of cases (**Table 2**).[55–59] The use of multilead defibrillating systems has also been shown to reduce the DFT compared with single-pathway shock.[3,60] Postshock virtual electrode polarization related to various electrode configurations, polarity, and pulsing pathways may explain the differences in the shock energy required to achieve the minimally effective current gradient over the entire myocardium and subsequent successful defibrillation.[61–63]

INTERACTIONS OF ANTIARRHYTHMIC DRUGS AND ICDs

It is important to understand the effects of antiarrhythmic drugs on the DFTs (**Box 2**). In general, membrane-active drugs such as Vaughan William class I and class III agents can affect the defibrillation energy requirement.[4,64] No consistent effect on DFT was observed with the use of class IA

Table 2
Reversal of shock polarity

Study	N	Mean DFT Reduction	RV+ Better	RV− Better	Same
Schauete 1997	27	17%	10	3	14
Shorofsky 1996	26	9%	—	—	—
Natale 1995	20	24%	12	2	6
Strickberger 1995	15	−4%	3	3	9
Keelan 1997	10	39%	7	0	3
Keelan 1997	12	26%	7	2	3
Overall	110	16%	39	10	35
% of patients	—	—	46%	12%	42%

Modified from Kroll M, Tchou P. Testing and programming of implantable defibrillator functions at implantation. In: Ellenbogen K, Kay G, Wilkoff B, editors. Clinical cardiac pacing and defibrillation. Philadelphia (PA): WB Saunders; 2000. p. 540–61; with permission.

<table>
<tr><td>

Box 2
Effects of antiarrhythmic drugs on DFTs

Class IA: minimal effect on DFT in therapeutic dosage

Class IB: mild increase of DFT

Class IC: significantly increase DFT

Class II: minimal effect on DFT

Class III: variable, chronic amiodarone: significantly increase DFT
</td></tr>
</table>

drugs in therapeutic dosages. Class IB drugs (lidocaine and mexiletine) can cause a reversible mild increase in DFTs. The use of class IC drugs is often associated with a significant increase in DFT in addition to proarrhythmia. The effects of class III drugs can be variable. It is generally accepted that amiodarone may lower the DFT when administered acutely (intravenous or orally), but chronic amiodarone exposure can significantly increase the DFT (>60%).[65–67] Therefore, repeated testing of ICD functions and DFT determination are recommended after initiation of antiarrhythmic drugs, particularly with amiodarone, to ensure an adequate margin of safety. Other drugs, including D-sotalol, N-acetylprocainamide (NAPA), and catecholamine may facilitate ventricular defibrillation and decrease the DFT (**Table 3**). Sildenafil citrate (Viagra) is a highly selective inhibitor of c-GMP–specific phosphodiesterase and has been

widely used for the treatment of erectile dysfunction. However, administration of sildenafil at a supratherapeutic level results in a significant increase in the DFT (∼38% by energy) in animal models.[68] The exact mechanism of sildenafil on cellular electrophysiology is unclear.

INCREASE OF DFTs

Clinically, a margin of greater than or equal to 10 J between the ICD energy output and the measured DFT should be maintained to assure defibrillation efficacy.[10] However, increase of defibrillation energy requirement may occur and represents a significant challenge. The true incidence in the current era of biphasic defibrillators is difficult to ascertain, but may be as high as 6.2% by one report. These patients tend to have a lower ejection fraction, large cardiac mass, large body size, wide QRS duration, less coronary artery disease, more heart failure, and are more likely to be taking

Table 3
Effects of drugs on DFTs

Increase DFT	Decrease DFT	Conflicting Reports
Encainide	Sotalol	Quinidine
Flecainide	NAPA	Mexiletine
Amiodarone (chronic)	Amiodarone (acute)?	Lidocaine
Sildenafil Citrate	Ibutilide	Bretylium
Cocaine?	Dofetilide	Amiodarone (acute)
Ajmaline	Tedisamil	Isoproterenol
Atropine		
Diltiazem		
Verapamil		
Carvedilol		

Adapted from Singer I, Lang D. The defibrillation threshold. In: Kroll M, Lehmann M, editors. Implantable cardioverter defibrillator therapy. Norwell (MA): Kluwer Academic Publishers; 1996. p. 89–130; with permission.

<table>
<tr><td>

Box 3
Management of high DFT

1. Modifications of ICD system:
   a. Optimize current vector/lead configurations:
      i. Apical-septal distal RV coil position
      ii. Innominate vein proximal coil location
      iii. Addition of subcutaneous (SQ) array
      iv. Removal of superior vena cava (SVC) coil
      v. Addition of coronary sinus/azygos vein coil
   b. High-output device
   c. Alternative shock waveform:
      i. Biphasic>monophasic
      ii. (RV+) polarity
      iii. Optimized waveform
2. Optimize testing protocol:
   a. Minimize VF induction, ULV protocol
3. Modifications of clinical variables:
   a. Antiarrhythmic drugs: reduction/discontinuation amiodarone
   b. Correct reversible causes: ischemia, hemodynamic, electrolytes
   c. Rule out pneumothorax
   d. Possible role for epicardial patches/mesh
</td></tr>
</table>

amiodarone.[69–71] Sudden death remains an important risk in patients with high DFTs, presumably caused by inadequate defibrillation safety margin.[72]

When confronted by a patient with insufficient energy margins for implantation, the influences of shock waveform, polarity, and current vectors/pathways must be considered, as well the interactions of antiarrhythmic drugs on defibrillation efficacy (**Box 3**).[57] Modification of the ICD system/leads, alteration of antiarrhythmic drug therapy, and correction of patients' underlying metabolic/respiratory/ischemic substrate may be required.[4,57,71,73,74]

Modification of the Defibrillator Lead System

Optimizing the current vectors and distributions of effective field gradient over the cardiac mass is essential. These maneuvers include (1) repositioning

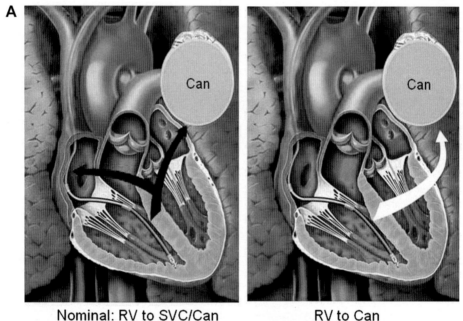

A

Nominal: RV to SVC/Can   RV to Can

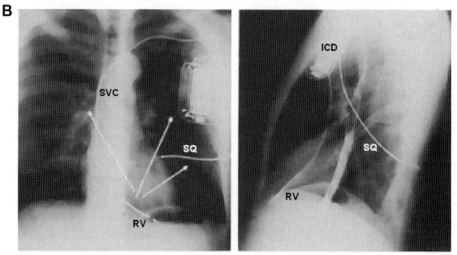

B

Frontal View   Lateral View

Fig. 12. Optimizing current vectors with modifications of ICD lead configurations. (*A*) Removal of SVC coil from the lead system improves current vector by minimizing shunting (blue) to right atrium and maximize current flow (yellow) to the left ventricle. (*B*) Radiographic image of the positions of the subcutaneous (SQ) coil, with the RV defibrillator lead and the ICD generator can. The overall lead impedance is lowered with greater current flow (*red arrows*). The outline of the esophagus is visible in the lateral view.

of RV coil, (2) removal of the SVC coil, (3) addition of a SQ array, (4) addition of a coronary sinus (CS) lead, and (5) azygos vein lead implant.

DFTs are significantly reduced with a more distal RV coil position compared with a proximal RV placement.[75] Such apical-septal lead positions probably induce a larger region of depolarization and refractoriness over the left ventricular mass. In patients with a dual-coil ICD lead system, with a distal RV coil and proximal coil near the SVC, the nominal lead configuration consists of RV to SVC/Can. Capping or removing the SVC defibrillating coil in selected patients can improve DFTs, and this strategy is particularly attractive in patients with a low shock lead impedance (<40 Ω). The mechanism consists primarily of maximizing current flow to the left ventricle and optimizing the lead impedance (**Fig. 12**A). This strategy was successful in 15% of patients with high DFTs by one report.[69]

Addition of a SQ lead/array further alters the current vectors and is a common strategy for lowering the DFTs. The SQ lead/array is inserted at the lateral edge of the pectoral pocket and tracked subcutaneously along the back to a position near the spine (see **Fig. 12**B). This lead position redirects the current flow posteriorly to encompass the left ventricular mass. In addition, the large surface area of the SQ lead reduces the overall shock lead impedance, increases current flow, and shortens the pulse width (see later discussion).[71] Other potential lead locations that provide such posterior current vector include the CS and the azygos vein.

The azygos vein is located along the thoracic column in the right posterior mediastinum (http://en.wikipedia.org/wiki/Vertebral_column) and provides an alternate path for blood to the SVC. A defibrillator coil positioned in the azygos vein provides stable current vectors that encompass the posterior portion of myocardium (**Fig. 13**).[76,77] The efficacy in improving DFTs is similar in both azygos vein lead and SQ lead implantation.[78]

Shock Waveform

The shock waveform is the parameter that most directly influences defibrillation efficacy. Biphasic shocks consistently show superior defibrillation efficacy compared with the monophasic waveform. Reversal of shock polarity improves DFTs in patients with the endocardial lead systems or patch-coil hybrid configurations, especially in those with high biphasic DFTs.

Although the tilt describes the shock waveform, it is not a measure of defibrillation efficacy. In addition to the shock voltage, which defines the spatial distribution of electrical field over the heart, waveform duration is also a critical parameter because the energy is delivered to the heart for the duration of the shock. Using passive resistor-capacitor modeling, a optimized, efficient defibrillation waveform can be predicted based on the charge-burping theory.[50,59,79,80] For capacitive-discharge

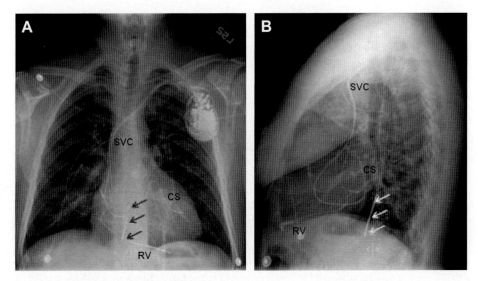

Posterior-Anterior View   Lateral View

Fig. 13. Fluoroscopic images of a defibrillating coil implant (*red arrows*) in the azygos vein. (*A*) The posterior to anterior (PA) view and (*B*) the lateral view. (*Adapted from* Kroll M, Schwab J. Achieving low defibrillation thresholds at implant: pharmacologic influences, RV coil polarity and position, SVC coil usage and positioning, pulse width settings, and the Azygous vein. Fundam Clin Pharmacol 2010;5:568; with permission.)

waveforms, effective defibrillation energy is minimized when the system time constant of the ICD equals the cell membrane time constant (**Fig. 14**). The shorter pulse width truncates phase 1 of the biphasic waveform at the peak of cellular membrane response, and phase-2 removes any residual membrane voltage and minimizes tissue electrical heterogeneity.

Most commercially available ICDs deliver fixed tilt waveforms between 50% and 65%. That is, the device truncates the capacitive discharge when a predetermined tilt is reached, with variable waveform durations depending on the

system capacitance and resistance. However, implantable defibrillators from St Jude Medical can deliver programmable shock pulse widths with variable tilt waveforms. Such tuned (optimized) waveform with shorter pulse width is associated with a modest reduction in the defibrillation energy requirement, especially in patients with increased DFTs, compared with the standard fixed tilt waveforms.[59,81,82] Optimizing the defibrillation waveform tilt should be considered in all patients when an adequate safety margin cannot be obtained with the nominal defibrillation waveform.

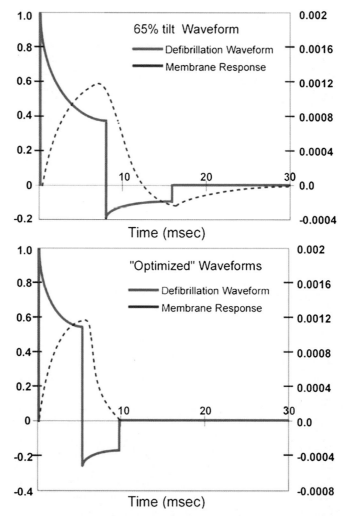

Fig. 14. Optimized pulse width compared with the standard biphasic waveform (*red curve*). The predicted optimal pulse duration for the optimal capacitance is equal to the cell membrane time constant. The capacity of the shock (phase 1) to charge the cell membrane (*blue curve*) is related to the peak voltage of the leading edge of phase 1. Energy applied after the maximum membrane response is wasted and may be counterproductive. The shorter pulse width truncates the phase 1 of the biphasic waveform at the peak of cellular membrane response. This duration is best approximated by the membrane time constant for any given capacitance. The phase 2 removes the residual membrane voltage left by phase 1 and minimizes postshock tissue electrical heterogeneity. Although the total energy (voltage×time) as area under the curve may be smaller, the waveform is more efficient.

Other Considerations

In addition to ICD system modifications, medication use, underlying metabolic derangement/ischemia must be considered in patients with increased DFTs. Antiarrhythmic drugs, particularly chronic amiodarone exposure, can significantly increase the DFTs (see **Box 2**, **Table 3**). Discontinuation of amiodarone or a switch to sotalol or dofetilide may reduce the DFTs. Pneumothorax is an unrecognized cause of high DFTs during device implantation, often associated with high lead impedance. Careful intraoperative fluoroscopic inspection of the thorax is recommended to assist early detection (Mainigi, 2006 #108)[73], (Kroll, 2007 #113).[59]

Prolonged DFT testing with anesthesia, multiple VF inductions, and shock deliveries may result in autonomic alterations, ischemia, and myocardial injury (Runsio, 1997 #47)[33], (Nikolski, 2005 #48)[34], (Tereshchenko, 2009 #41)[35], which can lead to an increased DFT, ventricular dysfunction, and electromechanical dissociation.[36] The ULV protocol provides a safe and more efficient method to determine the defibrillation efficacy by minimizing episodes of VF induction, particularly in patients with a reduced ejection fraction. The presence of epicardial patches from a prior ICD implantation may also affect DFTs. The epicardial patches may act as a shield that alters the current vector and gradient distribution over the heart.

A high-output generator may have achieved an adequate energy margin (E_{ICD}-DFT) in most patients.[70,73] However, empiric use of high-output devices in substitution of DFT testing is not recommended because system modifications are still often required.[69] If none of the considerations mentioned earlier result in a sufficient DFT, one can proceed to a surgical epicardial defibrillation implantation.

SUMMARY

Defibrillation efficacy is best measured by the sigmoidal dose-response curve that describes the probability for successful defibrillation versus shock energies. It provides an estimation of the energy margins between the defibrillator output and the energy required for successful defibrillation. Many methods are available to determine the DFT, which represents only a single value on the curve. The accuracy of DFT determinations to assess the defibrillation efficacy is dependent on the width of the curve. Despite the inherent variability and limitations, carefully measured DFT provides adequate estimate of the ability to defibrillate with a predictable relationship to the dose-response curve.

Complex electrophysiologic interactions exist between the cellular membrane potentials and shock-induced electrical field gradients that lead to either termination of fibrillation or reinitiation of reentry. Both the critical mass hypothesis and the ULV hypothesis may be involved, and successful defibrillation is critically dependent on both energy delivered and timing. The defibrillation efficacy is also influenced by the shock waveform, polarity, and current vectors/pathways, as well as the interactions of antiarrhythmic drugs, particularly amiodarone. In patients with increased DFTs, ICD system modification, alteration of drug therapy, and correction of patients' underlying substrate are required to achieve an adequate defibrillation margin of safety.

REFERENCES

1. Davy J, Fain E, Dorian P, et al. The relationship between successful defibrillation and delivered energy in open-chest dogs: reappraisal of the "defibrillation threshold" concept. Am Heart J 1987; 113(1):77–84.
2. McDaniel W, Schuder J. The cardiac ventricular defibrillation threshold: inherent limitations in its application and interpretation. Med Instrum 1987;21(3): 170–6.
3. Singer I, Lang D. Defibrillation threshold: clinical utility and therapeutic implications. Pacing Clin Electrophysiol 1992;15:932–49.
4. Singer I, Lang D. The defibrillation threshold. In: Kroll M, Lehmann M, editors. Implantable cardioverter defibrillator therapy. Norwell (MA): Kluwer Academic Publishers; 1996. p. 89–130.
5. Zipes D, Fischer J, King R, et al. Termination of ventricular fibrillation in dogs by depolarizing a critical amount of myocardium. Am J Cardiol 1975;36: 37–44.
6. Winkle R, Mead R, Ruder M, et al. Effect of duration of ventricular fibrillation on defibrillation efficacy in humans. Circulation 1990;81(5):1477–81.
7. Jones J, Jones R. Improved defibrillator waveform safety factor with biphasic waveforms. Am J Physiol 1983;245:H60–5.
8. Dillon S. The electrophysiology of ventricular defibrillation: today and yesterday. In: Allessie M, Fromer M, editors. Atrial and ventricular fibrillation: mechanisms and device therapy. Armonk (NY): Futura Publishing; 1997. p. 113–44.
9. Rattes M, Jones D, Sharma A, et al. Defibrillation threshold: a simple and quantitative estimate of the ability to defibrillate. Pacing Clin Electrophysiol 1987;1(Pt 1):70–7.
10. Marchlinski F, Flores B, Miller J, et al. Relation of the intraoperative defibrillation threshold to successful postoperative defibrillation with an automatic

implantable cardioverter defibrillator. Am J Cardiol 1988;62:393–8.

11. Wiggers C. Defibrillation of the ventricles. Circ Res 1953;1(3):191–9.

12. Wiggers C, Bell J, Paine M. Studies of ventricular fibrillation caused by electric shock: II. Cinematographic and electrocardiographic observations of the natural process in the dog's heart: its inhibition by potassium and the revival of coordinated beats by calcium. Ann Noninvasive Electrocardiol 2003;18(3):252–61.

13. Witkowski F, Penkoske P, Plonsey R. Mechanism of cardiac defibrillation in open-chest dogs with unipolar DC-coupled simultaneous activation and shock potential recordings. Circulation 1990;82(1):244–60.

14. Ideker R, Walcott G, Walcott K, et al. Mapping of ventricular fibrillation. In: Allessie M, Fromer M, editors. Atrial and ventricular fibrillation: mechanisms and device therapy. Armonk (NY): Futura Publishing; 1997. p. 63–79.

15. Tung L, Cysyk J. Imaging fibrillation/defibrillation in a dish. J Electrocardiol 2007;40:S62–5.

16. Nanthakumar K, Jalife J, Massé S, et al. Optical mapping of Langendorff-perfused human hearts: establishing a model for the study of ventricular fibrillation in humans. Am J Physiol Heart Circ Physiol 2007;293:H875–80.

17. Dosdall D, Huang J, Ideker R. Mechanism of defibrillation. In: Wang P, Hsia H, Al-Almad A, et al, editors. Ventricular arrhythmias and sudden cardiac death Malden (MA): Blackwell Futura; 2008. p. 277–88.

18. Ideker R, Zhou X, Knisley S. Correlation among fibrillation, defibrillation and cardiac pacing. Pacing Clin Electrophysiol 1995;18(Pt II):512–25.

19. Knisley S, Smith W, Ideker R. Effect of field stimulation on cellular repolarization in rabbit myocardium: implications for reentry induction. Circ Res 1992; 70(4):707–15.

20. Dillon S, Mehra R. Prolongation of ventricular refractoriness by defibrillation shocks may be due to additional depolarization of the action potential. J Cardiovasc Electrophysiol 1992;3(5):442–56.

21. Dillon S. Synchronized repolarization after defibrillation shocks: a possible component of the defibrillation process demonstrated by optical recordings in rabbit heart. Circulation 1992;85(5):1865–78.

22. Kwaku K, Dillon S. Shock-induced depolarization of refractory myocardium prevents wave-front propagation in defibrillation. Circ Res 1996;79(5):957–73.

23. Dillon S, Kwaku K. Progressive depolarization: a unified hypothesis for defibrillation and fibrillation induction by shocks. J Cardiovasc Electrophysiol 1998;9(5):529–52.

24. Chen P, Wolf P, Ideker R. Mechanism of cardiac defibrillation: a different point of view. Circulation 1991; 84(2):913–9.

25. Wang N, Lee M, Ohara T, et al. Optical mapping of ventricular defibrillation in isolated swine right ventricles: demonstration of a post-shock isoelectric window after near-threshold defibrillation shocks. Circulation 2001;104:227–33.

26. Link M, Wang P, Pandian N, et al. An experimental model of sudden death due to low-energy chest wall impact (commotio cordis). N Engl J Med 1998;33(25):1805–11.

27. Link M, Maron B, Wang P, et al. Upper and lower limits of vulnerability to sudden arrhythmic death with chest-wall impact (commotio cordis). J Am Coll Cardiol 2003;41(1):99–104.

28. Katz A, Sweeney R, Gill R, et al. Relation of atrial refractoriness to upper and lower limits of vulnerability for atrial fibrillation/flutter following implantable ventricular defibrillator shocks. Circulation 1999;100: 1125–30.

29. Frazier D, Wolf P, Wharton J, et al. Stimulus-induced critical point: mechanism for electrical initiation of reentry in normal canine myocardium. J Clin Invest 1989;83(3):1039–52.

30. Sweeney M, Sherfesee L, DeGroot P, et al. Differences in effects of electrical therapy type for ventricular arrhythmias on mortality in implantable cardioverter-defibrillator patients. Heart Rhythm 2010;7(3):353–60.

31. Daubert J, Zareba W, Cannom D, et al. Inappropriate implantable cardioverter-defibrillator shocks in MADIT II: frequency, mechanisms, predictors, and survival impact. J Am Coll Cardiol 2008;51(51):14.

32. Poole J, Johnson G, Hellkamp A, et al. Prognostic importance of defibrillator shocks in patients with heart failure. N Engl J Med 2008;359:1009–17.

33. Runsio M, Kallner A, Källner G, et al. Myocardial injury after electrical therapy for cardiac arrhythmias assessed by troponin-T release. Am J Cardiol 1997; 79:1241–5.

34. Nikolski V, Efimov I. Electroporation of the heart. Europace 2005;7:S146–54.

35. Tereshchenko L, Faddis M, Fetics B, et al. Transient local injury current in right ventricular electrogram after implantable cardioverter-defibrillator shock predicts heart failure progression. J Am Coll Cardiol 2009;54(9):822–8.

36. Mitchell L, Pineda E, Titus J, et al. Sudden death in patients with implantable cardioverter defibrillators: the importance of post-shock electromechanical dissociation. J Am Coll Cardiol 2002;39(8):1323–8.

37. Day J, Doshi R, Belott P, et al. Inductionless or limited shock testing is possible in most patients with implantable cardioverter-defibrillators/cardiac resynchronization therapy defibrillators: results of the multicenter ASSURE study (Arrhythmia Single Shock Defibrillation Threshold Testing Versus Upper Limit of Vulnerability: Risk Reduction Evaluation With Implantable Cardioverter-Defibrillator Implantations). Circulation 2007;115:2382–9.

38. Birgersdotter-Green U, Monir G, Ruetz L, et al. Automated vulnerability testing accurately identifies

patients with inadequate defibrillation safety margin. Circulation 2010;122:A20654 [abstract: 20654].

39. Chen P, Feld G, Kriett J, et al. Relation between upper limit of vulnerability and defibrillation threshold in humans. Circulation 1993;88(1):186–92.

40. Hwang C, Swerdlow C, Kass R, et al. Upper limit of vulnerability reliably predicts the defibrillation threshold in humans. Circulation 1994;90:2308–14.

41. Swerdlow C, Ahern T, Kass R, et al. Upper limit of vulnerability is a good estimator of shock strength associated with 90% probability of successful defibrillation in humans with transvenous implantable cardioverter-defibrillators. J Am Coll Cardiol 1996; 27(5):1112–8.

42. Swerdlow C, Davie S, Ahern T, et al. Comparative reproducibility of defibrillation threshold and upper limit of vulnerability. Pacing Clin Electrophysiol 1996;19:2103–11.

43. Martin D, Chen P, Hwang C, et al. Upper limit of vulnerability predicts chronic defibrillation threshold for transvenous implantable defibrillators. J Cardiovasc Electrophysiol 1997;8(3):241–8.

44. Birgersdotter-Green U, Undesser K, Fujimura O, et al. Correlation of acute and chronic defibrillation threshold with upper limit of vulnerability determined in normal sinus rhythm. J Interv Card Electrophysiol 1999;3:155–61.

45. Glikson M, Gurevitz O, Trusty J, et al. Upper limit of vulnerability determination during implantable cardioverter-defibrillator placement to minimize ventricular fibrillation inductions. Am J Cardiol 2004;94(11):1445–9.

46. Swerdlow C, Kass R, O'Connor M, et al. Effect of shock waveform on relationship between upper limit of vulnerability and defibrillation threshold. J Cardiovasc Electrophysiol 1998;9(4):339–49.

47. Gurevitz O, Friedman P, Glikson M, et al. Discrepancies between the upper limit of vulnerability and defibrillation threshold: prevalence and clinical predictors. J Cardiovasc Electrophysiol 2003;14(7): 728–32.

48. Hsia H, Chonielewski L, Coss'u S, et al. A practical application of upper limit of vulnerability for predicting defibrillation threshold in man. [Abstract]. Pacing Clin Electrophysiol 1996;19:656.

49. Blanchard S, Ideker R, Cooper R, et al. The defibrillation waveform. In: Kroll M, Lehmann M, editors. Implantable cardioverter defibrillator therapy. Norwell, (MA): Kluwer Academic Publishers; 1996. p. 147–61.

50. Swerdlow C, Fan W, Brewer J. Charge-burping theory correctly predicts optimal ratios of phase duration for biphasic defibrillation waveforms. Circulation 1996;94(9):2278–84.

51. Chapman P, Vetter J, Souza J, et al. Comparative efficacy of monophasic and biphasic truncated exponential shocks for non-thoracotomy internal defibrillation in dogs. J Am Coll Cardiol 1988;12(3): 739–45.

52. Bardy G, Ivey T, Allen M, et al. A prospective randomized evaluation of biphasic versus monophasic waveform pulses on defibrillation efficacy in humans. J Am Coll Cardiol 1989;14(3):728–33.

53. Winkle R, Mead R, Ruder M, et al. Improved low energy defibrillation efficacy in man with the use of a biphasic truncated exponential waveform. Am Heart J 1989;117:122–7.

54. Sims J, Miller A, Ujhelyi M. Disparate effects of biphasic and monophasic shocks on postshock refractory period dispersion. Am J Physiol 1998;43: H1943–9.

55. Thakur R, Souza J, Chapman P, et al. Electrode polarity is an important determinant of defibrillation efficacy using a nonthoracotomy system. Pacing Clin Electrophysiol 1994;17(5 Pt 1):919–23.

56. Shorofsky S, Gold M. Effects of waveform and polarity on defibrillation thresholds in humans using a transvenous lead system. Am J Cardiol 1996; 78(3):313–6.

57. Kroll M, Tchou P. Testing and programming of implantable defibrillator functions at implantation. In: Ellenbogen K, Kay G, Wilkoff B, editors. Clinical cardiac pacing and defibrillation. Philadelphia: WB Saunders; 2000. p. 540–61.

58. Rashba E, Shorofsky S, Peters R, et al. Effect of shock polarity on defibrillation thresholds with a hybrid patch-coil lead system. J Interv Card Electrophysiol 2003;9(3):391–6.

59. Kroll M, Swerdlow C. Optimizing defibrillation waveforms for ICDs. J Interv Card Electrophysiol 2007;18: 247–63.

60. Hsia H, Kleiman R, Flores B, et al. Comparison of simultaneous versus sequential defibrillation pulsing techniques using a nonthoracotomy system. Pacing Clin Electrophysiol 1994;17:1222–30.

61. Cheng Y, Mowrey K, Van Wagoner D, et al. Virtual electrode-induced reexcitation: a mechanism of defibrillation. Circ Res 1999;85(11):1056–66.

62. Eason J, Trayanova N. Phase singularities and termination of spiral wave reentry. J Cardiovasc Electrophysiol 2002;13(7):672–9.

63. Efimov I. Virtual electrodes in virtual reality of defibrillation. J Cardiovasc Electrophysiol 2002;13(7): 680–1.

64. Jung W, Manz M, Luderitz B. Effects of antiarrhythmic drugs on defibrillation threshold in patients with the implantable cardioverter defibrillator. Pacing Clin Electrophysiol 1992;15(part 3):645–8.

65. Fain E, Lee J, Winkle R. Effects of acute intravenous and chronic oral amiodarone on defibrillation energy requirements. Am Heart J 1987;114(1):8–17.

66. Jung W, Manz M, Pizzulli L, et al. Effects of chronic amiodarone therapy on defibrillation threshold. Am J Cardiol 1992;70(11):1023–7.

67. Pelosi F, Oral H, Kim M, et al. Effect of chronic amiodarone therapy on defibrillation energy requirements in humans. J Cardiovasc Electrophysiol 2000;11(7):736–40.

68. Shinlapawittayatorn K, Sungnoon R, Chattipakorn S, et al. Effects of sildenafil citrate on defibrillation efficacy. J Cardiovasc Electrophysiol 2006;17(3):292–5.

69. Russo A, Sauer W, Gerstenfeld E, et al. Defibrillation threshold testing: is it really necessary at the time of implantable cardioverter-defibrillator insertion? Heart Rhythm 2005;2(5):456–61.

70. Mainigi S, Cooper J, Russo A, et al. Elevated defibrillation thresholds in patients undergoing biventricular defibrillator implantation: incidence and predictors. Heart Rhythm 2006;3(9):1010–6.

71. Kroll M, Tchou P. Testing and programming of implantable defibrillator functions at implantation. In: Ellenbogen K, Kay G, Lau C, et al, editors. Clinical cardiac pacing, defibrillation and resynchronization therapy. Philadelphia: Saunders Elsevier; 2007. p. 531–57.

72. Epstein A, Ellenbogen K, Kirk K, et al. Clinical characteristics and outcome of patients with high defibrillation thresholds: a multicenter study. Circulation 1992;86(4):1206–16.

73. Mainigi S, Callans D. How to manage the patient with a high defibrillation threshold. Heart Rhythm 2006;3:492–5.

74. Kroll M, Schwab J. Achieving low defibrillation thresholds at implant: pharmacological influences, RV coil polarity and position, SVC coil usage and positioning, pulse width settings, and the azygous vein. Fundam Clin Pharmacol 2010;5:561–73.

75. Rashba E, Bonner M, Wilson J, et al. Distal right ventricular coil position reduces defibrillation thresholds. J Cardiovasc Electrophysiol 2003;14(10): 1036–40.

76. Cesario D, Bhargava M, Valderrábano M, et al. Azygos vein lead implantation: a novel adjunctive technique for implantable cardioverter defibrillator placement. J Cardiovasc Electrophysiol 2004; 15(7):780–3.

77. Kommuri N, Kollepara S, Saulitis E, et al. Azygos vein lead implantation for high defibrillation thresholds in implantable cardioverter defibrillator placement. Indian Pacing Electrophysiol J 2010;10(1): 49–54.

78. Cooper J, Latacha M, Soto G, et al. The Azygos defibrillator lead for elevated defibrillation thresholds: implant technique, lead stability, and patient series. Pacing Clin Electrophysiol 2008;31(11):1405–10.

79. Kroll M. A minimal model of the monophasic defibrillation pulse. Pacing Clin Electrophysiol 1993;16: 769–77.

80. Swerdlow C, Brewer J, Kass R, et al. Application of models of defibrillation to human defibrillation data: implications for optimizing implantable defibrillator capacitance. Circulation 1997;96(9):2813–22.

81. Mouchawar G, Kroll M, Val-Mejias J, et al. ICD waveform optimization: a randomized, prospective, pair-sampled multicenter study. Pacing Clin Electrophysiol 2000;11:1992–5.

82. Denman R, Umesan C, Martin P, et al. Does optimising an ICD's defibrillation waveform result in a lower defibrillation threshold (DFT)? Heart Rhythm 2004;(1, 1, May Supplement):S275–878.

Reducing ICD Shocks for Ventricular Arrhythmias

John A. Schoenhard, MD, PhD, Paul C. Zei, MD, PhD*

KEYWORDS

- Ventricular arrhythmia
- Implantable-cardioverter defibrillator • ICD shocks
- Defibrillation

Implantable cardioverter-defibrillators (ICDs) reduce mortality among high-risk patients with indication for primary or secondary prevention of sudden cardiac death.[1–3] Defibrillator shock therapy comes at a cost, however. Defibrillator shocks are acutely painful[4,5] and chronically detrimental to quality of life, due to diminished mental and physical well-being.[6–9] Both appropriate and inappropriate shocks are associated with subsequent mortality,[10–13] although causality has yet to be proved. Capacitor charging in anticipation of shock delivery results in considerable battery drain, decreased ICD longevity, and earlier ICD replacement. For all these reasons, reducing ICD shocks for ventricular arrhythmias is an important goal.

Current strategies aimed at reducing appropriate ICD shocks include device optimization, medical therapy, and catheter ablation. Device optimization may include programming changes to increase utilization of antitachycardia pacing (ATP), to increase the number of intervals to detect (NID) ventricular arrhythmia (VA), and to reconfirm VA immediately before shock delivery.

Device optimization may also include implantation of a left ventricular pacing lead for purposes of cardiac resynchronization therapy (CRT) and biventricular ATP in selected patients. Medical therapy may include β-blockers and amiodarone or class III antiarrhythmic drugs, whereas for drug-refractory patients, catheter ablation may achieve remission from ICD shocks.

ANTITACHYCARDIA PACING TO REDUCE ICD SHOCKS

ATP refers to the delivery of ventricular paced beats at coupling intervals slightly shorter than the ventricular tachycardia (VT) cycle length, with intent to penetrate an excitable gap in the VT circuit. Antidromic collision with the "head" of the VT wavefront and orthodromic block at the refractory "tail" of the VT may terminate tachycardia.

In slow VT, the excitable gap is typically large, so ATP more easily terminates the tachycardia. In fast VT, the excitable gap is shorter and ATP termination may be less reliable. Historically, this theoretic concern and fear of rate acceleration lead to underutilization of ATP for fast VT.

Prior to the Pacing Fast Ventricular Tachycardia Reduces Shock Therapies (PainFREE Rx) trials,[14,15] evidence for ATP safety was limited and mostly retrospective. For example, the Bilitch ICD Registry compared 1553 patients with shock-only ICDs to 550 patients with ATP-capable ICDs. After 24 months, survival was 89% in the shock-only group but improved to 94% in the ATP-capable group,[16] indicating potential survival benefit. Other early studies demonstrated that ATP successfully terminates 78% to 94% of slow VT (variably defined as <188 to 200 bpm), with only 2% to 4% risk of VT acceleration.[17–21]

The PainFREE Rx trials extended confidence in ATP as initial therapy to fast VT (defined as 188

Division of Cardiovascular Medicine, Stanford University Medical Center, 300 Pasteur Drive, H-2159, Stanford, CA 94305-5233, USA
* Corresponding author.
E-mail address: paulzei@stanford.edu

Card Electrophysiol Clin 3 (2011) 493–502
doi:10.1016/j.ccep.2011.05.013

to 250 bpm). Published in 2001, the PainFREE Rx I trial enrolled 220 patients with coronary artery disease and a secondary prevention indication for ICD implantation. Coronary artery disease was chosen as a prerequisite to increase the likelihood of macroreentrant VT in the study population, and a secondary prevention indication was necessary for ICD implantation because that was the standard of care at the time, pre–Multicenter Automatic Defibrillator Implantation Trial II (MADIT II). All patients received an ICD programmed to deliver ATP (2 bursts and 8 pulses; 88% of the VT cycle length minus 10 ms between bursts) as initial therapy after detection of fast VT, defined as 12 of 16 R-R intervals at 240 to 320 ms. During a mean follow-up period of 6.0 ± 3.6 months, 1100 episodes of VA occurred, of which 624 (57%) were slow VT, 446 (40%) were fast VT, and 30 (3%) were ventricular fibrillation (VF). Eighty-five percent of fast VT episodes were successfully treated by the first ATP attempt (77% when adjusted for multiple episodes per patient). ATP accelerated VT rarely (4%), and there were no episodes where shock therapy was not successful after failed ATP. The median duration of fast VT episodes was 6 seconds when ATP was successful, and 21 seconds when shock therapy was required, such that syncope was rare (2%). Limitations of the trial included its nonrandomized/no-comparator design, focus on coronary artery disease, and permissive 12 of 16 NID that may have deemed ATP successful in episodes that would otherwise have been nonsustained. Moreover, the study was limited to a single manufacturer's ICDs (Medtronic).

The PainFREE Rx II trial resolved many of these issues, with a randomized design comparing ATP (1 burst and 8 pulses; 88% of VT cycle length) with shock for initial therapy of fast VT, defined as 18 of 24 R-R intervals at 240 to 320 ms. Inclusion criteria were broader, excluding only patients believed unlikely to have monomorphic VT susceptible to ATP (eg, hypertrophic cardiomyopathy, long QT syndrome, and Brugada syndrome). A total of 634 patients were enrolled, with 313 patients randomized to the ATP arm and 321 to the shock arm. During a mean follow-up period of 11 ± 3 months, 1342 episodes of VA occurred, of which 777 (58%) were slow VT, 431 (32%) were fast VT, and 134 (10%) were VF. Eighty-one percent of fast VT episodes were successfully treated by ATP (72% when adjusted for multiple episodes per patient). When compared with the shock arm, programming ATP as initial therapy resulted in a relative shock reduction of 70%. On a per-patient basis, 80% of patients benefited from ATP. No significant differences were observed in acceleration (2% ATP arm and 1% shock arm),

median episode duration (10 seconds in ATP arm and 9.7 seconds in shock arm), syncope (2 episodes in ATP arm and 1 episode in shock arm), or sudden death (1 in ATP arm and 2 in shock arm). Taken together, PainFREE Rx II provided clear evidence that ATP is highly effective in treating fast VT.

The findings of PainFREE Rx II were subsequently confirmed in the Comparison of Empiric to Physician-Tailored Programming of Implantable Cardioverter-Defibrillators (EMPIRIC) trial,[22] which randomized 900 ICD patients to standardized (n = 445) or physician-tailored (n = 455) programming. Standardized programming was similar to the ATP arm of PainFREE Rx II, with ATP (1 burst and 8 pulses; 88% of VT cycle length) provided as initial therapy for fast VT, defined as 18 of 24 R-R intervals at 240 to 300 ms. In addition, burst then ramp ATP was enabled for slow VT, and Medtronic's proprietary supraventricular tachycardia discrimination algorithm was turned on. Although the EMPIRIC trial was not designed to compare specific programming options, the increased utilization of ATP on the standardized arm, when coupled with the high efficacy (92%) of ATP for VT, resulted in a significant reduction in shocked episodes of VT (13%) in the standardized arm compared with the physician-tailored arm (21%). This was accomplished with no significant differences in incidence of VT acceleration or syncope. Thus, it seems reasonable to program ATP as initial therapy for both slow and fast VT in all patients regardless of clinical presentation. For example, modeling of outcomes anticipated if EMPIRIC programming had been utilized in the Sudden Cardiac Death in Heart Failure Trial (SCD-HeFT) has suggested that the number of shocked VA episodes could have been reduced by 59% and the percentage of patients receiving shocks for VA could have been reduced from 31% to 26%.[23]

Increased utilization of ATP not only may reduce pain but also may reduce mortality. After pooling data from 2135 patients in 4 pivotal trials incorporating ATP to reduce shocks (PainFREE Rx,[14] PainFree Rx II,[15] EMPIRIC,[22] and Primary Prevention Parameters Evaluation [PREPARE][24]), predictors of mortality (n = 138; 6.5%) were identified.[13] Whereas ATP-terminated fast VT did not increase mortality, shocked fast VT increased risk by 32%. Survival rates were highest among patients with no VA (93.8%) or treated with ATP only (94.7%), and lowest for shocked patients (88.4%) over 10.8 ± 3.3 months' follow-up. Although this analysis could not exclude the possibility that ATP-refractory (and necessarily shocked) VT may be a marker for higher-mortality risk patients, the potential of ATP to prevent shock-mediated mortality is compelling and broadly applicable, in light of the high efficacy of ATP for both slow and fast VT (93.5% and 85.6%, respectively).

Given the many options available when programming ATP, it might be questioned which ATP scheme has the greatest likelihood of success. Although EMPIRIC programming is a reasonable choice,[22] other strategies have proved efficacy. For example, shorter bursts of more tightly coupled pulses (5 then 8 pulses; 84% of VT cycle length) were highly effective (89%) and rarely accelerated VT (2%) in a randomized trial of ATP versus shock as initial therapy for fast VT.[25] Alternatively, prolonged burst pacing (15 pulses; 88% of VT cycle length) was as effective as conventional burst pacing (8 pulses; 88% of VT cycle length) in the Antitachycardia Pacing (ATP) Delivery for Painless Implantable Cardioverter Defibrillator (ICD) Therapy (ADVANCE-D) trial and may be preferable for patients with preserved left ventricular ejection fraction (≥40%) and no history of heart failure.[26] Ramp pacing, however, is less effective than burst pacing for fast VT. This was demonstrated in the Project for the Investigation and Treatment of Ventricular Arrhythmias: a General Observational Registry on Antitachycardia Pacing Efficacy ICD trial,[27] which randomized 206 ICD patients in a 1:1 ratio to conventional burst pacing (8 pulses; 88% coupling interval) or ramp pacing (8 pulses; 91% coupling interval) for initial therapy of fast VT, defined as 18 of 24 R-R intervals at 240 to 320 ms. Although burst pacing successfully treated 75% of fast VT episodes, ramp pacing successfully treated only 54% (73% vs 52%, respectively, when adjusted for multiple episodes per patient). Burst ATP caused fewer accelerations than ramp (2% vs 7%), and VA-associated syncope was rare in both arms (1 patient each). Taken together, these results confirmed the superiority of burst over ramp ATP for termination of fast VT, as suggested in prior nonrandomized studies.[28–30]

INCREASING DETECTION INTERVALS TO REDUCE ICD SHOCKS

With current ICD battery and capacitor technology, charge times prior to shock delivery have been substantially reduced compared with a few years ago. Rapid delivery of ICD shocks, however, may overtreat potentially self-terminating arrhythmias. Overtreatment of nonsustained VA likely contributed to the excess number of shocks received by ICD recipients compared with the rate of sudden cardiac death among nonrecipients in pivotal trials of ICD versus medical therapy for primary or secondary prevention of sudden death. For example,

ICD recipients were 6.6-fold more likely to be shocked than nonrecipients to suffer sudden death in the Antiarrhythmics Versus Implantable Defibrillators (AVID) trial[1] and 5.7-fold more likely in SCD-HeFT.[3] One potential solution to this problem is to increase the NID VA, in order to allow self-terminating arrhythmias to extinguish prior to capacitor charging or therapy delivery. The safety of such a strategy is apparent when comparing outcomes in PainFREE Rx I with those in PainFREE Rx II. In PainFREE Rx I,[14] the NID for fast VT was programmed to 12 of 16 R-R intervals at 240 to 320 ms. In PainFREE Rx II,[15] the NID for fast VT was programmed to 18 of 24 R-R intervals at 240 to 320 ms. Extending the NID between the two studies, however, did not increase the rates of either arrhythmic syncope or sudden death. Rather, the fact that 34% of detected fast VT episodes in the shock arm of PainFREE Rx II terminated prior to therapy suggested that longer delay could further reduce unnecessary device detections.

Additional evidence supporting the extension of the NID from 12 of 16 to 18 of 24 was provided by retrospective analysis of stored intracardiac electrograms from the Gem DR trial, in which NID was programmed at the discretion of the investigator to either 12 of 16 (n = 305) or 18 of 24 (n = 570).[31] For patients programmed with NID 12/16, a 17% increased rate of unnecessary capacitor charging was observed, compared with the hypothetical scenario of these same patients programmed with NID 18/24. For patients programmed with NID 18/24, a 22% decreased rate of unnecessary capacitor charging was observed compared with the hypothetical scenario of these same patients programmed with NID 12/16. Programming NID 18/24 rather than 12/16 prevented unnecessary shocks in 10% of patients over 6 months. If patients programmed with NID 12/16 had been programmed with NID 18/24, the median incremental delay in detection time would have been 1.8 seconds (range 1.0–2.9 seconds). As a result, it can be strongly argued that increasing the NID from 12/16 to 18/24 results in fewer unnecessary capacitor charges and shocks with minimal incremental delay in detection. Nonetheless, in the EMPIRIC trial, clinicians decreased the nominal NID from 18/24 to 12/16 in 50% of patients randomized to physician-tailored programming.[22]

Subsequent trials have pushed the NID for fast VT and VF to 30 of 40 R-R intervals. The ongoing Avoid Delivering Therapies for Nonsustained Arrhythmias in ICD Patients III (ADVANCE III) trial will randomize 1915 ICD patients to either a conventional NID for fast VT of 18 of 24 intervals or a prolonged NID for fast VT of 30 of 40 intervals, targeting a 20% reduction in ICD therapies.[32] After 12 months' follow-up, the trial is expected to finish in December 2011. In the meantime, the PREPARE study has provided reasonable evidence, albeit nonrandomized, that increased the PREPARE study coupled with ATP can safely reduce shocks in patients receiving an ICD for primary prevention.[24] The PREPARE study followed a total of 700 biventricular and nonbiventricular ICD patients for 12 months and compared outcomes with a historical control group composed of the physician-tailored arm of the EMPIRIC trial and all patients in the Multicenter InSync Implantable Cardioverter Defibrillator Randomized Clinical Evaluation (MIRACLE ICD) trial. The PREPARE study cohort received standardized programming designed to detect only fast and sustained VA (30 out of 40 intervals <330 ms), with ATP (1 burst and 8 pulses; 88% of VT cycle length) provided as initial therapy for fast VT. The primary endpoint was a morbidity index composed of the combined incidence of device-delivered shocks, arrhythmic syncope, and untreated sustained symptomatic VA. Strategic programming in the PREPARE study resulted in a statistically significant 62% risk reduction in the primary endpoint compared with the control group. PREPARE patients were less likely to receive a shock (9% vs 17%), and arrhythmic syncope remained rare (1.6%). A major criticism of the PREPARE study was its usage of the physician-tailored rather than the standardized arm of the EMPIRIC trial, thereby enriching for inappropriate and unnecessary therapies. Still, physician-tailored programming does reflect real world practice.

Also nonrandomized, the Role of Long Detection Window Programming in Patients with Left Ventricular Dysfunction, Nonischemic Etiology in Primary Prevention Treated with a Biventricular ICD (RELEVANT) trial enrolled 324 primary prevention nonischemic heart failure patients implanted with biventricular defibrillators programmed to either a short NID of 12 out of 16 intervals less than 330 ms (n = 160) or a prolonged NID of 30 of 40 intervals less than 330 ms (n = 164). In both groups, ATP (1 burst and 8 pulses; 88% of VT cycle length) was programmed as initial therapy for fast VT. Although the incidences and rate distributions of VA were comparable between groups, 91% of VA episodes in the prolonged NID 30/40 cohort self-terminated in the interval between 13 and 29 beats, thereby avoiding unnecessary treatment. This markedly reduced the number of shocks delivered in the NID 30/40 arm compared with the NID 12/16 arm (22 vs 59, respectively). Although time to treatment was prolonged in the NID 30/40 compared with the NID 12/16 arm (9.3 vs 3.7 seconds), syncope and mortality were no more

frequent. There was a 60% risk reduction in heart failure hospitalizations for the NID 30/40 group. Taken together with the findings of prior trials, these results indicate that increasing detection intervals to reduce shocks is a safe and effective strategy in a majority of ICD patients. In rare patients who lose consciousness rapidly with VA or have clinically significant undersensing, however, a lower NID may be preferred.

BIVENTRICULAR PACING TO REDUCE ICD SHOCKS

Biventricular pacing may reduce the burden of VA and ICD shocks in selected patients with indications for CRT, namely symptomatic heart failure, severely depressed left ventricular ejection fraction, and wide QRS. Early randomized crossover studies of CRT found significantly less ventricular ectopy during Holter monitoring after 3 months with biventricular pacing turned on versus off[33] and significantly fewer VA episodes requiring ATP or shock during 3 months with biventricular pacing turned on versus off.[34] Similar results were obtained by two other studies that compared VA and shock burdens before and after CRT-D upgrade.[35,36] In the Cardiac Resynchronization in Heart Failure (CARE-HF) extension study, which followed patients for a median 37 ± 5 months, CRT without defibrillator backup significantly reduced the incidence of sudden death (25% CRT and 38% medical therapy) but only late in the course of the study.[37] This time-dependence suggested that reductions in sustained VA may be delayed and dependent on reverse anatomic remodeling.

Several pivotal studies of CRT have shown no reductions in VA or sudden death, potentially due to limited follow-up duration. In the Contak CD and MIRACLE ICD trials, which followed patients for 3 to 6 months and 6 months, respectively, similar rates of VA were observed regardless of whether CRT was programmed on or off.[38–40] In the Comparison of Medical Therapy, Pacing, and Defibrillation in Heart Failure (COMPANION) study, which followed patients for a mean of 16 months, no differences were observed in the rates of sudden death among CRT patients without defibrillator backup compared with those receiving optimal medical therapy alone.[41] But when other investigators have extended follow-up further, antiarrhythmic benefits of CRT have been observed. For example, in a case series by Desai and colleagues,[42] 209 CRT-D and 320 ICD patients were followed for a mean of 34 months. In that time, 25% of CRT-D patients and 35% of ICD patients received a shock for VA, with greater reduction in mortality (6% CRT-D and 16% ICD), despite less favorable baseline characteristics in the CRT-D group. In a case series by Nordbeck and colleagues,[43] 168 CRT-D and 561 ICD patients were followed for a mean of 41 months. In that time, only one CRT-D patient suffered electrical storm compared with 39 ICD patients (0.6% CRT-D and 7% ICD), whereas the overall proportions of patients with at least one treated VA episode were comparable between groups.

To test the hypothesis that an antiarrhythmic effect of CRT may follow reverse remodeling, several investigators compared the incidence of VA among echocardiographically defined high responders and low responders to CRT. In the InSync III Marquis study,[44] high responders were identified based on greater than or equal to 15% reduction in left ventricular end-systolic volume (LVESV) at 6 months. Over that time frame, high responders demonstrated 29% fewer single premature ventricular contractions, 48% fewer premature ventricular contraction runs, and 85% fewer treated episodes of VA than low responders. Only 6% of high responders but 15% of low responders experienced at least one treated episode of VA. In the InSync ICD Italian Registry,[45] high responders were identified based on greater than or equal to 10% reduction in LVESV at 6 months. Over 12 months, 37% of high responders and 46% of low responders experienced at least one treated episode of VA. Consistent with the time-dependent hypothesis that electric remodeling follows anatomic remodeling, reductions in VA episodes and shocks were observed only after the first month post implant.

Recently, the MADIT with Cardiac Resynchronization Therapy (MADIT-CRT) trial provided the first randomized controlled trial evidence that CRT prevents VA episodes and shocks, with high responders deriving greatest benefit. In brief, MADIT-CRT randomized 1820 patients with a left ventricular ejection fraction of 30% or less, a QRS duration of 130 ms or more, and New York Heart Association class I or II symptoms to either CRT-D (n = 1089) or an ICD only (n = 731).[46] High responders to CRT were identified based on greater than or equal to 25% reduction in LVESV at 12 months. Over a mean follow-up interval of 2.4 years, high responders experienced 55% reduction in the risk of VA compared with ICD-only patients, whereas the risk of VA was not significantly different between low responders and ICD-only patients.[47] Considering the entire CRT-D cohort, CRT-D significantly reduced the occurrence of VA (hazard ratio 0.81) and the risk of receiving a shock for VA (hazard ratio 0.68), with 16% of CRT-D patients and 21% of ICD only patients receiving at least one shock.[48] As a result,

it is reasonable to consider recommending implantation of a biventricular ICD in CRT-D eligible patients not only to reduce risk of heart failure but also to reduce risk of VA and shocks, although this recommendation is as yet not reflected in the current guidelines.

An additional benefit of left ventricular lead implantation is the availability of biventricular ATP. Early nonrandomized studies demonstrated the safety and efficacy of biventricular ATP. In one study with biventricular ATP programmed for all patients, spontaneous monomorphic VT was successfully treated with biventricular ATP in 88% of episodes.[38] In another study where biventricular versus right ventricular ATP was programmed at the discretion of the investigator, biventricular ATP was significantly more effective than right ventricular ATP for slow VT and showed a trend toward greater efficacy for fast VT, with fewer VA episodes accelerated by biventricular ATP.[49] To more rigorously compare biventricular and right ventricular ATP, the ADVANCE CRT-D study was performed.[50] ADVANCE CRT-D randomized 526 CRT-D patients to biventricular (n = 266) versus right ventricular (n = 260) ATP programming (1 burst and 8 pulses; 88% of VT cycle length). During 12 months' follow-up, 634 episodes of VA occurred, of which 363 (57%) were slow VT, 202 (32%) were fast VT, and 69 (11%) were VF. Comparable biventricular versus right ventricular ATP efficacy was observed for both slow VT (62% vs 71%) and fast VT (71% vs 61%), with a trend toward fewer fast VT episodes accelerated by biventricular ATP (4% vs 10%). No syncope occurred in the biventricular ATP group, whereas 4 syncope events occurred in the right ventricular ATP group. Among patients with coronary artery disease, biventricular ATP was significantly more effective for fast VT, whereas similar efficacy was seen for the two modalities among patients without coronary artery disease. Taken together, biventricular ATP is safe and effective and may be preferred for patients with ischemic cardiomyopathy, in whom stimulation of a larger area of myocardium may be advantageous to better advance the orthodromic wavefront of a macroreentrant VT into refractory tissue.[51]

Even as biventricular pacing benefits the majority of recipients, biventricular pacing can be proarrhythmic in rare cases. The potential mechanisms of this effect are twofold. First, epicardial left ventricular pacing increases transmural dispersion of repolarization, potentially creating the substrate for polymorphic VT similar to that seen in the long QT syndrome.[52] Second, biventricular pacing changes the activation pattern within and around myocardial scars, such that a propagating wavefront from left ventricular pacing may arrive earlier at a critical isthmus, encounter unidirectional block, and initiate reentry.[53] Two case series have considered the incidence and consequences of biventricular pacing–mediated VA. At one center, 5 of 145 patients (3.4%) developed recurrent VA within 1 week of initiation of biventricular pacing,[54] whereas at another, 8 of 191 patients (4.2%) developed recurrent VA a mean of 16 ± 12 days after initiation of biventricular pacing.[55] Both monomorphic and polymorphic VT were observed. In all but 3 cases, patients were able to be discharged with biventricular pacing programmed on after initiation or up-titration of antiarrhythmic drugs (n = 10), VT ablation (n = 5), left ventricular lead repositioning (n = 1), or decreased left ventricular lead output (n = 1). Therefore, although biventricular pacing may reduce VA and shocks over the long term in CRT high responders, close follow-up is indicated in the short-term after left ventricular lead implantation.

NONDEVICE THERAPY TO REDUCE ICD SHOCKS

Although ICD implantation has been shown superior to medical therapy alone for reduction of sudden death, adjuvant use of antiarrhythmic drugs is often necessary to further reduce potentially unnecessary shocks for VA. In the AVID trial,[1,50] 18% of patients in the ICD arm required antiarrhythmic drug therapy (amiodarone, 42%; sotalol, 21%; mexilitine, 20%; quinidine, 11%; and combination or other, 6%). Because antiarrhythmic drug therapy was considered a crossover, these percentages likely represent the absolute minimum number of ICD patients who may benefit from antiarrhythmic drug therapy. Among these crossover patients, the annual VA event rate was reduced from 90% to 64%, and the mean time to VA recurrence extended from 3.9 ± 0.7 to 11.2 ± 1.8 months. Benefit was primarily derived by reduction in shocks rather than ATP events.

Antiarrhythmic drugs reduce shocks by directly preventing VT, by slowing VT and thus rendering episodes more vulnerable to ATP, and by suppressing atrial tachyarrhythmias that may lead to inappropriate therapy or trigger VA. Some antiarrhythmic drugs also reduce the defibrillation threshold (DFT) and facilitate defibrillation of VA, whereas others increase the DFT. Antiarrhythmic drugs can be proarrhythmic, can slow VT below the detection rate cutoff, and can cause extracardiac side effects, such that caution is warranted.

Two studies have investigated the efficacy of racemic sotalol compared with placebo for reduction of ICD shocks. In a multicenter trial,[57] 302 ICD patients were randomized to sotalol (160–320 mg daily) or placebo and followed for 12 months. Treatment with sotalol was found to reduce the risk of death or all-cause shocks by 48%, risk of death or appropriate shock by 44%, and risk of death or inappropriate shock by 64%, irrespective of left ventricular ejection fraction or concomitant β-blocker usage. Sotalol also reduced the mean frequency of all-cause shocks (sotalol 1.4 ± 3.5; placebo 3.9 ± 10.7). Treatment was discontinued due to adverse events/side effects in 27% of patients receiving sotalol and 12% of patients receiving placebo and due to inefficacy in 3% of patients receiving sotalol and 14% of patients receiving placebo. Most of the side effects of sotalol were attributable to β-blocker effects, and torsades de pointes occurred only once in each group. Therefore, in ICD patients who tolerate β-blockers, sotalol is a safe and efficacious agent for reduction of ICD shocks. This conclusion was affirmed in a smaller study of 93 ICD patients randomized to sotalol (80–400 mg daily) or no antiarrhythmic drug,[58] in which sotalol was found to significantly reduce recurrent VA (sotalol, 32%; ICD only, 53%). Crossover to antiarrhythmic drug therapy was necessary for 25% of patients in the ICD-only arm, similar to the results in the ICD arm of AVID.[1,56]

Other investigators have suggested that metoprolol may be comparable with sotalol for reduction of ICD shocks. In a study of 100 ICD patients randomized to metoprolol or sotalol titrated to equivalent levels of β-blockade (metoprolol 108 ± 44 mg; sotalol 319 ± 91 mg), no significant differences were observed in the incidences of VA, shocks, or mortality.[59] In another study of 70 ICD patients randomized in similar fashion (metoprolol 104 ± 37 mg; sotalol 242 ± 109 mg), significantly fewer episodes of VA were observed in the metoprolol arm as compared with the sotalol arm, although the patients in this study were healthier in terms of their average left ventricular ejection fraction (40% ± 10%) than those in most other ICD trials.[60] Retrospective analyses of the MADIT-II and COMPANION trials also demonstrated significant reductions in risk of ICD therapy for VA for patients receiving β-blockers compared with patients not receiving β-blockers.[41,61] In addition, efficacy of ATP has been correlated with β-blocker usage.[62]

The Optimal Pharmacological Therapy in Cardioverter Defibrillator Patients (OPTIC) trial compared the efficacies of amiodarone plus β-blocker, sotalol alone, or a β-blocker alone for the prevention of ICD shocks.[63] Amiodarone without β-blockade was not tested, based on prior evidence for greater efficacy with the combination.[64] Over 1-year follow-up, amiodarone plus β-blocker was the most effective regimen for prevention of both appropriate and inappropriate shocks. Specifically, shocks occurred in 12 (10.3%) patients randomized to amiodarone plus β-blocker, 26 (24.3%) patients randomized to sotalol, and 41 (38.5%) patients randomized to β-blocker. Statistical significance was achieved by amiodarone plus β-blocker over both sotalol alone and β-blocker alone but not achieved by sotalol alone over β-blocker alone perhaps due to insufficient follow-up duration or the relatively low mean dose of sotalol provided (189 mg daily). Rates of study drug discontinuation were 18.2% for amiodarone, 23.5% for sotalol, and 5.3% for β-blocker, with bias toward less discontinuation of β-blocker because most patients had been tolerating β-blockers prior to study initiation. Adverse pulmonary, thyroid, and bradycardic events were more common with amiodarone treatment, but there were no events of torsades de pointes. Measured at baseline and after 8 to 12 weeks, amiodarone plus β-blocker therapy led to a small but statistically significant increase in mean DFT of 1.29 J, whereas sotalol alone and β-blocker alone were associated with decreases of 0.89 J and 1.67 J, respectively.[65] As a consequence, routine reassessment of DFT might not be necessary early after initiation of amiodarone or sotalol, except for patients with high DFT at baseline or for patients taking high-dose or long-term amiodarone therapy.[66] A subsequent metaanalysis has largely confirmed the conclusions of OPTIC.[67]

Other potential medical therapies to reduce ICD shocks include less extensively studied class III agents and lipid-altering therapies. Dofetilide has shown a trend toward reduced ICD shocks compared with placebo but also a high incidence of torsades de pointes.[68] Azimilide has shown dose-dependent reductions in VA episodes requiring ICD therapy[69,70] but awaits further testing prior to consideration for Food and Drug Administration approval. Statins have been associated with decreased risk of VA requiring ICD therapy in single-center retrospective studies[71,72] as well as in AVID[73] and MADIT-II[74] but not Defibrillators in Non-Ischemic Cardiomyopathy Treatment Evaluation (DEFINITE).[75] Omega-3 polyunsaturated fatty acids of various preparations have shown trends toward reduced incidence of VA in 3 of 4 randomized controlled trials but have yet to achieve statistical significance.[76–79]

Catheter ablation has emerged as an effective therapy for treating drug-refractory VA. The Substrate Mapping and Ablation in Sinus Rhythm to Halt Ventricular Tachycardia (SMASH-VT) study randomized 128 patients with an ICD for secondary prevention or an appropriate shock from a primary prevention ICD to undergo either catheter ablation or no additional therapy.[80] Over a mean follow-up interval of 23 ± 5 months, those who underwent catheter ablation had a 65% reduction in appropriate ICD therapies compared with the control group, and that reduction was 73% when ATP therapies were excluded from the analysis. No significant difference in mortality was observed (ablation, 9%; control, 17%).

SUMMARY

There is substantial evidence that ICD therapy provides significant reduction in mortality risk in appropriate patient populations. Not all ventricular arrhythmias, however, require treatment specifically with cardioversion or defibrillation, because many episodes can be terminated with ATP therapy or may self-terminate before the onset of symptoms. Several innovations in device programming described in this article have been shown to reduce the number of ICD shocks without compromising safety. The authors recommend that in appropriate patients, these interventions should be implemented. When ICD shocks continue despite these programming interventions, pharmacologic and ablative therapies should be pursued.

REFERENCES

1. The Antiarrhythmics versus Implantable Defibrillators (AVID) Investigators. A comparison of antiarrhythmic-drug therapy with implantable defibrillators in patients resuscitated from near-fatal ventricular arrhythmias. N Engl J Med 1997;337:1576–84.
2. Moss AJ, Zareba W, Hall WJ, et al. Prophylactic implantation of a defibrillator in patients with myocardial infarction and reduced ejection fraction. N Engl J Med 2002;346:877–83.
3. Bardy GH, Lee KL, Mark DB, et al. Amiodarone or an implantable cardioverter-defibrillator for congestive heart failure. N Engl J Med 2005;352:225–37.
4. Dunbar SB, Warner CD, Purcell JA. Internal cardioverter defibrillator device discharge: experiences of patients and family members. Heart Lung 1993;22:494–501.
5. Ahmad M, Bloomstein L, Roelke M, et al. Patients' attitudes toward implanted defibrillator shocks. Pacing Clin Electrophysiol 2000;23:934–8.
6. Schron EB, Exner DV, Yao Q, et al. Quality of life in the Antiarrhythmics versus Implantable Defibrillators trial: impact of therapy and influence of adverse symptoms and defibrillator shocks. Circulation 2002;105:589–94.
7. Passman R, Subacius H, Ruo B, et al. Implantable cardioverter defibrillators and quality of life: results from the Defibrillators in Nonischemic Cardiomyopathy Treatment Evaluation study. Arch Intern Med 2007;167:2226–32.

8. Mark DB, Anstrom KJ, Sun JL, et al. Quality of life with defibrillator therapy or amiodarone in heart failure. N Engl J Med 2008;359:999–1008.

9. Noyes K, Corona E, Veazie P, et al. Examination of the effect of implantable cardioverter-defibrillators on health-related quality of life: based on results from the Multicenter Automatic Defibrillator Trial II (MADIT II). Am J Cardiovasc Drugs 2009;9:393–400.

10. Moss AJ, Greenberg H, Case RB, et al. Long-term clinical course of patients after termination of ventricular tachyarrhythmias by an implanted defibrillator. Circulation 2004;110:3760–5.

11. Daubert JP, Zareba W, Cannom DS, et al. Inappropriate implantable cardioverter-defibrillator shocks in MADIT II: frequency, mechanisms, predictors, and survival impact. J Am Coll Cardiol 2008;51:1357–65.

12. Poole JE, Johnson GW, Hellkamp AS, et al. Prognostic importance of defibrillator shocks in patients with heart failure. N Engl J Med 2008;359:1009–17.

13. Sweeney MO, Sherfesee L, DeGroot PJ, et al. Differences in effects of electrical therapy type for ventricular arrhythmias on mortality in implantable cardioverter-defibrillator patients. Heart Rhythm 2010;7:353–60.

14. Wathen MS, Sweeney MO, DeGroot PJ, et al. Shock reduction using antitachycardia pacing for spontaneous rapid ventricular tachycardia in patients with coronary artery disease. Circulation 2001;104:796–801.

15. Wathen MS, DeGroot PJ, Sweeney MO, et al. Prospective randomized multicenter trial of empirical antitachycardia pacing versus shocks for spontaneous rapid ventricular tachycardia in patients with implantable cardioverter-defibrillators: Pacing Fast Ventricular Tachycardia Reduces Shock Therapies (PainFREE Rx II) trial results. Circulation 2004;110:2591–6.

16. Gross JR, Sackstein RD, Song SL, et al. The antitachycardia pacing ICD: impact on patient selection and outcome. Pacing Clin Electrophysiol 1993;16:165–9.

17. Yee R, Klein GJ, Guiraudon GM, et al. Initial clinical experience with the pacemaker-cardioverter-defibrillator. Can J Cardiol 1990;6:147–56.

18. Luceri RM, Salem MH, David IB, et al. Changing trends in therapy delivery with a third generation noncommitted implantable defibrillator: results of a large single center clinical trial. Pacing Clin Electrophysiol 1993;16:159–64.

19. Trappe HJ, Klein H, Fieguth HG, et al. Clinical efficacy and safety of the new cardioverter defibrillator systems. Pacing Clin Electrophysiol 1993;16:153–8.

20. Peinado R, Almendral JM, Rius T, et al. Randomized, prospective comparison of four burst pacing algorithms for spontaneous ventricular tachycardia. Am J Cardiol 1998;82:1422–5.

21. Schaumann A, von zur Muhlen F, Herse B, et al. Empirical versus tested antitachycardia pacing in implantable cardioverter defibrillators: a prospective study including 200 patients. Circulation 1998;97:66–74.

22. Wilkoff BL, Ousdigian KT, Sterns LD, et al. A comparison of empiric to physician-tailored programming of implantable cardioverter-defibrillators: results from the prospective randomized multicenter EMPIRIC trial. J Am Coll Cardiol 2006;48:330–9.

23. Volosin KJ, Exner DV, Wathen MS, et al. Combining shock reduction strategies to enhance ICD therapy: a role for computer modeling. J Cardiovasc Electrophysiol 2011;22:280–9.

24. Wilkoff BL, Williamson BD, Stern RS, et al. Strategic programming of detection and therapy parameters in implantable cardioverter-defibrillators reduces shocks in primary prevention patients: results from the PREPARE (Primary Prevention Parameters Evaluation) Study. J Am Coll Cardiol 2008;52:541–50.

25. Jimenez-Candil J, Arenal A, Garcia-Alberola A, et al. Fast ventricular tachycardias in patients with implantable cardioverter-defibrillators: efficacy and safety of antitachycardia pacing. J Am Coll Cardiol 2005;45:460–1.

26. Santini M, Lunati M, Defaye P, et al. Prospective multicenter randomized trial of fast ventricular tachycardia termination by prolonged versus conventional anti-tachycardia burst pacing in implantable cardioverter-defibrillator patients—Atp DeliVery for pAiNless ICD therapy (ADVANCE-D) Trial results. J Interv Card Electrophysiol 2010;27:127–35.

27. Gulizia MM, Piraino L, Scherillo M, et al. A randomized study to compare ramp versus burst antitachycardia pacing therapies to treat fast ventricular tachyarrhythmias in patients with implantable cardioverter defibrillators: the PITAGORA ICD trial. Circ Arrhythmia Electrophysiol 2009;2:146–53.

28. Gillis AM, Leitch JW, Sheldon RS, et al. A prospective randomized comparison of autodecrement pacing to burst pacing in device therapy for chronic ventricular tachycardia secondary to coronary artery disease. Am J Cardiol 1993;72:1146–51.

29. Schaumann A, Poppinga A, von zur Muehlen F. Antitachycardia pacing for ventricular tachycardias above and below 200 beats/min: a prospective study for ramp versus can mode [abstract]. Pacing Clin Electrophysiol 1997;20:1108.

30. Peters RW, Zhang X, Gold MR. Clinical predictors and efficacy of antitachycardia pacing in patients with implantable cardioverter defibrillators: the importance of the patient's sex. Pacing Clin Electrophysiol 2001;24:70–4.

31. Gunderson BD, Abeyratne AI, Olson WH, et al. Effect of programmed number of intervals to detect ventricular fibrillation on implantable cardioverter-defibrillator

aborted and unnecessary shocks. Pacing Clin Electrophysiol 2007;30:157–65.

32. Schwab JO, Gasparini M, Lunati M, et al. Avoid delivering therapies for nonsustained fast ventricular tachyarrhythmia in patients with implantable cardioverter/defibrillator: the ADVANCE III trial. J Cardiovasc Electrophysiol 2009;20:663–6.

33. Walker S, Levy TM, Rex S, et al. Usefulness of suppression of ventricular arrhythmia by biventricular pacing in severe congestive cardiac failure. Am J Cardiol 2000;86:231–3.

34. Higgins SL, Yong P, Scheck D, et al. Biventricular pacing diminishes the need for implantable cardioverter defibrillator therapy. J Am Coll Cardiol 2000;36:824–7.

35. Kies P, Bax JJ, Molhoek SG, et al. Effect of left ventricular remodeling after cardiac resynchronization therapy on frequency of ventricular arrhythmias. Am J Cardiol 2004;94:130–2.

36. Ermis C, Seutter R, Zhu AX, et al. Impact of upgrade to cardiac resynchronization therapy on ventricular arrhythmia frequency in patients with implantable cardioverter-defibrillators. J Am Coll Cardiol 2005; 46:2258–63.

37. Cleland JGF, Daubert J-C, Erdmann E, et al. Longer-term effects of cardiac resynchronization therapy on mortality in heart failure [the CArdiac REsynchronization-Heart Failure (CARE-HF) trial extension phase]. Eur Heart J 2006;27:1928–32.

38. Higgins SL, Hummel JD, Niazi IK, et al. Cardiac resynchronization therapy for the treatment of heart failure in patients with intraventricular conduction delay and malignant ventricular tachyarrhythmias. J Am Coll Cardiol 2003;42:1454–9.

39. Young JB, Abraham WT, Smith AL, et al. Combined cardiac resynchronization and implantable cardioversion defibrillation in advanced chronic heart failure: the MIRACLE ICD trial. JAMA 2003;289: 2685–94.

40. McSwain RL, Schwartz RA, DeLurgio DB, et al. The impact of cardiac resynchronization therapy on ventricular tachycardia / fibrillation: an analysis from the combined Contak-CD and InSync-ICD studies. J Cardiovasc Electrophysiol 2005;16: 1168–71.

41. Saxon LA, Bristow MR, Boehmer J, et al. Predictors of sudden cardiac death and appropriate shock in the comparison of medical therapy, pacing, and defibrillation in heart failure (COMPANION) trial. Circulation 2006;114:2766–72.

42. Desai H, Aronow WS, Ahn C, et al. Incidence of appropriate cardioverter-defibrillator shocks and mortality in patients with heart failure treated with combined cardiac resynchronization plus implantable cardioverter-defibrillator therapy versus implantable cardioverter-defibrillator therapy. J Cardiovasc Pharmacol Ther 2010;15:37–40.

43. Nordbeck P, Seidl B, Fey B, et al. Effect of cardiac resynchronization therapy on the incidence of electrical storm. Int J Cardiol 2010;143:330–6.

44. Markowitz SM, Lewen JM, Wiggenhorn CJ, et al. Relationship of reverse anatomical remodeling and ventricular arrhythmias after cardiac resynchronization. J Cardiovasc Electrophysiol 2009;20: 293–8.

45. Di Biase L, Gasparini M, Lunati M, et al. Antiarrhythmic effect of reverse ventricular remodeling induced by cardiac resynchronization therapy: the InSync ICD (implantable cardioverter-defibrillator) Italian registry. J Am Coll Cardiol 2008;52:1442–9.

46. Moss AJ, Hall WJ, Cannom DS, et al. Cardiac-resynchronization therapy for the prevention of heart-failure events. N Engl J Med 2009;361:1329–38.

47. Barsheshet A, Wang PJ, Moss AJ, et al. Reverse remodeling and the risk of ventricular arrhythmias in MADIT-CRT [abstract]. J Am Coll Cardiol 2011; 57:E14.

48. Evans JC, Al-Ahmad A, McNitt S, et al. Cardiac resynchronization reduces risk of shock in the MADIT-CRT trial [abstract]. Heart Rhythm 2011;8:S63.

49. Kühlkamp V, for the InSync 7272 ICD World Wide Investigators. Initial experience with an implantable cardioverter-defibrillator incorporating cardiac resynchronization therapy. J Am Coll Cardiol 2002; 39:790–7.

50. Gasparini M, Anselme F, Clementy J, et al. Biventricular versus right ventricular antitachycardia pacing to terminate ventricular tachyarrhythmias in patients receiving cardiac resynchronization therapy: the ADVANCE CRT-D trial. Am Heart J 2010;159: 1116.e2–23.e2.

51. Byrd IA, Rogers JM, Smith WM, et al. Comparison of conventional and biventricular antitachycardia pacing in a geometrically realistic model of the rabbit ventricle. J Cardiovasc Electrophysiol 2004;15:1066–77.

52. Fish JM, Di Diego JM, Nesterenko V, et al. Epicardial activation of left ventricular wall prolongs QT interval and transmural dispersion of repolarization: implications for biventricular pacing. Circulation 2004;109: 2136–42.

53. Robertson JF, Cain ME, Horowitz LN, et al. Anatomic and electrophysiologic correlates of ventricular tachycardia requiring left ventricular stimulation. Am J Cardiol 1981;48:263–8.

54. Shukla G, Chaudhry GM, Orlov M, et al. Potential proarrhythmic effect of biventricular pacing: fact or myth? Heart Rhythm 2005;2:951–6.

55. Nayak HM, Verdino RJ, Russo AM, et al. Ventricular tachycardia storm after initiation of biventricular pacing: incidence, clinical characteristics, management, and outcome. J Cardiovasc Electrophysiol 2008;19:708–15.

56. Steinberg JS, Martins J, Sadanandan S, et al. Antiarrhythmic drug use in the implantable defibrillator

arm of the Antiarrhythmics Versus Implantable Defibrillators (AVID) study. Am Heart J 2001;142:520–9.

57. Pacifico A, Hohnloser SH, Williams JH, et al. Prevention of implantable-defibrillator shocks by treatment with sotalol. N Engl J Med 1999;340:1855–62.

58. Kühlkamp V, Mewis C, Mermi J, et al. Suppression of sustained ventricular tachyarrhythmias: a comparison of d, l-sotalol with no antiarrhythmic drug treatment. J Am Coll Cardiol 1999;33:46–52.

59. Kettering K, Mewis C, Dörnberger V, et al. Efficacy of metoprolol and sotalol in the prevention of recurrences of sustained ventricular tachyarrhythmias in patients with an implantable cardioverter defibrillator. Pacing Clin Electrophysiol 2002;25:1571–6.

60. Seidl K, Hauer B, Schwick NG, et al. Comparison of metoprolol and sotalol in preventing ventricular tachyarrhythmias after the implantation of a cardioverter/defibrillator. Am J Cardiol 1998;82:744–8.

61. Brodine WN, Tung RT, Lee JK, et al. Effects of beta-blockers on implantable cardioverter defibrillator therapy and survival in the patients with ischemic cardiomyopathy (from the Multicenter Automatic Defibrillator Implantation Trial-II). Am J Cardiol 2005;96:691–5.

62. Kouakam C, Lauwerier B, Klug D, et al. Effect of elevated heart rate preceding the onset of ventricular tachycardia on antitachycardia pacing effectiveness in patients with implantable cardioverter defibrillators. Am J Cardiol 2003;92:26–32.

63. Connolly SJ, Dorian P, Roberts RS, et al. Comparison of β-blockers, amiodarone plus β-blockers, or sotalol for prevention of shocks from implantable cardioverter defibrillators: the OPTIC study: a randomized trial. JAMA 2006;295:165–71.

64. Boutitie F, Boissel JP, Connolly SJ, et al. Amiodarone interactions with β-blockers: analysis of the merged EMIAT and CAMIAT databases. Circulation 1999;99:2268–75.

65. Hohnloser SH, Dorian P, Roberts R, et al. Effect of amiodarone and sotalol on ventricular defibrillation threshold: the optimal pharmacological therapy in cardioverter defibrillator patients (OPTIC) trial. Circulation 2006;114:104–9.

66. Wood MA, Ellenbogen KA. Follow-up defibrillator testing for antiarrhythmic drugs: probability and uncertainty. Circulation 2006;114:98–100.

67. Ferreira-González I, Dos-Subirá L, Guyatt GH. Adjunctive antiarrhythmic drug therapy in patients with implantable cardioverter defibrillators: a systematic review. Eur Heart J 2007;28:469–77.

68. O'Toole M, O'Neill PG, Kluger J, et al. Efficacy and safety of oral dofetilide in patients with an implanted defibrillator: a multicenter study [abstract]. Circulation 1999;100:S794.

69. Singer I, Al-Khalidi H, Niazi I, et al. Azimilide decreases recurrent ventricular tachyarrhythmias in patients with implantable cardioverter defibrillators. J Am Coll Cardiol 2004;43:39–43.

70. Dorian P, Borggrefe M, Al-Khalidi HR, et al. Placebo-controlled, randomized clinical trial of azimilide for prevention of ventricular tachyarrhythmias in patients with an implantable cardioverter defibrillator. Circulation 2004;110:3646–54.

71. Chiu JH, Abdelhadi RH, Chung MK, et al. Effect of statin therapy on risk of ventricular arrhythmia among patients with coronary artery disease and an implantable cardioverter-defibrillator. Am J Cardiol 2005;95:490–1.

72. Beri A, Contractor T, Gardiner JC, et al. Reduction in the intensity rate of appropriate shocks for ventricular arrhythmias with statin therapy. J Cardiovasc Pharmacol 2010;56:190–4.

73. Mitchell LB, Powell JL, Gillis AM, et al. Are lipid lowering drugs also antiarrhythmic drugs? An analysis of the Antiarrhythmics versus Implantable Defibrillators (AVID) trial. J Am Coll Cardiol 2003;42:81–7.

74. Vyas AK, Guo H, Moss AJ, et al. Reduction in ventricular tachyarrhythmias with statins in the multicenter automatic defibrillator implantation trial (MADIT)-II. J Am Coll Cardiol 2006;47:769–73.

75. Goldberger JJ, Subacius H, Schaechter A, et al. Effects of statin therapy on arrhythmic events and survival in patients with nonischemic dilated cardiomyopathy. J Am Coll Cardiol 2006;48:1228–33.

76. Leaf A, Albert CM, Josephson M, et al. Prevention of fatal arrhythmias in high-risk subjects by fish oil n-3 fatty acid intake. Circulation 2005;112:2762–8.

77. Raitt MH, Connor WE, Morris C, et al. Fish oil supplementation and risk of ventricular tachycardia and ventricular fibrillation in patients with implantable defibrillators: a randomized controlled trial. JAMA 2005;293:2884–91.

78. Brouwer IA, Zock PL, Camm AJ, et al. Effect of fish oil on ventricular tachyarrhythmias and death in patients with implantable cardioverter defibrillators: the Study on Omega-3 Fatty Acids and Ventricular Arrhythmia (SOFA) randomized trial. JAMA 2006;295:2613–9.

79. Finzi AA, Latini R, Barlera S, et al. Effects of n-3 polyunsaturated fatty acids on malignant ventricular arrhythmias in patients with chronic heart failure and implantable cardioverter-defibrillators: a substudy of the Gruppo Italiano per lo Studio della Sopravvivenza nell'Insufficienza Cardiaca (GISSI-HF) trial. Am Heart J 2011;161:338,e1–43.

80. Reddy VY, Reynolds MR, Neuzil P, et al. Prophylactic catheter ablation for the prevention of defibrillator therapy. N Engl J Med 2007;357:2657–65.

New Developments in ICD Leads and ICD Lead Configurations

Paul J. Wang, MD

KEYWORDS

• ICD leads • ICD connectors • Coil coating
• Lead configurations

Since the first transvenous implantable cardio-verter-defibrillator (ICD) systems were developed, ICD lead design has continuously evolved and advanced. Some fundamental changes have been made in ICD connectors, new outer insulation, and novel coil coating, with the potential to substantially improve lead function.[1]

ICD LEAD 4-POLE CONNECTORS

One of the major advances in ICD lead design was the introduction of a new international standard for a 4-pole connector (**Box 1**). Since the introduction of the first several ICD lead generations, the connectors consisted of 3 separate terminal pins, 1 for the low-voltage bipole for pacing and sensing and 1 each for the high-voltage shock coil electrodes. In the ICD header were 3 corresponding ports. Having a single port for the ICD lead terminal pin results in a significant reduction in the header size, which represents a significant proportion of the ICD size, particularly because the generator size itself has gradually decreased.[1] The 4-pole connector obviates the need for 3 separate connectors on the ICD lead, substantially reducing the bulk of the terminal portion of the ICD lead. Bulk of the ICD lead in the pocket results in a larger pocket formed and may increase the likelihood of skin erosion due to outward pressure of the leads within the pocket (**Figs. 1** and **2**). The bulk of the ICD leads with 3 separate terminal connectors may result in increased wear on the insulation of the ICD lead within the pocket, eventually resulting in lead failure, oversensing with inappropriate shocks, and failure to pace.

The 4-pole connector fits into a single port, preventing reversal of the 2 separate ICD shock lead terminal pins in the header. The inadvertent reversal of the ICD shock terminal pins has been reported as a potential cause of increased defibrillation thresholds. Specifically, because the proximal coil is usually tied to the ICD can as a single electrode, reversal of the ICD terminal pins would result in a configuration in which the distal coil is tied to the ICD can as a single electrode pole and the proximal coil as the other electrode. This shock vector is thought to be less optimal in achieving defibrillation and should generally be avoided.[2] The 4-pin connector has only 1 terminal pin; thus, its use probably results in a lower likelihood of a loose terminal pin, which may result in shock failure, failure to pace, or oversensing.

Box 1
Advantages of international standard for 4-pole connector

Smaller header with 1 port

Decreased bulk of having 1 terminal pin compared with 3 terminal pins

Decreased lead body interaction with decreased lead insulation erosion

Preventing reversal of leads

Probable reduced likelihood of loose terminal pin

Creating interchangeability among manufacturers

Department of Medicine, Stanford University School of Medicine, 300 Pasteur Drive, Stanford, CA 94305-5233, USA
E-mail address: Paul.J.Wang@stanford.edu

Card Electrophysiol Clin 3 (2011) 503–506
doi:10.1016/j.ccep.2011.05.014
1877-9182/11/$ – see front matter © 2011 Elsevier Inc. All rights reserved.

cardiacEP.theclinics.com

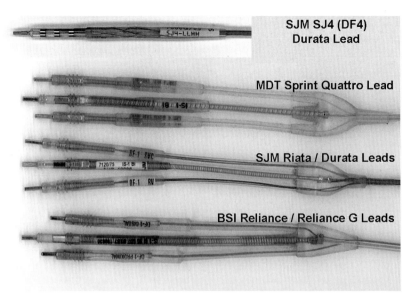

Fig. 1. The 4-pole connector lead (SJ4) (*top*). Examples of the terminal pins of standard high-voltage and low-voltage connectors (*bottom*). Sprint Quattro (Medtronic, Minneapolis, MN, USA), Riata (St. Jude Medical), Reliance (Boston Scientific, Inc. Natick, MA, USA).

Creation of an international standard is critical in permitting the interchangeability of manufacturers' ICD leads. The ability to use a 4-pole connector with a range of ICDs from different manufacturers increases the simplicity and flexibility in planning a generator change.

The international standard for the 4-pole connector has a high-voltage configuration and a low-voltage configuration. This discussion focuses only on the high-voltage configuration because the 4-pole low-voltage connector is designed for a 4-electrode pacing lead, such as for left ventricular pacing. The international standard, however, creates a lockout design that prevents the 4-pole low-voltage connector from contacting the high-voltage electrode contacts within the high-voltage port (**Fig. 3**). The high-voltage connector may have either 1 or 2 high-voltage contacts combined with the 2 low-voltage contacts (**Fig. 4**). The 1 high-voltage contact is used for a single-coil ICD lead and the 2 high-voltage contacts for a dual-coil ICD lead. The design of the international standard 4-pole connector incorporates sealing rings inside the connector cavity so that during generator

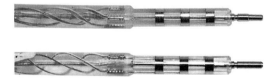

Fig. 2. The 4-pole DF4 connector with 2 high-voltage and 2 low-voltage conductors (*top*). The 4-pole IS4 connector for 4 low-voltage conductors (*bottom*).

changes, new sealing rings result. The sealing rings play a critical role in achieving electrical isolation between the high-voltage and-low voltage terminal pins.

MULTILUMINAL ICD LEAD DESIGN

Current-generation ICD leads have a multiluminal design in which the electrode conductors are within their own lumens. The primary insulator is silicone. The tip cathode electrode has a coil structure with a central lumen, which also may be used for the lead stylet. There may be additional lumens that are used to absorb any compression pressures (**Fig. 5**).[1]

Outer Insulation

Silicone rubber is the most commonly used insulating material for ICD leads. Silicone rubber may become abraded or layers of silicone rubber may be moved to the side, creating a denuded area of conductor coil. A copolymer hybrid, called Elast-Eon (AorTech Biomaterials, Clayton, Victoria, Australia), has been developed to provide strength along with softness and stability. This copolymer is a combination of polyurethane and silicone, providing the strength of 55D polyurethane while maintaining the softness and stability of silicone rubber. This copolymer is used in the St. Jude Optim Insulation and exhibits one-quarter of the friction of silicone. The material has a flexibility that is similar to silicone and much greater than polyurethane.

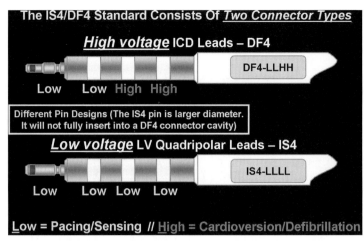

Fig. 3. The 4-pole DF4 connector with 2 high-voltage (H) and 2 low-voltage (L) conductors (DF4-HHLL) (*top*). The 4-pole IS4 connector for 4 low-voltage conductors (IS4-LLLL) (*bottom*).

ICD Coil Coating

ICD leads with a bare metal coil structure exhibit an exuberant fibrous reaction in the body, particularly at points of contact with the endocardium and endothelium. Extraction of these leads is particularly difficult because of ingrowth of fibrous tissue between the turns of the coil of the ICD lead. A common solution to this problem is to fill the spaces between the coils with silicone, a process called backfilling. There is still some fibrous tissue ingrowth around the area of the coils that are exposed, however. A flat coil design with backfilling of silicone results in a flat surface with minimal

areas for ingrowth. The coils may also be nearly flat with a minimal curve of the coils. Expanded polytetrafluoroethylene Gore-Tex (W. L. Gore and Associates, Flagstaff, Arizona) may be placed over the coils and may reduce any fibrous tissue ingrowth (**Fig. 6**).[3–6] In a study by Di Cori and colleagues,[3] 17 Endotak Reliance G (Boston Scientific, Inc.) dual-coil ICD leads, with mean implantation time of 23 ± 26 months, were removed with manual retraction in 29% of patients compared with 0%

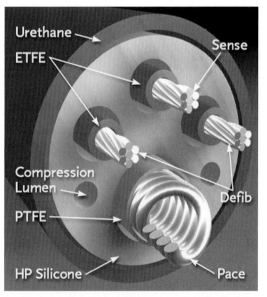

Fig. 5. Example of a current generation (Medtronic) ICD lead with multiple lumens, including lumens to relieve compression. Defib, defibrillation connector; ETFE, ethylene tetrafluoroethylene; PTFE, polytetrafluoroethylene; HP Silicone, high performance silicone. (*Courtesy of* Medtronic, Inc., Minneapolis, Minnesota; with permission.)

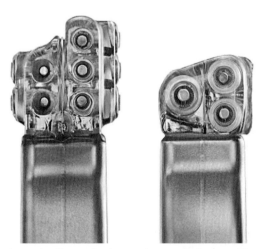

Fig. 4. (*Left*) Standard ports for CRT-D device with 3 low-voltage (right atrial, right ventricular, and left ventricular) terminal ports and 2 high-voltage terminal ports. (*Right*) DF4 connector for CRT-D device with 1 port for right atrial terminal pin, 1 port for left ventricular terminal pin, and 1 port for DFT4 connector.

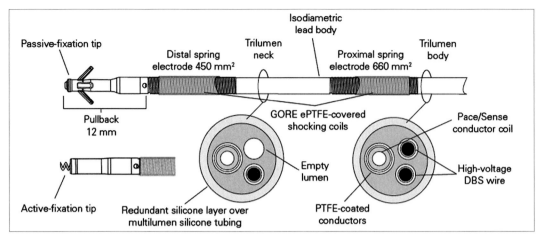

Fig. 6. Expanded polytetrafluoroethylene-covered ICD lead coils. ePTFE, expanded polytetrafluoroethylene; PFTE, polytetrafluoroethylene; DBS, drawn brazed strand. (*Courtesy of* Boston Scientific, Inc., Natick, Massachusetts; with permission.)

of patients with Sprint Quattro (Medtronic) and 3% of patients with St. Jude Riata leads. Similarly, this group had shorter extraction time, 5 ± 11 minutes, compared with 21 ± 22 minutes in the Sprint Quattro and 16 ± 22 minutes for the St. Jude Riata 1570 leads. In addition, there is some evidence that the expanded polytetrafluoroethylene-covered leads may prevent chatter on an integrated bipolar ICD lead.

SUMMARY

ICD leads continue to advance in important ways, addressing issues of lead bulk, reversal of terminal pins, fibrous ingrowth around ICD coils, and erosion of ICD lead insulation.

REFERENCES

1. Haqqani HM, Mond HG. The implantable cardioverter-defibrillator lead: principles, progress, and promises. Pacing Clin Electrophysiol 2009;32:1336–53.

2. Chawla P, Hanon S, Lam P, et al. An uncommon cause of myopotentisl. Pacing Clin Electrophysiol 2009;32:1584–6.

3. Di Cori A, Bongiorni MG, Zucchelli G, et al. Transvenous extraction performance of expanded polytetrafluoroethylene covered ICD leads in comparison to traditional ICD leads in humans. Pacing Clin Electrophysiol 2010;33:1376–81.

4. Hackler JW, Sun Z, Lindsay BD, et al. Effectiveness of implantable cardioverter-defibrillator lead coil treatments in facilitating ease of extraction. Heart Rhythm 2010;7:890–7.

5. Wilkoff BL, Belott PH, Love CJ, et al. Improved extraction of ePTFE and medical adhesive modified defibrillation leads from the coronary sinus and great cardiac vein. Pacing Clin Electrophysiol 2005;28:205–11.

6. Koplan BA, Weiner S, Gilligan D, et al. Clinical and electrical performance of expanded polytetrafluoroethylene-covered defibrillator leads in comparison to traditional leads. Pacing Clin Electrophysiol 2008;31:47–55.

Index

Note: Page numbers of article titles are in **boldface** type.

Card Electrophysiol Clin 3 (2011) 507–510
doi:10.1016/S1877-9182(11)00056-6
1877-9182/11/$ – see front matter © 2011 Elsevier Inc. All rights reserved.

cardiacEP.theclinics.com